A Practical Approach to Cancer Imaging

Contents

Permissions

List of Contributors

Index

Preface

Cancer is one of the leading causes of death in the world today. The lethality of the disease can be attributed to its ability to divide uncontrollably, and infiltrate and destroy normal body tissue. The best chance for a cure lies in its diagnosis in the early stages. Cancer imaging allows the examination of the body and other internal organs in a noninvasive manner. Various imaging tests can aid in the diagnosis of cancer at all stages, such as X-ray, MRI, CT scan, mammogram, PET scan, ultrasound and bone scan, etc. X-rays use invisible electromagnetic beams for producing images of bones, organs and internal tissues. CT scan integrates X-rays and computer technology to produce axial or horizontal images of the body. This facilitates detailed images of the bones, fat, muscles and organs. A mammogram can help to detect breast cancers, while tumors in the abdomen, kidney and liver can be detected through sonography. MRI facilitates the visual assessment of soft tissues, particularly the brain, heart, pancreas, liver, reproductive organs, etc. A PET scan holds valuable insights into the metabolism, physiology and biochemical properties of an organ or tissue, as well as the progress of the treatment. This book contains some path-breaking studies in the field of cancer imaging. It outlines the diverse techniques of cancer imaging and their applications in detail. It is appropriate for students and experts seeking detailed information in oncology and medical imaging.

The researches compiled throughout the book are authentic and of high quality, combining several disciplines and from very diverse regions from around the world. Drawing on the contributions of many researchers from diverse countries, the book's objective is to provide the readers with the latest achievements in the area of research. This book will surely be a source of knowledge to all interested and researching the field.

In the end, I would like to express my deep sense of gratitude to all the authors for meeting the set deadlines in completing and submitting their research chapters. I would also like to thank the publisher for the support offered to us throughout the course of the book. Finally, I extend my sincere thanks to my family for being a constant source of inspiration and encouragement.

Editor

Utility of SUV$_{max}$ on ^{18} F-FDG PET in detecting cervical nodal metastases

Rebecca S. M. Lim[1,2,6*], Shakher Ramdave[3], Paul Beech[3,4], Baki Billah[5], Md Nazmul Karim[5], Julian A. Smith[2], Adnan Safdar[1,2] and Elizabeth Sigston[1,2]

Abstract

Background: The presence of cervical lymph node metastasis is an important prognostic factor for patients with head and neck squamous cell carcinomas (HNSCC). Accurate assessment of lymph node metastasis in these patients is essential for appropriate prognostic and management purposes. Here, we evaluated the effectiveness of the maximum standardized uptake value (SUV$_{max}$) on positron emission tomography (PET) in assessing lymph node metastasis in HNSCC prior to surgery.

Methods: A retrospective review of 74 patients with HNSCC who underwent PET/CT prior to neck dissection were examined. Pre-operative PET/CT scans were reviewed by two experienced nuclear medicine physicians and SUV$_{max}$ of the largest node in each nodal basin documented. These were compared with the histology results of the neck dissection.

Results: A total of 359 nodal basins including 86 basins with metastatic nodes were evaluated. A nodal SUV$_{max}$ ≥3. 16 yielded a sensitivity of 74.4 % and specificity of 84.9 % in detecting metastatic nodes. The nodal SUV$_{max}$/Liver SUV$_{max}$ ratio was found on receiver operating characteristic (ROC) to be effective in detecting metastatic nodes with an area under ROC curve of 0.90. A nodal SUV$_{max}$/Liver SUV$_{max}$ ratio ≥0.90 yielded a sensitivity of 74.1 % and specificity of 93.4 %. By comparison, visual inspection yielded sensitivities of 66.3 and 61.6 % in observers 1 and 2 respectively. The corresponding specificities were 77.7 and 86.5 %.

Conclusions: Nodal SUV$_{max}$ and nodal SUV$_{max}$/liver SUV$_{max}$ are both useful in the pre-operative detection of metastatic nodes with the latter being superior to visual inspection. The ratio is likely to be more useful as it corrects for inter-scanner variability.

Keywords: Lymphadenopathy, Metastasis, Positron emission tomography (PET), Standardized uptake value, Squamous cell carcinoma

Background

Accurate nodal staging of the neck is essential in guiding management and predicting prognosis for patients with head and neck squamous cell carcinoma (HNSCC). A single nodal metastasis reduces a patient's survival rate by 50 %–this is further halved with bilateral lymphadenopathy [1–3]. The use of ^{18}F-fluorodeoxyglucose positron emission tomography (^{18} F-FDG PET) in the workup of HNSCC has allowed non-invasive, quantitative assessment

of a tissue by analysing the 3-dimensional distribution of radioactivity based on the annihilation photons that are emitted by labelled tracer [4]. PET scans are superior to computed tomography (CT) and magnetic resonance imaging (MRI) because metabolic changes resulting from malignancies precede structural changes [5]. However, while providing metabolic information about tissues, PET scans offer poor visualization of anatomic structures, thereby limiting their use. This shortcoming has been overcome by integrated ^{18}F-FDG PET/CT scanners and has improved the nodal staging of the neck [6, 7].

At present, there have been only two studies that have examined the relationship between the maximum standardized uptake value (SUV$_{max}$) of a node and the

* Correspondence: rebecca1188@gmail.com
[1]Department of Otolaryngology and Head & Neck Surgery, Monash Medical Centre, 823-865 Centre Rd, Bentleigh East, VIC 3165, Australia
[2]Department of Surgery, School of Clinical Sciences, Monash University, 246 Clayton Rd, Clayton, VIC 3168, Australia
Full list of author information is available at the end of the article

presence of nodal metastasis [8, 9]. Both studies used nodal SUV_{max} in conjunction with nodal size measured from the CT images to predict nodal metastasis. There have been no studies using nodal SUV_{max} alone or using a ratio nodal SUV_{max} and background tissue SUV_{max} to negate variables that could cause different SUV_{max} readings between patients and between institutions.

The aims of this study were to define a nodal SUV_{max} cut-off with the greatest sensitivity and specificity for the detection of nodal metastasis, as well as to determine if a ratio between nodal SUV_{max} and each of aortic blood pool SUV_{max}, liver SUV_{max} and primary tumour SUV_{max} could be used as a universal predictor of cervical lymph node metastasis.

Methods

Study population

This retrospective single tertiary centre study identified 74 patients from January 2011 to December 2014 with newly diagnosed HNSCC who had undergone elective neck dissection with curative intent at the Department of Otolaryngology and Head & Neck Surgery, Monash Health, Melbourne.

The exclusion criteria included the following: patients who had previous chemotherapy or radiotherapy for any malignancy; patients who did not undergo pre-operative [18] F-FDG PET/CT or had [18] F-FDG PET/CT scans performed external to our institution; patients whose neck dissection specimens were not clearly divided into the individual levels; and patients who did not have a HNSCC, were excluded. The study protocol was approved by the ethics committee at Monash Health.

PET/CT imaging and SUV measurements

[18] F-FDG PET/CT scans were obtained with an advanced integrated PET/CT scanner (Siemens Biograph™ TruePoint™). All patients were fasted for at least six hours prior to the PET/CT examination. A standard dose of 300 MBq [18] F-FDG tracer was used for all patients. In the period between injection of [18] F-FDG tracer and image acquisition, the patient was instructed to remain seated or recumbent and silent in order to minimize muscular [18] F-FDG uptake. Patients were kept warm 30–60 min prior to tracer injection and throughout the uptake period in order to minimize [18] F-FDG accumulation in brown fat. Blood glucose was measured for all diabetic patients to ensure that it was within acceptable limits. Patients with blood glucose >10 mmol/L were rescheduled. Image acquisition was performed 53 to 124 min after tracer injection. Dual time point imaging was not used in this study.

A standard scan for suspected HNSCC at our institution covered vertex to upper thighs. The CT images were acquired without contrast and comprised of a topogram and the helical CT scan. The reconstruction parameters used for a standard scan were 168matrix, True D reconstruction, FWHM 5.0, 3 iterations, 21 subsets and 1.0 zoom.

After the acquisition, SUV_{max} was assessed on the Siemens syngo MultiModality WorkPlace (MMWP) system by a single nuclear medicine physician. SUV_{max} was determined by manually placing a cylindrical region of interest (ROI) over the largest lymph node in each nodal basin of interest, as well as the primary tumour site, the descending aorta and liver. This was done on trans-axial images by an experienced nuclear medicine physician. Node SUV_{max} values were divided by the SUV_{max} of the primary tumour, descending aorta and liver to calculate the following:

- nodal SUV_{max}/primary tumour SUV_{max}
- nodal SUV_{max}/aortic SUV_{max}
- nodal SUV_{max}/liver SUV_{max}

The short and long axis of the largest node in each nodal basin were also recorded.

Only cervical nodal levels 1 to 5 were examined in this study as these were the most common levels removed in a neck dissection.

Two nuclear medicine physicians then systematically examined each PET/CT scan visually and determined which cervical nodal levels had metastatic nodes. This was compared to the pathology results. A nodal basin with at least one metastatic node was deemed to be a 'metastatic basin', regardless of the number of metastatic nodes within the basin or the size of the metastatic deposit(s).

Histopathological analysis

Neck dissection specimens were either removed level by level or enbloc and then divided into the individual nodal levels. Nodal evaluation was performed by dedicated head and neck pathologists at our institution, in accordance with the guidelines issued by the Royal College of Pathologists in the United Kingdom. The specimens were inspected and palpated and each discrete palpable node was dissected out with attached peri-capsular adipose tissue. These nodes were then placed in a cassette which was then stained and serially sliced prior to being loaded onto pathology slides for viewing under the microscope. Pathologic findings on the lymph nodes were recorded at each anatomic level. Only lymph nodes in cervical levels one to five were examined—intra-parotid, occipital or pre-auricular nodes were excluded.

The pathology reports were reviewed by the investigators to determine if the nodal basin contained any metastatic nodes.

Table 1 Primary Sites

Primary site	Frequency	Percent
Oral cavity	43	58.1
Larynx	13	17.6
Cutaneous	10	13.5
UNPHNC	5	6.8
Hypopharynx	3	4.1
Total	74	100

Statistical analysis

All statistical analyses were performed using IBM SPSS version 22 by two bio-statisticians. The pathologic status and SUV_{max} of cervical lymph nodes were collected for calculating the receiver operating characteristic (ROC) curve and Youden's Index for determining the cut-off value for SUV_{max}. The Youden index, which is a comprehensive measurement for the performance of a diagnostic test, was generated considering every possible cut-off point. The value that generates the highest Youden's Index for the particular ratio is considered as the best cut-off for that ratio, as it provides highest discrimination between pathology and no pathology. A p-value of 0.05 or less was considered statistically significant.

Binary logistic regression was applied to assess the association of individual predictor with chance of metastasis adjusting for all possible confounding. For choosing the most suitable predictor for metastatic node a backward logistic regression was fitted including all plausible predictors. $P < 0.05$ was considered as significant.

Results

Patient demographics

The study cohort consisted of 74 patients with HNSCC, including 57 males and 17 females. The median patient age was 64 (range 35–89). Primary sites included the oral cavity, hypopharynx, larynx and skin. Five patients had no primary site found (Table 1).

Type of neck dissection

A total of 95 neck-sides, including 359 nodal basins, were dissected (Table 2). Metastatic nodes were found in 86 of 359 levels (24.0 %). The most common neck

dissection performed was a selective neck dissection of levels I to IV (33.7 %) followed by a selective neck dissection of levels II to IV (21.1 %), supra-omohyoid neck dissection of levels I to III (SOHND) (17.9 %) modified radical neck dissection of levels I to V (MRND) (13.7 %), selective neck dissection of levels II to V (8.4 %) and radical neck dissection of levels I to V (5.3 %).

SUV_{max} for pathologically positive and negative lymph nodes and the cut-off value for diagnosis

SUV_{max} was measured for the largest lymph node in each level and compared with the results of histopathologic examination. The median SUV_{max} values of pathologically negative and positive nodes were 1.55 (range 0.58–5.2) and 5 (range 0.91–23.49) respectively. The median primary tumour SUV_{max} was 14.26 (range 3.89–36.69). The median aortic SUV_{max} was 2.70 (range 1.79–4.68). The median liver SUV_{max} was 3.38 (range 2.27–5.51).

A Receiver Operating Characteristic (ROC) curve was drawn and the Youden's Index used to determine the cut-off value for SUV_{max} at which sensitivity and specificity were the highest (Table 3). The best nodal SUV_{max} cut-off was found to be 3.16. This yielded a sensitivity of 74.4 % and specificity of 84.9 %.

SUV_{max} ratios for pathologically positive and negative lymph nodes and the cut-off value for diagnosis

A ROC analysis was employed to evaluate usefulness of three different ratios in determining the presence or absence of metastatic nodes:

- nodal SUV_{max}/primary tumour SUV_{max}
- nodal SUV_{max}/aortic SUV_{max}
- nodal SUV_{max}/liver SUV_{max}

The results are shown in Fig. 1 and Table 4.

ROC analysis of Nodal SUV_{max}/Primary SUV_{max} ratio, Nodal SUV_{max}/Aorta SUV_{max} ratio and Nodal SUV_{max}/Liver SUV_{max} ratio confirms that the latter two ratios are good predictors of nodal metastasis (Fig. 1). Nodal SUV_{max}/Primary SUV_{max} ratio was a poorer predictor than the other two ratios. To choose the best predictor

Table 2 Nodal Basins Dissected

Nodal basin	Dissection frequency	No. of positive basins	% of tumours ipsilateral to the positive node	% of tumours contralateral to the positive node	% of tumours midline to the positive node	% of positive nodes with unknown primaries
Level I	70	18	10/18 (55.6 %)	1/18 (5.6 %)	3/18 (16.7 %)	4/18 (22.2 %)
Level II	95	33	18/33 (54.5 %)	3/33 (9.1 %)	5/33 (15.1 %)	7/33 (21.2 %)
Level III	95	21	12/21 (57.1 %)	1/21 (4.8 %)	6/21 (28.6 %)	2/21 (9.5 %)
Level IV	77	10	6/10 (60.0 %)	0/10 (0 %)	3/10 (30.0 %)	1/10 (10.0 %)
Level V	27	4	2/4 (50.0 %)	0/4 (0 %)	2/4 (50.0 %)	0/4 (0 %)
Total	364	86	48/86 (55.8 %)	5/86 (5.8 %)	19/86 (22.1 %)	14/86 (16.3 %)

Table 3 ROC analysis for generating nodal SUV_{max} Cut-off with maximum sensitivity and specificity

	Highest Youden's Index	Cut-off[a]	Sensitivity	Specificity	Likelihood Ratio Pos. Test	Likelihood Ratio Neg. Test
Nodal SUV_{max}	0.693	3.16	0.744	0.849	14.57	0.270

[a]Positive if greater Than or Equal To

of nodal metastasis adjusting for all possible confounding factors a stepwise backward elimination multivariable logistic regression analysis was performed on all the potential PET predictors of nodal metastasis. After each step, the predictor with the lowest p-value was removed. By the end of the analysis, nodal SUV_{max}/liver SUV_{max} ratio was found to be the best predictor for nodal metastasis (Table 4).

The optimal cut-off value for nodal SUV_{max}/liver SUV_{max} ratio is 0.903. This means that a node with a nodal SUV_{max}/liver SUV_{max} of greater than or equal to 0.903 is considered metastatic with a sensitivity of 74.1 % and specificity of 93.4 % (Table 5).

Comparing visual detection of metastatic nodes, nodal SUV_{max} and nodal SUV_{max}/liver SUV_{max}

ROC analysis of visual detection of metastatic nodes, nodal SUV_{max} and nodal SUV_{max}/liver SUV_{max} ratio found that while visual detection demonstrated good discrimination between metastatic and benign nodes, the use of nodal SUV_{max} and nodal SUV_{maz}/liver SUV_{max} had better discrimination. The area under the curves for visual observer 1 was 0.737 and 0.703 for visual observer 2. In contrast, the area under the curve was 0.883 for both nodal SUV_{max} and nodal SUV_{maz}/liver SUV_{max} (Table 6

and Fig. 2). Observer 1 detected metastatic nodes with a sensitivity of 66.3 % and a specificity of 77.7 %, while the corresponding values for Observer 2 were 61.6 and 86.5 %. Using a Nodal SUV_{max}/Liver SUV_{max} ratio of >0.903 yielded a sensitivity of 72.8 % and specificity of 93.8 %.

Short and long nodal diameters had no statistically significant impact on predicting nodal basin metastasis

The short and long axis of the largest node in each nodal basin were recorded. Neither diameter was a statistically significant predictor of a metastatic basin (Table 7).

Multi-variable analysis of various indicators of metastatic nodes

Multivariable logistic regression was conducted with plausible indicators of metastatic nodes. Adjusting for all possible confounders and indicators entered in the model nodal SUV_{max} appeared as significant indicator of metastatic nodes. (OR 3.275; 95%CI: 2.018–5.317; $P < 0.000$). None of the other factors 'primary tumour SUV_{max}' ($p > 0.05$), 'extra-capsular spread' ($p > 0.05$), 'nodal necrosis' ($p > 0.05$), largest nodal diameter ($p > 0.05$) and smallest nodal diameter ($p > 0.05$) appeared to be significant indicators of metastatic nodes (Table 8).

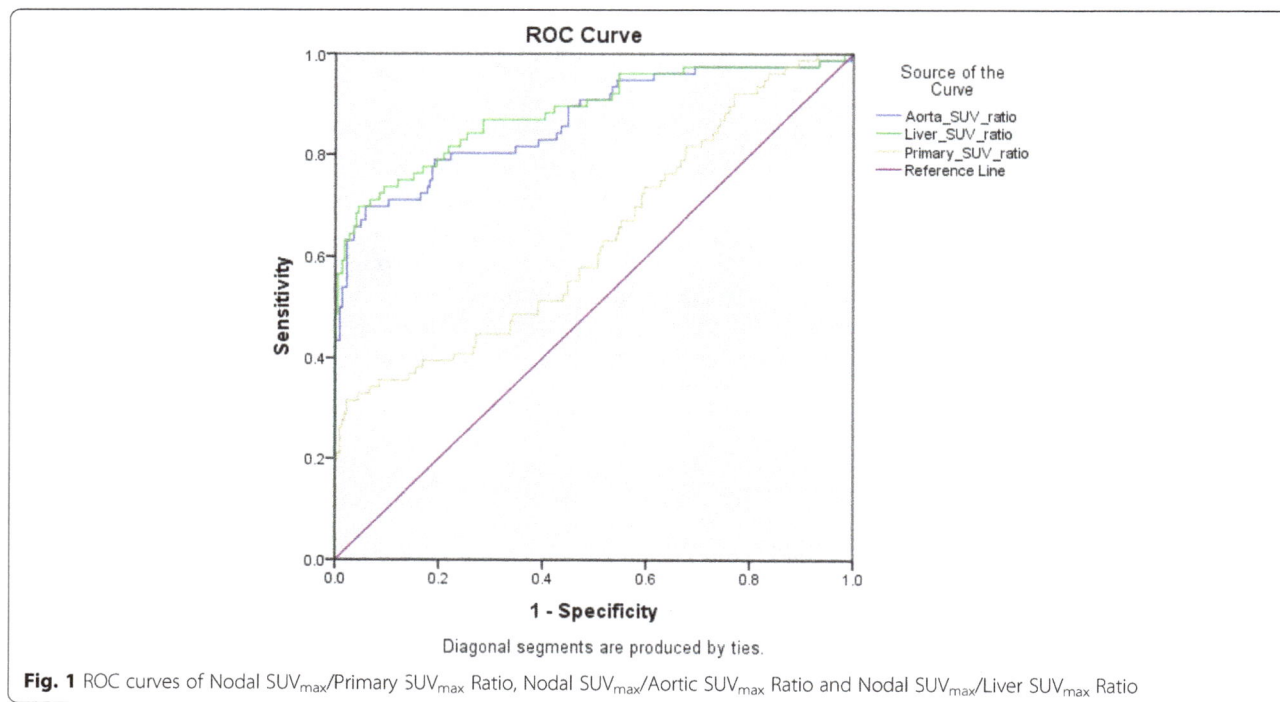

Fig. 1 ROC curves of Nodal SUV_{max}/Primary SUV_{max} Ratio, Nodal SUV_{max}/Aortic SUV_{max} Ratio and Nodal SUV_{max}/Liver SUV_{max} Ratio

Table 4 Stepwise multi-variable logistic regression analysis

Predictor	B	S.E.	P Value	OR	95 % C.I. for OR	
					Lower	Upper
Nodal SUV_{max}/Liver SUV_{max}	4.114	0.556	.000*	61.1	20.2	185.6
Constant	−4.642	0.496	.000	0.010		

*Statistically significant

Discussion

The introduction of ^{18} F-FDG PET/CT has greatly improved preoperative staging of HNSCC. As the presence of nodal metastasis is one of the most important prognostic factors for patients with HNSCC, accurate nodal staging of these patients is essential for both appropriate management and prognostic purposes [2, 7, 10].

For malignancies with a high risk of occult nodal metastasis, such as oral cavity SCC, elective neck dissections are routinely performed on patients with clinically negative necks. This serves staging as well as therapeutic purposes. However, for patients in whom an elective dissection is not planned based on the site and histological grade of the primary tumour, nodal staging is based solely on clinical examination and radiological imaging. In these cases, the use of SUV_{max} can aid in distinguishing between metastatic and benign nodes, and thus in deciding whether an elective neck dissection should be undertaken.

The standardized uptake value (SUV) is the most widely used method for the quantification of ^{18} F-FDG uptake [11]. The SUV of a target can be expressed as SUV_{mean} or SUV_{max}. SUV_{mean} is the average SUV calculated from multiple voxels, while SUV_{max} is the highest voxel SUV reading in the region of interest. [12] The SUV_{max} is the more common method of reporting SUV, due to the fact that it is more reproducible and less observer-dependent than SUV_{mean} [12, 13]. The SUV_{max} is used at our institution for this reason. In our study, we have also decided to perform a per-nodal-level analysis as this analysis is commonly presented in the literature and allows comparison with other studies.

The use of SUV_{max} to detect nodal metastases has been studied extensively in lung cancers, but not in head and neck malignancies. A study by Bryant et al. included 397 patients with non-small cell lung cancer and found that the median SUV_{max} of metastatic mediastinal lymph nodes was significantly higher than that of benign nodes. Indeed, when a SUV_{max} cutoff of 5.3 was used instead of the traditional value of 2.5, the accuracy of ^{18} F-FDG-PET/CT for detecting mediastinal lymph node metastasis increased to 92 % [14]. Another study by Ela Bella et al. looked at the ideal SUV_{max} cutoff for identification of metastatic mediastinal lymph nodes and found SUV_{max} of 4.1 to be ideal. This cut-off yielded a sensitivity of 80 % and specificity of 92 % [15]. A similar SUV_{max} cut-off for identifying metastatic mediastinal lymph nodes was reported by Vansteenkiste et al. [16].

The use of SUV_{max} to detect nodal metastases in the head and neck has only been reported in two studies. In 2012, Matsubara et al. looked at 38 patients with oral SCC and compared their pre-operative ^{18} F-FDG-PET/CT scan results with histopathological findings [8]. The authors reported that nodes with a SUV_{max} of more than 4.5 were all pathologically confirmed as being metastatic, but for nodes with $SUV_{max} \leq 4.5$, it was not possible to distinguish between true positives and false positives. Hence, the long and short axis diameters were measured for those nodes and the long-axis diameter was found to be significantly longer in the true positive nodes. No significant difference between the true positive and false positive nodes were found in the short-axis diameter.

Murakami et al. studied 23 patients with HNSCC and found that SUV_{max} accurately characterized lymph nodes >15 mm in diameter, but was not reliable with respect to nodes <15 mm. Thus, size based SUV_{max} cut-offs were used in this study: they were 1.9 for nodes less than 10 mm in diameter, 2.5 for those 10–15 mm, and 3.0 for nodes more than 15 mm. These values yielded 79 % sensitivity and 99 % specificity [9].

The limitations of these studies are the small sample sizes and the lack of accounting for other variables that could influence SUV readings. These include the blood sugar level of the patient at the time of PET scanning, the presence of an inflammatory process near the tumour, patient movement and the interval between injection of ^{18} F-FDG and acquisition of PET.

In our study, we have found that nodal SUV_{max} was a statistically significant predictor of metastatic nodes ($p < 0.001$), and that a nodal SUV_{max} cut-off of ≥ 3.16 yielded a sensitivity of 74.4 % and specificity of 84.9 %. We

Table 5 Optimal nodal SUV_{max}/liver SUV_{max} ratio for generating Cut-off with maximum sensitivity and specificity

	Highest Youcen's Index	Cut-off[a]	Sensitivity	Specificity	Likelihood Ratio Pos. Test	Likelihood Ratio Neg. Test
Nodal SUV_{max}/Liver SUV_{max} ratio	0.675	0.903	0.741	0.934	11.266	0.277

[a]Positive if greater Than or Equal To

Table 6 Receiver operating characteristics of visual detection and nodal SUV_{max}/liver SUV_{max} ratio

	Sensitivity	Specificity	PPV	NPV	AUC (95 % CI)
Observer 1	61.63	86.45	58.89	87.73	0.703 (0.633, 0.772)
Observer 2	66.28	77.66	48.31	87.97	0.737 (0.667, 0.807)
N/L SUV (≥0.903)	72.84	93.78	81.94	89.91	0.883 (0.772, 0.894)

then hypothesized that a ratio of SUV_{max} values (ie, nodal SUV_{max}/background SUV_{max}) may be one way to negate these inherent differences between PET centres and standardize the measurement. Thus we measured the SUV_{max} of the liver parenchyma, aortic blood pool and primary tumour to see if these ratios could improve the detection of metastatic nodes. Multi-variable logistic regression analysis found the nodal SUV_{max}/liver SUV_{max} ratio to be able to distinguish, with statistical significance, between metastatic and benign nodes. This ratio offered a similar sensitivity as nodal SUV_{max} alone (74.1 % compared to 74.4 %). The significance of our results are that the nodal SUV_{max}/liver SUV_{max} is able to negate inherent differences between patients and PET centres and therefore standardize the measurement.

This is the first study to propose using a SUV ratio to detect metastatic cervical nodes. Currently, the lack of literature on this matter means that arbitrary SUV_{max} cut-off values are used. These vary significantly between institutions and the evidence for their use is lacking. Using the nodal SUV_{max} cut-off and/or the SUV_{maz} ratio cut-off proposed in this study, in addition to the usual methods of detecting a nodal metastasis, might improve

the overall sensitivity and specificity of PET/CT for the detection of metastatic nodes.

Improving the pre-operative detection of nodal metastasis is important as it has the potential to alter surgical management. In patients for whom an elective dissection is not planned based on the site and histological grade of the primary tumour, nodal staging is based mainly on clinical examination and radiological imaging. In these cases, the use of nodal SUV_{max} alone or nodal SUV_{max}/liver SUV_{max} can aid in distinguishing between metastatic and benign nodes, and thus in deciding whether an elective neck dissection should be undertaken.

Using a nodal SUV_{max}/liver SUV_{max} ratio also allows comparison of nodal tracer uptake between PET scans performed using different scanners. Currently, a comparison is not meaningful due to differences in scanner calibration and thus SUV readings. However, a ratio would negate inherent differences between scanners, making it possible to compare a pre-treatment PET scan with a post-treatment PET scan performed at a different centre to assess treatment response.

While we think the use of nodal SUV_{max}/liver SUV_{max} ratio is promising, there are a few caveats in the use of

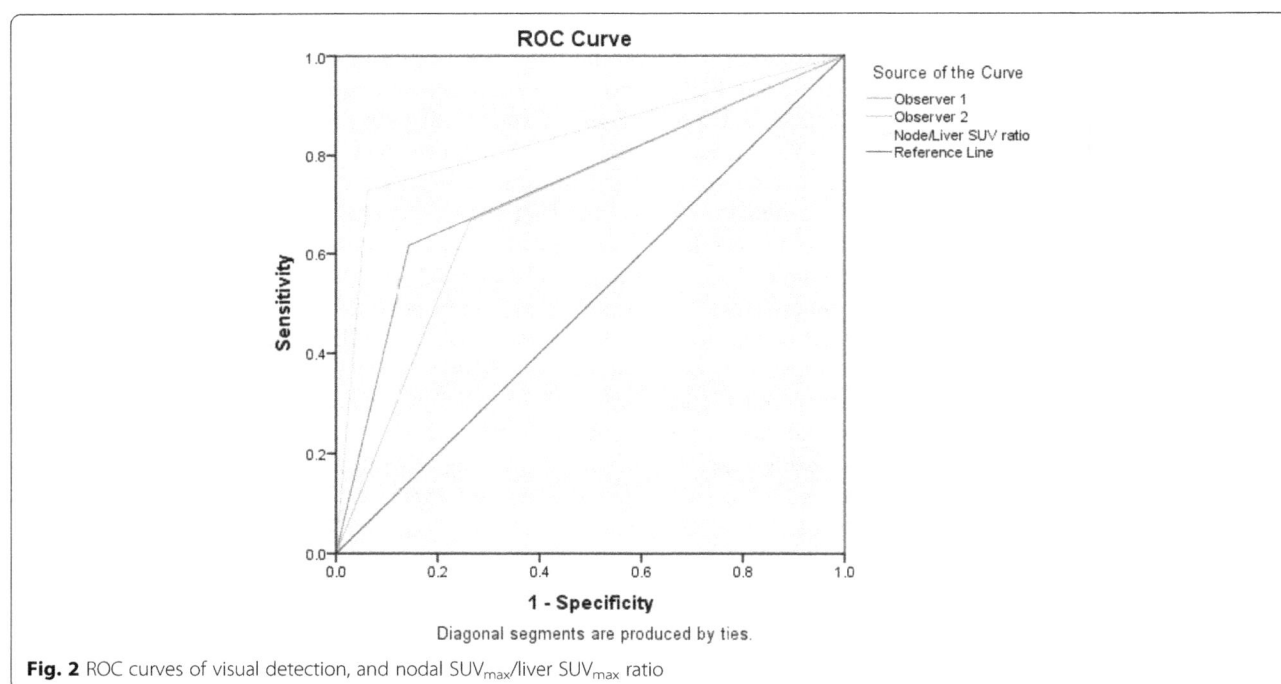

Fig. 2 ROC curves of visual detection, and nodal SUV_{max}/liver SUV_{max} ratio

Table 7 Binary logistic regression illustrating predictors of a metastatic basin

	B	S.E.	P Value	OR	95 % C.I. for OR	
					Lower	Upper
PET nodal SUVmax	1.215	.241	.000*	3.369	2.101	5.402
Largest nodal diameter	0.045	.128	.724	1.046	.814	1.344
Smallest nodal diameter	−0.110	.164	.500	.896	.650	1.234

*Statistically significant at P < 0.001

liver SUV as a proxy for background SUV_{max}. The first is that the liver has an abundance of glucose-6-phosphatase, which could cause continuous glycolysis and reduce its measured SUV more rapidly compared to other tissues. However, a prospective study by Laffon et al. performed PET acquisition at two time points on the same day and reported that the decay-corrected SUV of the liver remains nearly constant if the time delay between tracer injection and PET acquisition is in the range of 50–110 min. [17] This suggests that in clinical practice, liver SUV can be used for comparison with SUV of suspected malignant lesions, if comparison is made within this timeframe.

Another caveat of using liver SUV is in the presence of fatty liver. This has been suggested to result in a slightly decreased metabolic activity [18], while another study reported no significant difference in SUV_{max} [19]. The presence of liver tumours or metastatic disease would also give spurious liver SUV readings [20].

The main drawback of using nodal SUV_{max} is that this measurement might be spuriously low in necrotic nodes. In these cases, correlation with CT findings is essential.

Another limitation of this study is the time lapse between the PET/CT scan and surgery. The median time between a patient in our study having the PET/CT scan and the neck dissection was 27 days (range 1–62). Disease progression could have occurred during this time and what was initially a benign node at the time of scanning could have turned malignant by the time of surgery.

Despite these limitations, our study has shown nodal SUV_{max} and nodal SUV_{max}/liver SUV_{max} ratio to be

better detectors of metastatic nodes than visual inspection. This is surprising as visual interpretation integrates more information than the nodal SUV_{max} or SUV_{max} ratio measurements, in particular the distribution pattern, size, number and relative intensity of lesions and the relationship of the lesions with the primary tumour, to determine the probability of these foci of uptake representing metastatic disease. A meta-analysis by Sun et al. published in 2015 included 19 studies that performed a per-nodal-level analysis and found that the pooled sensitivity and specificity was 80 % (range 0 %–96.3 %) and 96 % (range 73.4 %–98.9 %) respectively [21]. We acknowledge that our sensitivities and specificities for visual inspection were somewhat lower than this but when a Nodal SUV_{max}/Liver SUV_{max} ratio of >0.903 was used the sensitivity and specificity yielded was comparable.

A few reasons may account for the difference. Firstly, selective reporting bias may have contributed to the high reported sensitivities and specificities of ^{18}FDG-PET/CT in the meta-analysis. Furthermore, 12 of the 19 studies that were included in the meta-analysis had either CT and/or MRI performed in addition to the ^{18}FDG-PET/CT. Thus, it is possible that the imaging observers might have known the diagnostic outcome of other conventional imaging methods before assessing the results of ^{18}FDG-PET/CT imaging, resulting in a spuriously high sensitivity and specificity for ^{18}FDG-PET/CT.

Conclusions

This preliminary study has identified two predictors of metastatic nodes on PET scans–nodal SUV_{max} and nodal SUV_{max}/liver SUV_{max} ratio. It is the first study examining the utility of a SUV ratio in detection of metastatic cervical lymph nodes and more data are needed from a larger number of patients from multiple centres. Further research could examine prospectively if these predictors, combined with conventional visual detection methods, are able to improve the overall accuracy of detecting metastatic cervical lymph nodes.

Abbreviations
^{18}F-FDG: 18F-fluorodeoxyglucose; HNSCC: Head and neck squamous cell carcinoma; MRND: Modified radical neck dissection; PET: Positron emission tomography; ROC: Receiver operating characteristic; SCC: Squamous cell carcinoma; SUV: Standardized uptake value

Acknowledgements
Mr. Jason Bradley, Charge Technologist of Nuclear Medicine and PET (Monash Imaging), who kindly helped with the technical retrieval of PET/CT scans for viewing by our nuclear medicine physicians and with the technical aspects of the PET scanning protocol.

Funding
Statistical analysis funded by Monash University Department of Surgery. Monash University played no role in the actual design of the study and collection.

Table 8 Binary logistic regression illustrating indicators of metastatic nodes

Indicators	B	OR	95 % C.I. for OR		P Value
Nodal SUVmax	1.186	3.275	2.018	5.317	**<0.000***
Primary tumour SUVmax	−0.052	0.949	0.877	1.027	0.194
Extra-capsular spread	−1.595	5.50	0.14	2.900	0.240
Nodal necrosis	−0/718	1.104	0.056	4.245	0.515
Largest nodal diameter	−0.079	1.082	0.824	1.402	0.571
Smallest nodal diameter	−0.104	0/901	0.643	1.263	0.545
Constant	0.546	1.726	-	-	0.799

*Statistically significant at P < 0.001

Authors' contributions

RSL, MBBS (Hons). Study design, data collection and writing of manuscript. SR, MBBS, MD, FRACP. Study design, data collection, interpretation of PET scans, reviewing of manuscript. PB, MBBS, FRANZCR, FAANMS. Data collection, interpretation of PET scans. BB, BSc (Hons), MAS, PhD. Statistical analysis. MdNK MSc, MBBS. Statistical analysis. JAS, MBBS, MS, FRACS. Supervised the study design, and facilitated data collection and reviewed manuscript. AS, MBBS, FRCS, FRACS (ORL-HNS). Supervised the study design, and facilitated data collection and reviewed manuscript. ES, MBBS, FRACS. Supervised the study design, and facilitated data collection and reviewed manuscript. All authors read and approved the final manuscript.

Competing interests

The authors declare that they have no competing interests.

Author details

[1]Department of Otolaryngology and Head & Neck Surgery, Monash Medical Centre, 823-865 Centre Rd, Bentleigh East, VIC 3165, Australia. [2]Department of Surgery, School of Clinical Sciences, Monash University, 246 Clayton Rd, Clayton, VIC 3168, Australia. [3]Department of Nuclear Medicine & PET, Monash Medical Centre, 823-865 Centre Rd, Bentleigh East, VIC 3165, Australia. [4]Department of Nuclear Medicine, The Alfred, First Floor, East Block, Commercial Road, Melbourne, VIC 3004, Australia. [5]School of Public Health, Monash University, The Alfred Centre, 99 Commercial Road, Melbourne, VIC 3004, Australia. [6]Department of Radiology, Westmead Hospital, Cnr Hawkesbury Road and Darcy Road, Westmead, NSW 2145, Australia.

References

1. Mukherji SK, Armao D, Joshi VM. Cervical nodal metastases in squamous cell carcinoma of the head and neck: what to expect. Head Neck. 2001;23(11):995–1005.
2. Nguyen A, Luginbuhl A, Cognetti D, Van Abel K, Bar-Ad V, Intenzo C, et al. Effectiveness of PET/CT in the preoperative evaluation of neck disease. Laryngoscope. 2014;124(1):159–64.
3. Walden MJ, Aygun N. Head and neck cancer. Semin Roentgenol. 2013;48(1):75–86.
4. Boellaard R, O'Doherty MJ, Weber WA, Mottaghy FM, Lonsdale MN, Stroobants SG, et al. FDG PET and PET/CT: EANM procedure guidelines for tumour PET imaging: version 1.0. Eur J Nucl Med Mol Imaging. 2010;37(1):181–200.
5. Muylle K, Castaigne C, Flamen P. 18F-fluoro-2-deoxy-D-glucose positron emission tomographic imaging: recent developments in head and neck cancer. Curr Opin Oncol. 2005;17(3):249–53.
6. Kyzas PA, Evangelou E, Denaxa-Kyza D, Ioannidis JP. 18F-fluorodeoxyglucose positron emission tomography to evaluate cervical node metastases in patients with head and neck squamous cell carcinoma: a meta-analysis. J Natl Cancer Inst. 2008;100(10):712–20.
7. Yongkui L, Jian L, Wanghan, Jingui L. 18FDG-PET/CT for the detection of regional nodal metastasis in patients with primary head and neck cancer before treatment: a meta-analysis. Surg Oncol. 2013;22(2):e11–6.
8. Matsubara R, Kawano S, Chikui T, Kiyosue T, Goto Y, Hirano M, et al. Clinical significance of combined assessment of the maximum standardized uptake value of F-18 FDG PET with nodal size in the diagnosis of cervical lymph node metastasis of oral squamous cell carcinoma. Acad Radiol. 2012;19(6):708–17.
9. Murakami R, Uozumi H, Hirai T, Nishimura R, Shiraishi S, Ota K, et al. Impact of FDG-PET/CT imaging on nodal staging for head-and-neck squamous cell carcinoma. Int J Radiat Oncol Biol Phys. 2007;68(2):377–82.
10. Agarwal V, Branstetter BF, Johnson JT. Indications for PET/CT in the head and neck. Otolaryngol Clin N Am. 2008;41(1):23–49. v.
11. Siddiqui F, Faulhaber PF, Yao M, Le Q-T. The Application of FDG-PET as Prognostic Indicators in Head and Neck Squamous Cell Carcinoma. PET Clinics. 2012;7(4):381–94.
12. Adams MC, Turkington TG, Wilson JM, Wong TZ. A systematic review of the factors affecting accuracy of SUV measurements. AJR Am J Roentgenol. 2010;195(2):310–20.
13. Lee JR, Madsen MT, Bushnel D, Menda Y. A threshold method to improve standardized uptake value reproducibility. Nucl Med Commun. 2000;21(7):685–90.
14. Bryant AS, Cerfolio RJ, Klemm KM, Ojha B. Maximum standard uptake value of mediastinal lymph nodes on integrated FDG-PET-CT predicts pathology in patients with non-small cell lung cancer. Ann Thorac Surg. 2006;82(2):417–22. discussion 22–3.
15. Ela Bella AJ, Zhang YR, Fan W, Luo KJ, Rong TH, Lin P, et al. Maximum standardized uptake value on PET/CT in preoperative assessment of lymph node metastasis from thoracic esophageal squamous cell carcinoma. Chin J Cancer. 2014;33(4):211–7.
16. Vansteenkiste JF, Stroobants SG, De Leyn PR, Dupont PJ, Bogaert J, Maes A, et al. Lymph node staging in non-small-cell lung cancer with FDG-PET scan: a prospective study on 690 lymph node stations from 68 patients. J Clin Oncol. 1998;16(6):2142–9.
17. Laffon E, Adhoute X, de Clermont H, Marthan R. Is liver SUV stable over time in (1)(8)F-FDG PET imaging? J Nucl Med Technol. 2011;39(4):258–63.
18. Qazi F, Oliver D, Nguyen N, Osman M. Fatty liver: Impact on metabolic activity as detected with 18F FDG-PET/CT. J Nucl Med. Meeting Abstracts. 2008;49(MeetingAbstracts_1):263P-c-.
19. Abele JT, Fung CI. Effect of hepatic steatosis on liver FDG uptake measured in mean standard uptake values. Radiology. 2010;254(3):917–24.
20. Wahl RL, Jacene H, Kasamon Y, Lodge MA. From RECIST to PERCIST: Evolving Considerations for PET response criteria in solid tumors. J Nucl Med. 2009;50 Suppl 1:122S–50S.
21. Sun R, Tang X, Yang Y, Zhang C. (18)FDG-PET/CT for the detection of regional nodal metastasis in patients with head and neck cancer: a meta-analysis. Oral Oncol. 2015;51(4):314–20.

2

Identification of the pericardiacophrenic vein on CT

Yoshiyuki Ozawa[1*], Ritsuko Suzuki[1], Masaki Hara[2] and Yuta Shibamoto[1]

Abstract

Background: To evaluate the depictability of pericardiacophrenic veins (PCPV) as landmarks for the location of the phrenic nerves on multi-detector-row computed tomography (MDCT), and to investigate the usefulness of depicting the PCPV to aid differential diagnosis of anterior mediastinal lesions.

Methods: Fifty-six patients with anterior mediastinal lesions (Fifty lesions originated from the thymus, six were of non-thymic origin) were evaluated. Contrast-enhanced CT scans of the chest were performed in all cases before diagnosis, and 22 of these scans were performed with electrocardiographic (ECG) gating. Two chest radiologists assessed the depictability of the PCPV and the positional relationship between the center of each anterior mediastinal lesion and the ipsilateral PCPV.

Results: The use of ECG gating increased the PCPV depiction rate in the lower left part of the mediastinum. The depiction rate of the left PCPV was significantly higher than that of the right PCPV. All 50 tumors of thymic origin and 3 of the 6 tumors of non-thymic origin were located on the medial side of the ipsilateral PCPV. The 3 lesions located on the lateral side of the ipsilateral PCPV were of non-thymic origin ($p = 0.0007$).

Conclusion: The use of ECG gating during MDCT may improve the depictability of the PCPV in the lower left section of the anterior mediastinum. Solitary anterior mediastinal lesions located on the lateral side of the ipsilateral PCPV are likely to be of non-thymic origin.

Keywords: Anterior mediastinum, Tumor, Phrenic nerve, Ct, Thymoma

Background

The phrenic nerves are small and difficult to detect on computed tomography (CT), and no previous studies have examined the positional relationship between anterior mediastinal tumors and the phrenic nerves, or the clinical significance of identifying the phrenic nerves in such cases.

Anterior mediastinal tumors, such as thymic epithelial tumors, mediastinal lymphomas, and germ cell tumors, mainly arise from the thymus [1]. However, some non-thymic lesions also develop in the anterior mediastinum, and it is sometimes difficult to diagnose these anterior mediastinal lesions based on morphological information alone. To identify additional sources of information that can facilitate the diagnosis of such tumors, we hypothesized that identifying the pericardiacophrenic veins (PCPV), which run parallel to the phrenic nerves [2–4], would aid the differentiation of thymic and non-thymic tumors because the phrenic nerves may be used as a landmark to locate the border of the thymus [5].

The purpose of this study was: 1) to evaluate PCPV depictability as landmarks to locate the phrenic nerves on multi-detector-row CT (MDCT) with or without ECG gating; and 2) to investigate the usefulness of identifying the PCPV to aid the differential diagnosis of anterior mediastinal lesions.

Methods

Subjects

Consecutive 56 patients (34 males and 22 females; age range: 15–80 years, median age: 53 years) with a pathologically confirmed anterior mediastinal lesion seen between 2004 and 2011 were included in this study. All of the CT images were evaluable, so no patients were

* Correspondence: ykiooster@gmail.com
[1]Department of Radiology, Nagoya City University, Graduate School of Medical Sciences, 1 Kawasumi, Mizuho-cho, Mizuho-ku, Nagoya 467-8601, Japan
Full list of author information is available at the end of the article

excluded. Fifty lesions originated from the thymus (33 thymomas, 11 thymic carcinomas, 3 germ cell tumors, 2 malignant lymphomas, and 1 thymolipoma), and 6 lesions were of non-thymic origin (2 sarcomas, a metastatic tumor from renal cell carcinoma, a tuberculoma, Castleman's disease, and an aneurysm). We used Felson's classification to define the mediastinal compartment of the lesions. The institutional review board approved this retrospective study and no individual patient consent was required.

CT acquisition

Contrast-enhanced CT of the chest was performed in all cases before surgical resection (47 cases) or image-guided percutaneous biopsy (9 cases). Twenty-four patients were scanned with a 16-row MDCT scanner (IDTI6; Philips Medical Systems, Cleveland, OH), and 32 were scanned with a 64-slice dual source (DS) CT scanner (Somatom Definition, Siemens Medical Systems, Erlangen, Germany). Our institution introduced the DSCT in 2006, and thereafter, the majority of data for this study were obtained with the DSCT. In all cases, contrast-enhanced CT scans were obtained in the craniocaudal direction during inspiratory breath holding. During the scans, 100 mL of contrast medium (300 mgI/mL) were injected into the antecubital vein at a rate of 2 mL/s using a power injector. The CT data were acquired after a scan delay of 100 s. Of the 56 patients, 22 were scanned using the ECG-gating method and the 64-slice DSCT scanner. The CT scan parameters were as follows: for the non-ECG-gated 16-row MDCT ($n = 24$): mAs, 200; tube voltage, 120 kVp; collimation, 16 × 0.75 mm; rotation time, 0.5 s/rotation; and pitch, 0.9; for the non-ECG-gated 64-slice DSCT ($n = 10$): single source mode; reference mAs, 215; tube voltage, 120 kVp; collimation, 64 × 0.6 mm; rotation time, 0.33 s/rotation; and pitch, 1; and for the ECG-gated 64-slice DSCT ($n = 22$): dual source mode; reference mAs, 320/rotation; tube voltage,

120 kVp; collimation, 64 × 0.6 mm; rotation time, 0.33 s/rotation; and pitch, variable depending on the patient's heart rate. A retrospective ECG-gating method was used for the ECG-gated CT, and the cardiac phase that exhibited the fewest motion artifacts was selected for the mediastinal tumor evaluations. We did not use ECG gating when the anterior mediastinal lesions did not seem to clearly invade the adjacent organs. Axial CT images were reconstructed using gapless 3-mm-thick slices and a smooth kernel for soft tissue, and were displayed at a window width of 300 Hounsfield Unit (HU) and a level of 30 HU for the mediastinum and a window width of 1500 HU and a level of −550 H.U for the lung. The Volume CT Dose Index (CTDIvol) was recorded in 32 of the 56 cases. Mean ± standard deviation of CTDIvol of CT examination with and without ECG gating was 53.5 ± 16.6 and 12.8 ± 3.08, respectively.

Image interpretation

Two chest radiologists (observers 1 and 2 with 28 and 10 years of experience, respectively), blinded to the patients' histopathological diagnoses, assessed the CT scans independently. We divided the mediastinum into 4 sections; i.e., into the cranial and caudal parts on each side of the superior margin of each auricle. We named the right upper part section 1, the right lower part section 2, the left upper part section 3, and the left lower part section 4.

The PCPV depiction rate in each of the four sections and the spatial relationship between the center of each anterior mediastinal lesion on the trans-axial image where the lesion was the largest and the ipsilateral PCPV, were assessed on each scan. The center of the mediastinal lesion was determined as a point at which the longest axis and the maximum minor axis vertical to the longest axis crossed. The borderline between the medial and lateral sides was determined as a line from the PCPV, which ran vertical to the mediastinal plane (Fig. 1). The PCPV

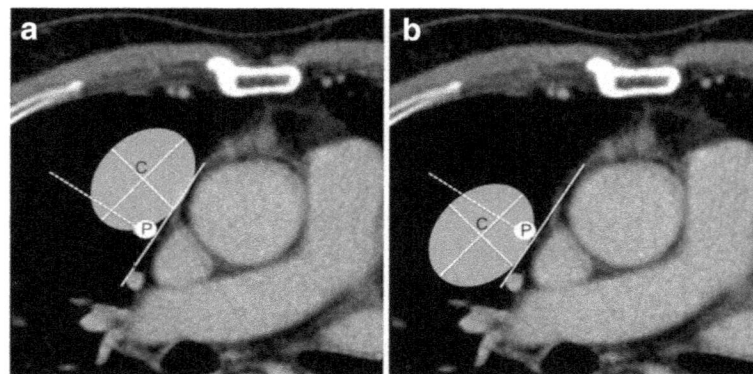

Fig. 1 The positional relationships between the center of each anterior mediastinal lesion and the ipsilateral PCPV. We evaluated whether the center of the lesion (C) was located on the medial or lateral side of the ipsilateral PCPV (P). The borderline (dotted line) between the medial and lateral sides was determined as a line vertical to the mediastinal plane. **a** Schema of the center of the lesion located on the medial side of the ipsilateral PCPV. **b** Schema of the center of the lesion located on the lateral side of the ipsilateral PCPV

depiction rate was visually scored using a 4-point scale: detectable in <25% of slices: 1; 25–50%: 2; 50–75%: 3; and 75–100%: 4. The differences in the PCPV depiction rate between ECG-gated and non-ECG-gated CT were assessed statistically. The two radiologists learned the anatomy and typical CT images of the PCPV before-hand. Any difference in interpretation was solved by consensus of the two observers. When PCPV depiction was poor around the anterior mediastinal mass, we determined the relationship between the locations of the lesion and PCPV, to complement the PCPV, by the detectable parts of the PCPV located at the cranial and caudal portions of the invisible area.

Evaluation of phrenic nerve resection and palsy

Frequency of phrenic nerve conservation and resection at surgery and occurrence of phrenic nerve palsy after surgery were evaluated from the medical record.

Statistical analysis

We used the Wilcoxon rank sum test for comparisons of the PCPV depiction rates obtained for each section with and without ECG-gating. The Wilcoxon signed-ranked test was used to compare the PCPV depiction rates for the left and right sides. These two tests were carried out using a software MEPHAS on the web (http://www.gen-info.osaka-u.ac.jp/MEPHAS/). Fisher's exact test was used to assess the relationships between the location of each anterior mediastinal lesion relative to the PCPV and the histological diagnosis, with a software js-STAR (http://www.kisnet.or.jp/nappa/software/star/). P-values of less than 0.05 were considered to indicate significant differences.

Results

PCPV depiction rate for each region

The PCPV depiction rates for each mediastinal section obtained by each observer are shown in Table 1. When a depiction rate score of 3 or more on both the right and left sides was defined as indicating overall good depiction of the PCPV, 20/56 (36%) on the right side and 28/56 (50%) on the left side were judged as good depiction by observer 1, and 17/56 (30%) and 28/56 (50%), respectively, by observer 2. The differences in each PCPV depiction rate between non-ECG-gated and ECG-gated CT are shown in Table 2. Regarding the PCPV depiction rates obtained with or without ECG gating by observer 1, the PCPV depiction rate for the lower left section of the mediastinum was significantly higher when ECG gating was used ($p = 0.0032$) (Fig. 2). During the evaluations performed by observer 2, the PCPV depiction rate for the lower left section of the mediastinum tended to increase during ECG gating ($p = 0.069$).

Table 1 PCPV depiction rates for each part of the mediastinum

	PCPV depiction rate score			
Observer 1	1	2	3	4
Section 1	14 (25)	15 (27)	16 (29)	11 (20)
Section 2	8 (14)	13 (23)	17 (30)	18 (32)
Section 3	4 (7)	8 (14)	15 (27)	29 (52)
Section 4	10 (18)	14 (25)	17 (30)	15 (27)
Observer 2				
Section 1	17 (30)	17 (30)	10 (18)	12 (21)
Section 2	10 (18)	10 (18)	25 (45)	11 (20)
Section 3	6 (11)	8 (14)	14 (25)	28 (50)
Section 4	14 (25)	9 (16)	18 (32)	15 (27)

The figures in parentheses are percentages
PCPV pericardiacophrenic veins

Table 2 Differences in the PCPV depiction rates for each part of the mediastinum between non-ECG gated and ECG gated CT

	PCPV depiction rate score				
Observer 1	1	2	3	4	*p*-value
Section 1					
Non-ECG gated	11 (32)	10 (29)	6 (18)	7 (21)	0.14
ECG gated	3 (14)	5 (23)	10 (45)	4 (18)	
Section 2					
Non-ECG gated	5 (15)	9 (26)	11 (32)	9 (26)	0.35
ECG gated	3 (14)	4 (18)	6 (27)	9 (41)	
Section 3					
Non-ECG gated	3 (9)	5 (15)	8 (24)	18 (53)	0.96
ECG gated	1 (5)	3 (14)	7 (32)	11 (50)	
Section 4*					
Non-ECG gated	9 (26)	10 (29)	10 (29)	5 (15)	0.0032
ECG gated	1 (5)	4 (18)	7 (32)	10 (45)	
Observer 2					
Section 1					
Non-ECG gated	11 (32)	12 (35)	3 (9)	8 (24)	0.54
ECG gated	6 (27)	5 (23)	7 (32)	4 (18)	
Section 2					
Non-ECG gated	7 (21)	7 (21)	14 (41)	6 (18)	0.34
ECG gated	3 (14)	3 (14)	11 (50)	5 (23)	
Section 3					
Non-ECG gated	3 (9)	6 (18)	9 (26)	16 (47)	0.69
ECG gated	3 (14)	2 (9)	5 (23)	12 (55)	
Section 4					
Non-ECG gated	11 (32)	6 (18)	10 (29)	7 (21)	0.069
ECG gated	3 (14)	3 (14)	8 (36)	8 (36)	

ECG electrocardiographic, *PCPV* pericardiacophrenic veins
* The differences between the data obtained using non-ECG gated and ECG gated CT were statistically significant ($p < 0.05$). The figures in parentheses are percentages

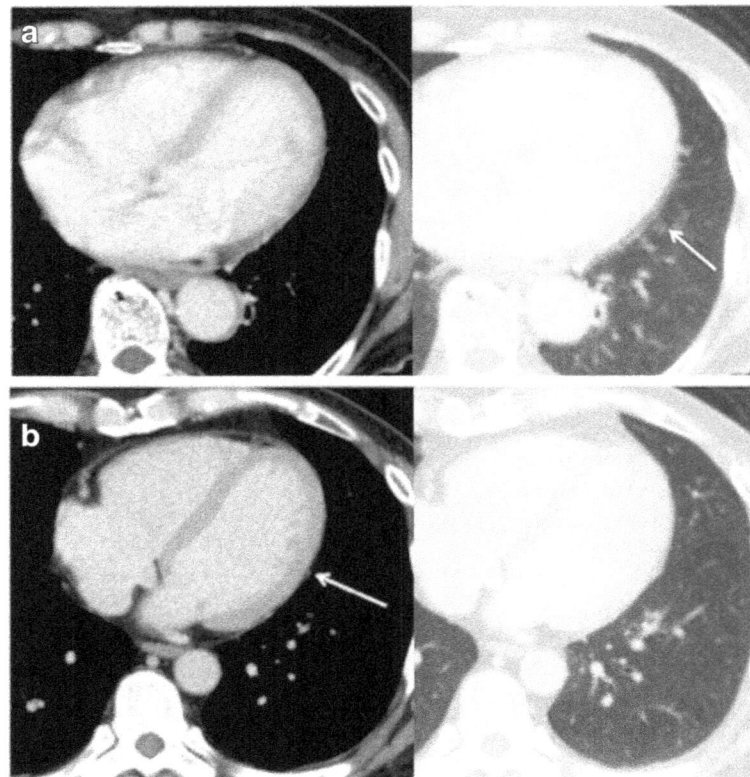

Fig. 2 a Axial non-ECG-gated CT scan obtained in a case with a PCPV depiction rate score of 1. The PCPV was not detectable in the left lower part of the mediastinum because of cardiac motion artifacts (arrow). **b** Axial ECG-gated CT scan obtained in a case with a PCPV depiction rate score of 4. The PCPV was clearly depicted in the left lower part of the mediastinum (arrow)

Relationships between the location of each anterior mediastinal lesion relative to the PCPV and the histological diagnosis

All 50 thymic tumors and 3 of the 6 non-thymic lesions were located on the medial side of the ipsilateral PCPV (Fig. 3). The 3 lesions located on the lateral side of the ipsilateral PCPV were confirmed to be non-thymic (Castleman's disease, a metastatic tumor from renal cell carcinoma (Fig. 4), and a tuberculoma) ($p = 0.0007$) (Table 3).

Phrenic nerve resection and palsy

Nine of the 56 (16%) cases underwent phrenic nerve resection due to tumor invasion to the nerve, which resulted in postoperative phrenic nerve palsy in all cases. On the other hand, the phrenic nerves could be preserved in 4 of the 56 (7%) cases despite that they were surrounded by the tumors. In one of the 4 cases, mild phrenic nerve palsy developed even after preservation of the nerve at surgery.

Discussion

Our results indicate the depictability of the PCPV, which runs parallel to the phrenic nerves, on MDCT. Relatively good depiction of the PCPV was obtained in the left upper part of the mediastinum. The PCPV depiction rate

in the left lower part of the mediastinum was improved significantly by the ECG-gating technique. All 3 lesions located on the lateral side of the ipsilateral PCPV were diagnosed as non-thymic tumors based on the spatial relationship between their centers and the ipsilateral

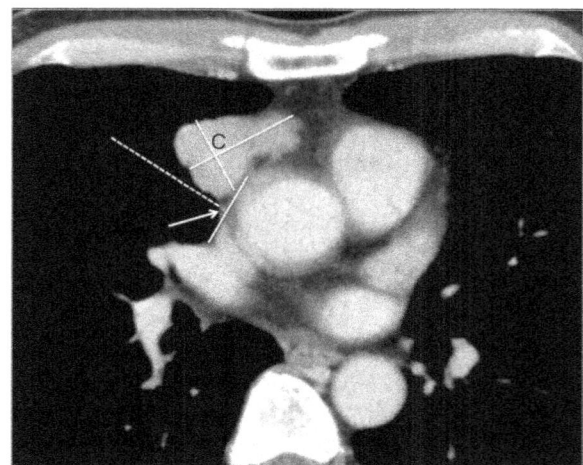

Fig. 3 Axial CT detected a thymoma in the anterior mediastinum. The center of the tumor (C) was located on the medial side of the ipsilateral PCPV (arrow)

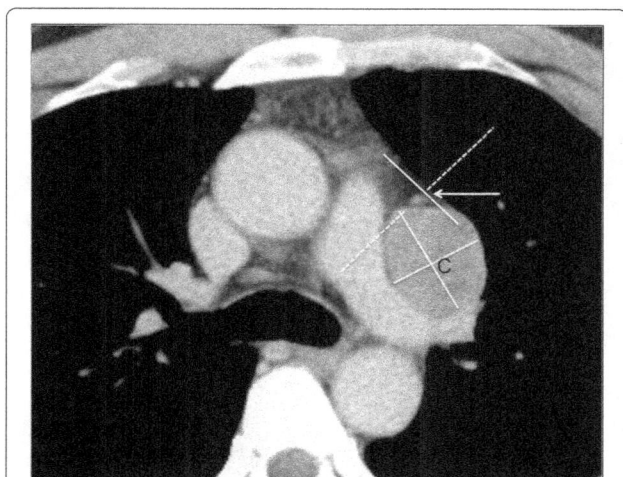

Fig. 4 A case involving a metastatic tumor derived from renal cell carcinoma. The center of the lesion (C) was located on the lateral side of the ipsilateral PCPV (arrow)

PCPV. These results indicate that the locations of the bilateral phrenic nerves can be determined by identifying the PCPV on MDCT. ECG-gated CT may reduce cardiac motion artifacts in the left lower part of the heart, resulting in better depiction of the PCPV. When the center of an anterior mediastinal lesion is located on the lateral side of the PCPV, non-thymic lesions should be considered during diagnosis.

The phrenic nerves innervate the diaphragm to provide motor functions and the central intrathoracic and peritoneal surfaces of the diaphragm to provide sensory functions [6]. The phrenic nerves originate from the cervical C3-C5 nerves and run from the thoracic inlet to the diaphragm along the lateral part of the mediastinum [6, 7]. The right phrenic nerve lies laterally to the right brachiocephalic vein and the superior vena cava, while the left phrenic nerve runs laterally to the aortic arch. Both phrenic nerves then pass anteriorly to their respective pulmonary hila and inferiorly in a broad vertical plane along the margin of the heart between the fibrous (parietal) pericardium and the mediastinal pleura (Fig. 5) [6]. The PCPV, which have connections to the pericardium, pleura, and diaphragm, ascend towards the phrenic nerves between the parietal pericardium and mediastinal pleura. The PCPV are sometimes connected

Table 3 Relationships between the location of the center of each anterior mediastinal lesion relative to the ipsilateral PCPV and lesion type

	Medial	Lateral	Total
Thymic origin	50	0	50
Non-thymic origin	3	3	6
	53	3	56

PCPV pericardiacophrenic veins

superiorly to the internal thoracic, left superior intercostal, and brachiocephalic veins. The left PCPV feeds into the left brachiocephalic vein via an opening opposite the orifice for the left jugular vein, while the right PCPV feeds into the ipsilateral brachiocephalic vein at a more proximal site. In cases involving the occlusion of the superior vena cava and azygos vein, the PCPV can increase in diameter due to the development of collateral blood vessels [2–4]. This anatomical information regarding the PCPV can help clinicians to identify the location of the phrenic nerves.

There have been a few papers about the depiction of the PCPV or the phrenic nerves on CT [3, 4, 6–10], but no previous studies have examined the relationship between the locations of the phrenic nerves and anterior mediastinal lesions. It is difficult to visualize the phrenic nerves on CT, as they are encased in folds of the parietal pleura and mediastinal fat, but the PCPV can be used as landmarks to locate the phrenic nerves [8]. The pericardiacophrenic artery (PCPA) also runs parallel to the phrenic nerve, but the PCPA is usually smaller than the PCPV in diameter, and we used images at the delayed contrast enhancement phase. So, we evaluated the PCPV rather than the PCPA. In a previous study, the phrenic nerve depiction rate on CT images with a slice thickness of 8 mm was 85% (11/13) on the left side, 8% (1/13) on the right side, and 8% (1/13) for the bilateral nerves [9]. A study based on coronary 64-row MDCT indicated that the phrenic nerves were detected in 78 of 106 cases (74%) on the left side and 50 cases (47%) on the right side [10]. The PCPV depiction rate on the left side was also higher in our study than on the right side. It might be due to the location of the upper part of the right phrenic nerve that runs closely to the right brachiocephalic vein and superior vena cava. It would be difficult to separate these veins and the right phrenic nerve. On the other hand, the upper part of the left phrenic nerve tends to separate from the subaortic arch, leading to the difference in detectability between the right and left phrenic nerves. The phrenic nerve is a tiny structure with a diameter of 1–3 mm [9]. So, high spatial resolution of CT could help detect the nerve. We did not employ thin slice images, and evaluated 3-mm-thick images for routine clinical use. The ECG gating technique might be useful for lesions located at the left lower part (Section 4), since the region is usually most affected by cardiac motion. In this section, the PCPV depiction rate improved by ECG gating in observer 1 ($p = 0.0032$) and tended to improve in observer 2 ($p = 0.069$). The difference between the two observers may be due to the differences in their experience with chest radiology and the ECG-gating technique. The ECG-gating technique is rather unusual as a preoperative examination. So, we think that the ECG-gating technique might be useful for

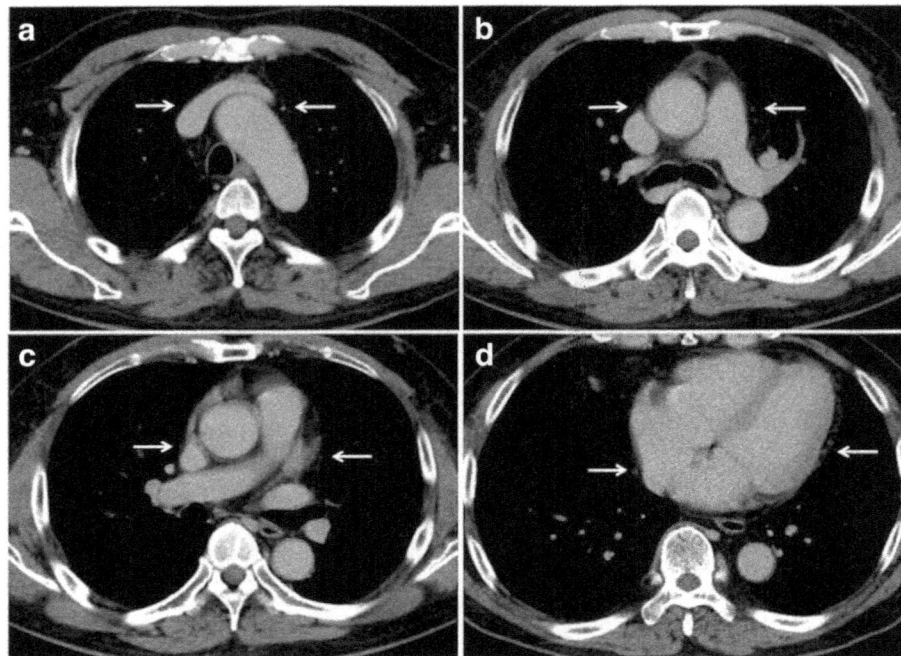

Fig. 5 Representative location of the bilateral PCPV, which runs parallel to the phrenic nervesThe PCPV on each CT slice is shown as dotted structures (arrows). **a** On the right side, the phrenic nerve lies laterally to the right brachiocephalic vein and the superior vena cava, while the left phrenic nerve runs laterally to the aortic arch. **b-d** The bilateral phrenic nerves pass anteriorly to the respective pulmonary hila and inferiorly in a broad vertical plane along the margin of the heart between the parietal pericardium and the mediastinal pleura.

patients with an anterior mediastinal lesion, especially adjacent to the left ventricle of the heart, and for whom evaluation of anatomical relationship between the phrenic nerves and mediastinal lesion is considered clinically important.

Thymoma, thymic carcinoma, thymic cyst, mature teratoma, malignant germ cell tumor, and malignant lymphoma are representative anterior mediastinal tumors [11, 12]. However, other lesions such as metastases and tuberculosis infections also occur in the anterior mediastinum [12]. Identifying the phrenic nerves and evaluating the positional relationships between anterior mediastinal lesions and the phrenic nerves may aid the differentiation of anterior mediastinal lesions; i.e., it could help to determine whether a lesion is of thymic origin. The 3 lesions located on the lateral side of the ipsilateral PCPV were of non-thymic origin in this study. Of these lesions, the treatment strategy for the metastasis from renal cell carcinoma and tuberculoma might have been changed to a non-surgical one if these lesions had been diagnosed preoperatively.

It is clinically important to detect the phrenic nerves during preoperative CT evaluations. Combined resection of the phrenic nerves and mediastinal tumors could impair respiratory function and cause severe postoperative complications. Preoperative evaluations to determine whether a tumor has invaded the phrenic nerves are

clinically important because patients with thymomas that have invaded the phrenic nerves may be candidates for neoadjuvant chemotherapy in order to prevent phrenic nerve resection. Conservation of the phrenic nerves could result in better postoperative respiratory function and prognosis. In the present study, the phrenic nerve could be preserved in 4 patients despite the tumors surrounding the nerve, and only one of them developed mild phrenic nerve palsy. Thus, clinical outcome of the patients could be improved by preoperatively evaluating the relationship between the phrenic nerve and mediastinal tumor and determining the strategy for manipulation of the phrenic nerve. In addition, during extended thymectomy for thymoma combined with myasthenia gravis the lateral resection border is basically defined by the phrenic nerves. Therefore, the detection of the phrenic nerves on CT is useful to determine the surgical field preoperatively [5]. It may also be useful to detect extensions of the phrenic nerves in order to diagnose neurogenic tumors derived from the phrenic nerves and identify the cause of cases of phrenic nerve paralysis.

The main limitation of this study was that it did not include many non-thymic tumors. However, we assume that the information regarding the positional relationships between the phrenic nerves and anterior mediastinal tumors obtained in this study may aid decisions as to whether anterior mediastinal tumors are thymic in origin. So, further investigations of such tumors are desirable. In addition, we did not evaluate relationship between the amount of mediastinal fat and PCPV depiction; the depiction rate might become higher if the mediastinal fat is rich, because the PCPV would separate from the heart.

Conclusions

We evaluated the PCPV depiction rate, and it was suggested that the use of the ECG-gating technique during MDCT improves the depictability of the PCPV in the left lower section of the anterior mediastinum. Solitary anterior mediastinal lesions located on the lateral side of the ipsilateral PCPV are likely to be non-thymic.

Abbreviations
CT: computed tomography; DS: dual source; ECG: electrocardiographic; MDCT: multi-detector-row computed tomography; PCPV: pericardiacophrenic veins

Acknowledgments
Not applicable.

Funding
Not applicable.

Authors' contributions
Study concepts: MH. Study design: YO, MH, RS. Data acquisition: YO, MH. Data analysis and interpretation: YO, RS. Manuscript preparation: YO, YS. Manuscript editing: YS, YO. Manuscript review: YS, YO, RS, MH. All authors read and approved the final manuscript.

Competing interests
The authors declare that they have no competing interests.

Author details
[1]Department of Radiology, Nagoya City University, Graduate School of Medical Sciences, 1 Kawasumi, Mizuho-cho, Mizuho-ku, Nagoya 467-8601, Japan. [2]Department of Radiology, Nagoya City West Medical Center, Nagoya, Japan.

References
1. Travis WD, Brambilla E, Müller-Hermelik HK, Harris CC. Pathology and genetics of Tumours of the lung, pleura, thymus and heart. Lyon: IARC Press; 2004.
2. Godwin JD, Chen JTT. Thoracic venous anatomy. AJR. 1986;147:674–84.
3. Lawler LP, Fishman EK. Pericardial varices: depiction on three-dimensional CT angiography. AJR. 2001;177:202–4.
4. Pineda V, Andreu J, Cáceres J, Merino X, Varona D, Domínguez-Oronoz R. Lesions of the cardiophrenic space: findings at cross-sectional imaging. Radiographics. 2007;27:19–32.
5. Masaoka A, Yamakawa Y, Niwa H, Fukai I, Kondo S, Kobayashi M, et al. Extended thymectomy for myasthenia gravis patients: a 20- year review. Ann Thorac Surg. 1996;62:853–9.
6. Aquino SL, Duncan GR, Hayman LA. Nerves of the thorax: atlas of normal and pathologic findings. Radiographics. 2001;21:1275–81.
7. Nalson LK, Walker CM, McNeeley MF, Burivong W, Fligner CL, Godwin JD. Imaging of the diaphragm: anatomy and function. Radiographics. 2012;32:E51–70.
8. Berkmen YM, Davis SD, Kazam E, Auh YH, Yankelevitz D, Girgis FG. Right phrenic nerve: anatomy, CT appearance, and differentiateon from the pulmonary ligament. Radiology. 1989;173:43–6.
9. Taylor GA, Fishman EK, Kramer SS, Siegelman SSCT. Demonstration of the phrenic nerve. J Comput Assist Tomogr. 1983;7:411–4.
10. Matsumoto Y, Krishnan S, Fowler SJ, Saremi F, Kondo T, Ahsan C, et al. Detection of phrenic nerves and their relation to cardiac anatomy using 64-slice multidetector computed tomography. Am J Cardiol. 2007;100:133–7.
11. Tomiyama N, Honda O, Tsubamoto M, Inoue A, Sumikawa H, Kuriyama K, et al. Anterior mediastinal tumors: diagnostic accuracy of CT and MRI. Eur J Radiol. 2009;69:280–8.
12. Tecce PM, Fishman EK, Kuhlman JECT. Evaluation of the anterior mediastinum: spectrum of disease. Radiographics. 1994;14:973–90.

3

Evaluation of metabolic response with ^{18}F- FDG PET-CT in patients with advanced or recurrent thymic epithelial tumors

Sabrina Segreto[1], Rosa Fonti[2], Margaret Ottaviano[3], Sara Pellegrino[1], Leonardo Pace[4], Vincenzo Damiano[3], Giovannella Palmieri[3] and Silvana Del Vecchio[1,2*]

Abstract

Background: Patients with advanced or recurrent thymic epithelial tumors (TETs) often need several consecutive lines of chemotherapy. The aim of this retrospective monocentric study was to test whether ^{18}F-Fluorodeoxyglucose positron emission tomography-computed tomography (^{18}F-FDG PET-CT) is able to monitor standard chemotherapy efficacy in those patients and whether metabolic response correlates with morphovolumetric response as assessed by Response Evaluation Criteria in Solid Tumor (RECIST).

Methods: We evaluated 27 consecutive patients with advanced (16 patients) or recurrent (11 patients) TETs. All patients underwent ^{18}F-FDG PET-CT before and after at least 3 cycles of chemotherapy. Maximum standardized uptake value (SUV_{max}) of all detected lesions was recorded and the most ^{18}F-FDG avid lesion in each patient was selected for determination of percentage change of SUV_{max} (ΔSUV_{max}) in pre- and post-treatment scans. Tumor response was assessed by contrast-enhanced computed tomography (CE-CT) using RECIST criteria. Receiver operating characteristic (ROC) curve analysis was performed to define the optimal threshold of ΔSUV_{max} discriminating responders from non-responders.

Results: Metabolic response expressed as ΔSUV_{max} was significantly correlated with morphovolumetric response (Spearman's rank correlation, $r = 0.64$, $p = 0.001$). ROC curve analysis showed that a ΔSUV_{max} value of -25% could discriminate responders from non-responders with a sensitivity of 88% and a specificity of 80%. Conversely, basal SUV_{max} values were not predictive of morphovolumetric tumor response.

Conclusions: Our findings indicate that metabolic response assessed by ^{18}F-FDG PET-CT, through evaluation of ΔSUV_{max}, may allow identification of responders and non-responders thus guiding adaptation of therapy in patients with advanced or recurrent TETs.

Keywords: Thymoma, Thymic carcinoma, ^{18}F-FDG PET-CT, Tumor response, RECIST

Background

Thymic epithelial tumors (TETs) are rare malignancies arising in the anterior mediastinum showing a high variable biological behaviour, from slow-growing benign lesions to highly aggressive carcinomas [1, 2]. According to the histological classification of the World Health Organization (WHO), TETs are subdivided into type A, AB, B1, B2, B3 and thymic carcinomas, characterized by an increasing degree of malignancy [1]. Thymic epithelial tumors are routinely staged according to Masaoka-Koga staging system, that considers the integrity of the thymic capsule (stage I), the micro or macroscopic invasion of surrounding tissues and organs (stage II and III), the presence of pleural or pericardial metastasis (stage IVA) and the lymphogenous or haematogenous metastatic spread (stage IVB) [3, 4]. Although both WHO classification and Masaoka-Koga staging system contribute to risk stratification of patients with TETs, therapeutic decisions are essentially taken on the basis of disease stage [5, 6] since WHO classification appeared to have a limited clinical predictive value [7].

* Correspondence: delvecc@unina.it
[1]Department of Advanced Biomedical Sciences, University of Naples Federico II, Via Pansini 5, Edificio 10, 80131 Naples, Italy
[2]Institute of Biostructures and Bioimaging, National Research Council, Via T. De Amicis 95, 80145 Naples, Italy
Full list of author information is available at the end of the article

The treatment strategy for thymic epithelial tumour is primarily based on whether the tumor can be radically resected or not at diagnosis [8–10]. Although surgery remains the treatment of choice, most of these tumors are unresectable or in advanced stages at diagnosis and require chemotherapy, eventually followed by surgery if tumors become resectable after the planned regimen. Furthermore, despite radical resection, recurrence is quite common in those patients and, although recurrent lesions are managed with the same approach used for newly diagnosed TETs, multi-course therapy is often necessary [8–10]. Cisplatin-based combination regimens are usually administered to patients candidate for both neoadjuvant and palliative chemotherapy [11–14]. Several consecutive lines of chemotherapy are also available for patients presenting tumor progression.

In this clinical context imaging modalities are of primary importance in the assessment of tumor resectability and for the evaluation of tumor response to chemotherapy. Contrast-enhanced computed tomography (CE-CT) is the routinely used imaging modality for diagnosis, staging and follow-up of TETs [15–19]. Furthermore in patients with advanced disease undergoing primary or definitive chemotherapy, CE-CT is usually performed to reassess resectability or to determine tumor response using Response Evaluation Criteria in Solid Tumor (RECIST) [20, 21].

Functional imaging with ^{18}F-Fluorodeoxyglucose positron emission tomography (^{18}F-FDG PET) with its ability to identify more aggressive and invasive subtypes of TETs provides useful information for the biologically characterization of thymic masses [22–25] and for disease stage [26–29]. Furthermore, ^{18}F-FDG PET-CT has been performed to monitor the efficacy of targeted therapy in patients with advanced TETs and a reduction of ^{18}F-FDG uptake higher than 30% closely correlated with objective tumor response [30]. Despite the wide use of ^{18}F-FDG PET-CT in the assessment of metabolic response to standard chemotherapy in many solid tumors [31, 32], only few studies tested the ability of ^{18}F-FDG PET-CT to identify responders and non-responders to standard chemotherapy in small series of patients with TETs [33–36]. Since metabolic response usually precedes the morphovolumetric reduction of tumor burden, the early detection of treatment failure may indicate the need to adopt alternative regimens [32, 37, 38]. The aim of the present study is to test whether ^{18}F-FDG PET-CT performed in patients with advanced or recurrent TETs before and after standard chemotherapy may discriminate responders from non-responders and whether metabolic response correlates with morphovolumetric RECIST criteria of tumor response.

Methods

Patients and treatment

In this retrospective monocentric study we evaluated the medical records of twenty-seven consecutive patients, 18 male (mean age ± SD, 56 ± 12 y) and 9 female (mean age ± SD, 57 ± 11 y), with advanced (16 patients) or recurrent (11 patients) thymic epithelial tumors who had undergone whole-body ^{18}F-FDG PET-CT before and after standard chemotherapy regimens. Histopathological diagnosis was obtained in all patients and, based on WHO classification, 1 B1, 7 B2 and 7 B3 TETs along with 12 thymic carcinoma were included in the study. All patients were staged using the Masaoka-Koga staging system based on CE-CT findings at presentation: 3 patients had unresectable stage III, 5 were in stage IVA and 19 patients had stage IVB which included a high percentage of thymic carcinomas (11 patients).

Among the 27 patients, 16 had no chemotherapy before the basal ^{18}F-FDG PET-CT whereas 5 patients received prior adjuvant or neoadjuvant chemotherapy and 6 were treated with definite chemotherapy for advanced, unresectable TET (Table 1). Furthermore, 5 patients underwent radiation therapy after surgery or in combination with chemotherapy. After the basal ^{18}F-FDG PET-CT scan, platinum-based chemotherapy was administered to 23 patients (3-8 cycles, median 5); four additional patients with advanced disease who were in progression after platinum-based chemotherapy were treated with gemcitabine-capecitabine (at least 7 cycles).

Response evaluation

Contrast-enhanced CT scan of skull, neck, chest, abdomen and pelvis was performed at baseline and at the end of the planned regimen and the effects of chemotherapy were assessed using the RECIST version 1.1 [21]. Tumor response was defined as: complete response (CR) when there was disappearance of all lesions; partial response (PR) if there was ≥ 30% reduction in lesion size; progressive disease (PD) if there was increase of more than 20% in lesion size or appearance of a new lesion; stable disease (SD) when no PR and no PD occurred. For statistical purposes patients with CR and PR were grouped in the class of responders whereas patients with SD and PD were considered non-responders.

^{18}F-FDG PET-CT Study

^{18}F-FDG PET-CT scans were acquired after fasting for 8 h and 60 min after intravenous administration of ^{18}F-FDG (350–370 MBq). The blood glucose level, measured just before tracer administration, was < 120 mg/dL in all patients. Dual-modality imaging was performed with a PET-CT Discovery LS scanner (GE Healthcare, Milan, Italy) consisting of a PET scanner and a four-row multidetector computed tomography (MDCT) system. MDCT scan was acquired using the following

Table 1 Clinical characteristics of patients ($N = 27$)

Characteristics	N_0	%
Age (yr)		
Mean ± SD* (range)	56 ± 11 (36–82)	
Gender		
Male	18	67
Female	9	33
Histopathology (WHO[a] classification)		
B1	1	4
B2	7	26
B3	7	26
Thymic carcinoma	12	44
Stage at presentation (Masaoka-Koga)		
III	3	11
IV A	5	19
IV B	19	70
Platinum-based regimen		
Yes	23	85
No	4	15
Prior chemotherapy		
Prior therapy for advanced TETs[b]	6	22
Prior adjuvant/neoadjuvant therapy	5	19
No prior therapy	16	59
Prior surgical resection of primary tumor		
Yes	11	41
No	16	59
Prior radiotherapy		
Yes	5	19
No	22	81

*SD Standard Deviation
[a]WHO World Health Organization
[b]TETs Thymic epithelial tumors

parameters: 4×5 mm collimation (140 kV, 80 mAs), 0.8 s rotation time, pitch of 1.5; when indicated, a fully diagnostic contrast-enhanced CT was performed. PET scan was subsequently performed in 2-dimensional mode using 4 min per bed position and six to eight bed positions per patient, depending on patient height. Iterative images reconstruction was completed with an ordered subsets-expectation maximization algorithm (2 iterations, 28 subsets). Attenuation corrected emission data were obtained using filtered back projection CT reconstructed images (Gaussian filter with 8 mm full width half maximum) to match the PET resolution. Transaxial, sagittal, and coronal images as well as coregistered images were examined using Xeleris software and then transferred in DICOM format to an OsiriX workstation (Pixmeo, Switzerland). All areas of focal ^{18}F-FDG uptake visible on 2 contiguous PET slices at least and not

corresponding to physiological tracer uptake were considered to be positive [39]. The SUV_{max} values of all lesions in the pre- and post-treatment scan were recorded by two board-certified nuclear medicine physicians and discrepancies between their assessments were resolved by consensus through discussion. The SUV_{max} value of the most metabolically active lesion in each examination was used to define the ΔSUV_{max} as follows: $\Delta SUV_{max} = [(SUV_{max} \text{ post} - SUV_{max} \text{ pre})/SUV_{max} \text{ pre}] \times 100$.

Statistical analysis

Statistical analysis was performed using the software MedCalc for Windows, version 10.3.2.0, (MedCalc Software, Mariakerke, Belgium). Data are expressed as mean ± SD if not differently indicated. Unpaired Student's t test was used to compare means of normally distributed data sets as assessed by Kolmogorov-Smirnov test. Spearman's rank correlation was used to examine the association between ΔSUV_{max} and tumor response. Receiver operating characteristic (ROC) curve analysis was performed to estimate the best value of ΔSUV_{max} capable of discriminating responders from non-responders. A p value < 0.05 was considered statistically significant.

Results

Patient characteristics are summarized in Table 1. Pre-treatment ^{18}F-FDG PET-CT scan showed abnormal ^{18}F-FDG uptake in all patients detecting a total of 77 lesions, including 18 mediastinal masses, 15 lymph nodes, 23 pleura/pericardial implants, 16 visceral lesions and 5 bone lesions, with an average of 2.85 ± 2.03 lesions per patient (range 1-8). The lesion with the highest SUV_{max} value in each patient was selected as the target lesion for the assessment of metabolic response; these 27 target lesions showed a mean size of 52.90 mm ± 21.24 mm. The SUV_{max} values of those lesions ranged between 3.3 (pleural implant) and 20 (thymic carcinoma) with a mean of 8.67 ± 4.89 (Table 2). Post-treatment ^{18}F-FDG PET-CT showed reduction of FDG uptake in the target lesion of 19 patients and an increase of tracer accumulation in 8 patients (Table 2). None of the patients showing reduction of ^{18}F-FDG in the target lesion showed the appearance of new site of abnormal ^{18}F-FDG uptake whereas new metabolically active lesions (3 metastatic lymph nodes, 1 lung lesion, 3 pleural implants and 1 large vessel infiltration) were found in 5 out of 8 patients showing increased ^{18}F-FDG accumulation in the target lesion.

After treatment with standard chemotherapy, morphovolumetric tumor response was assessed by contrast-enhanced CT. Based on RECIST criteria, an objective tumor response was observed in 17 patients (2 CR and 15 PR) whereas in the remaining patients, 8 showed SD and 2 had PD (Table 2).

Table 2 Pre- and post-treatment SUV$_{max}$ and ΔSUV$_{max}$ values compared to morphovolumetric tumor response assessed by RECIST

Patient	Target lesion	SUV$_{max}$ pre[a]	SUV$_{max}$ post[b]	ΔSUV$_{max}$ (%)	RECIST[d]
1	Mediastinal mass	10.00	7.50	−25	PR
2	Mediastinal mass	6.60	3.50	−47	PR
3	Mediastinal mass	13.00	6.20	−52	SD
4	Pleural implant	9.23	0.00	−100	CR
5	Mediastinal mass	4.10	3.00	−27	PR
6	Lung lesion	18.70	17.00	−9	SD
7	Lymph node	12.00	11.50	−4	SD
8	Pleural implant	5.80	2.10	−64	PR
9	Pleural implant	7.60	1.70	−78	PR
10	Lymph node	3.70	8.20	120	PD
11	Mediastinal mass	4.19	5.30	26	SD
12	Mediastinal mass	8.40	11.30	35	SD
13	Lung lesion	19.70	5.70	−71	PR
14	Mediastinal mass	4.20	4.60	10	PR
15	Mediastinal mass	5.00	3.00	−40	PR
16	Mediastinal mass	8.40	0.00	−100	CR
17	Pleural implant	4.00	4.80	20	PD
18	Mediastinal mass	15.60	18.5	19	PR
19	Mediastinal mass	7.70	2.20	−71	PR
20	Lung lesion	8.80	14.40	64	SD
21	Mediastinal mass	8.30	5.70	−31	PR
22	Lymph node	8.50	5.40	−36	PR
23	Pleural implant	3.30	1.90	−42	PR
24	Mediastinal mass	7.00	4.50	−36	SD
25	Mediastinal mass	5.60	1.80	−68	PR
26	Mediastinal mass	20.00	15.00	−25	PR
27	Mediastinal mass	4.80	6.70	40	SD

[a]SUV$_{max}$ pre: pre-treatment maximum Standardized Uptake Value
[b]SUV$_{max}$ post: post-treatment maximum Standardized Uptake Value
[c]ΔSUV$_{max}$: percentage change in maximum Standardized Uptake Value
[d]RECIST Response Evaluation Criteria in Solid Tumors, CR Complete response, PR Partial response, SD Stable disease, PD, Progressive disease

Normally distributed SUV$_{max}$ values of pre- and post-treatment ^{18}F-FDG PET-CT scan in responders and non-responders were expressed as mean ± SD and compared. SUV$_{max}$ values of pre-treatment ^{18}F-FDG PET-CT scan were not significantly different between responders and non-responders (8.80 ± 5.04 vs 8.45 ± 4.88, p = 0.8645). Conversely SUV$_{max}$ values of post-treatment ^{18}F-FDG PET-CT scan were significantly lower in responders as compared to non-responders (3.94 ± 3.62 vs 8.99 ± 4.34, p = 0.0038).

The change of ^{18}F-FDG uptake between baseline and post-treatment scan was -46.82% ± 8.10% (SE) in responders, indicating a reduction of tracer uptake, whereas non-responders showed an increase of ^{18}F-FDG uptake with a ΔSUV$_{max}$ of 20.40% ± 15.75% (SE). The normally distributed values of ΔSUV$_{max}$ were significantly different in responders and non-responders (p = 0.0003, unpaired t-test) and were significantly correlated with morphovolumetric response (Spearman's rank correlation, r = 0.64, p = 0.001). Fig. 1 shows the distribution of ΔSUV$_{max}$ values in responders and non-responders.

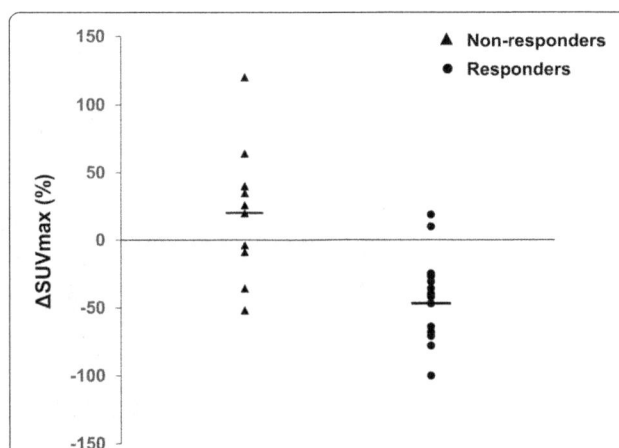

Fig. 1 Distribution of ΔSUV$_{max}$ values in patients allocated in the class of responders and non-responders by RECIST criteria. Responders showed ΔSUV$_{max}$ values significantly lower than those of non-responders (p = 0.0003, unpaired t-test) and a significant correlation was found between ΔSUV$_{max}$ values and morphovolumetric response (Spearman's rank correlation, r = 0.64, p = 0.001). Horizontal bar indicates mean

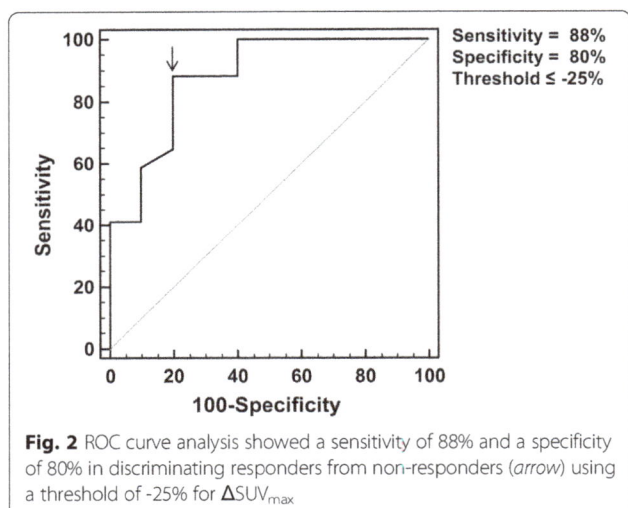

Fig. 2 ROC curve analysis showed a sensitivity of 88% and a specificity of 80% in discriminating responders from non-responders (*arrow*) using a threshold of -25% for ΔSUV_{max}

ROC curve analysis showed that a ΔSUV_{max} value of -25% could discriminate responders from non-responders with a sensitivity of 88% and a specificity of 80% (Fig. 2).

Figures 3 and 4 show representative ^{18}F-FDG PET-CT images of baseline and post-treatment scans in a patient with metabolic response and a patient with metabolic progression of the disease, respectively. The responding patient of Fig. 3 was allocated in the class of PR using RECIST and showed a 47% reduction of tracer uptake indicating a concordance between morphologic and metabolic tumor response. Conversely the non-responding patient of Fig. 4 was judged to have stable disease by RECIST but he showed a 64% increase of ^{18}F-FDG uptake indicating a metabolic progression.

Discussion

The present study showed that ^{18}F-FDG PET-CT may be used to monitor tumor response to standard chemotherapy in patients with advanced or recurrent TETs. The percentage change of ^{18}F-FDG uptake between baseline and post-treatment scans was indeed able to discriminate responders from non-responders and significantly correlated with tumor response assessed by RECIST criteria. In particular, a 25% reduction of ^{18}F-FDG uptake identified responders with a sensitivity of 88% and a specificity of 80%. Our findings are in agreement with previous studies evaluating early metabolic response in patients with TETs mainly treated with targeted therapy [30]. All patients in our study received conventional chemotherapy for advanced or recurrent disease and, being potentially candidate to several consecutive lines of chemotherapy, tumor response was carefully assessed to guide subsequent therapeutic options.

Assessment of tumor response in patients with TETs is usually performed using RECIST criteria in which unidimensional tumor measurements are obtained from pre-- and post-treatment CT scans to evaluate changes of tumor burden in response to therapy [20, 21]. Although RECIST criteria are widely accepted as the standard method to evaluate tumor response in solid tumors, they have some limitations in TETs. In fact, TETs differ from other solid tumors in terms of growth and dissemination patterns especially in advanced stages. They are often large masses with indefinite borders encasing mediastinal structures and infiltrating adjacent tissues. Furthermore non-contiguous pleural metastases are common in these patients and measurements of these lenticular lesions may be difficult. In order to overcome these limitations, International Thymic Malignancy Interest Group proposed modified RECIST criteria for the assessment of tumor response in TETs taking into account the peculiar growth and dissemination patterns of the disease [40–44].

Although standard criteria for the assessment of objective tumor response remain based on anatomical measurements, functional imaging with ^{18}F-FDG-PET-CT has been used for the evaluation of metabolic response to therapy in many solid tumors. Previous

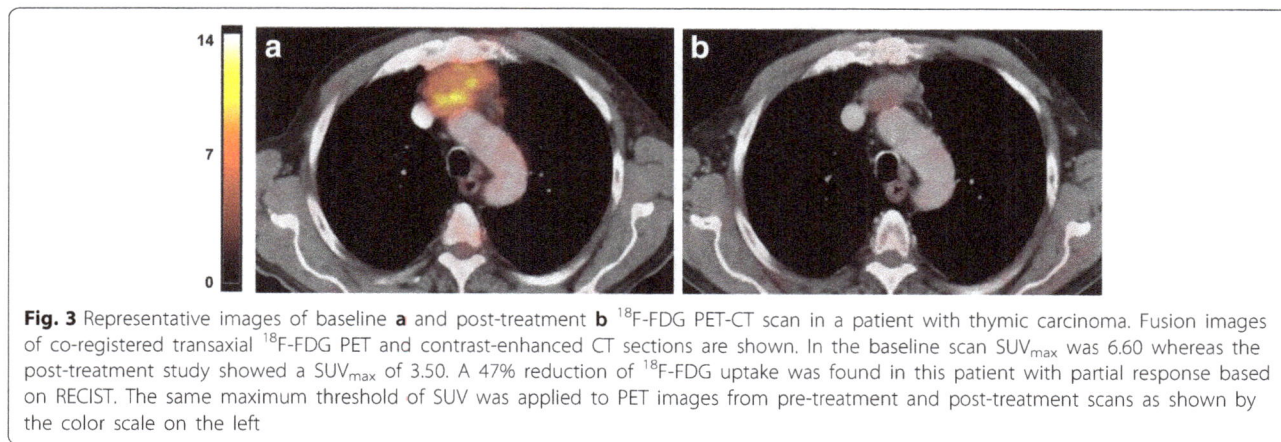

Fig. 3 Representative images of baseline **a** and post-treatment **b** ^{18}F-FDG PET-CT scan in a patient with thymic carcinoma. Fusion images of co-registered transaxial ^{18}F-FDG PET and contrast-enhanced CT sections are shown. In the baseline scan SUV$_{max}$ was 6.60 whereas the post-treatment study showed a SUV$_{max}$ of 3.50. A 47% reduction of ^{18}F-FDG uptake was found in this patient with partial response based on RECIST. The same maximum threshold of SUV was applied to PET images from pre-treatment and post-treatment scans as shown by the color scale on the left

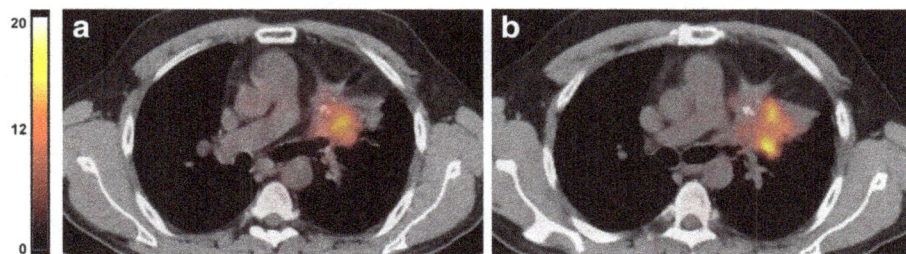

Fig. 4 Representative images of baseline **a** and post-treatment **b** ^{18}F-FDG PET-CT scan in a patient with thymic carcinoma. Fusion images of co-registered transaxial ^{18}F-FDG PET and CT sections are shown. In the baseline scan SUV$_{max}$ was 8.80 whereas the post-treatment study showed a SUV$_{max}$ of 14.40. A 64% increase of ^{18}F-FDG uptake was found in this patient with stable disease based on RECIST. The same maximum threshold of SUV was applied to PET images from pre-treatment and post-treatment scans as shown by the color scale on the left

studies showed indeed that conventional cytotoxic agents, by inducing tumor cell death, cause a reduction of cell viability and glucose demand with a consequent decrease of ^{18}F-FDG uptake that may precede tumor shrinkage as assessed by anatomical measurements [32, 37, 38, 45, 46]. Due to the consistent results of a number of studies, recommendations on the use of ^{18}F-FDG-PET for monitoring efficacy of therapy have been published and include EORTC (European Organization for Research and Treatment of Cancer) and PERCIST (PET Response Criteria in Solid Tumors) criteria which are based on changes of tracer uptake in response to treatment [31, 47]. Although clinically relevant thresholds have been proposed to classify metabolic response [48, 49] the optimal cut-off to discriminate responders and non-responders may vary among different malignancies depending on their tracer uptake patterns and dynamics during therapy. In our study, the optimal threshold that identifies responding and non-responding TETs is in agreement with the values proposed by both EORTC and PERCIST recommendations.

Despite the large use of ^{18}F-FDG in the evaluation of metabolic response of solid tumors to therapy, it is still not clear how many lesions should be included in the analysis of pre and post-treatment PET scans especially in advanced stages. Previous studies reported analysis of both single and multiple lesions and both approaches resulted to be predictive of morphovolumetric response or outcome [48, 50]. Considering the potential association between ^{18}F-FDG uptake and degree of invasiveness of TETs and the possible coexistence of different WHO histotypes in the same tumor mass, we decide to analyse the most ^{18}F-FDG avid lesion in pre and post-treatment scans in order to derive the percentage change of tracer uptake, after ensuring that no new lesions were found or metabolic progression occurred in all other lesions in post-treatment ^{18}F-FDG PET-CT. This simplified approach may be easily employed to evaluate metabolic response in patients with TETs in daily clinical practice

although we are aware that other volume-based metabolic parameters, such as metabolic tumor volume (MTV) and total lesion glycolysis (TLG) may better reflect metabolic response in all lesions and be more reliable predictive markers of survival [51].

Limitations of our monocentric study are the retrospective analysis of imaging findings and the relatively limited series of patients. Therefore further studies are needed to confirm our findings in a larger population of patients and, since TETs are rare tumors, this may require the involvement of several institutions.

Conclusions

Our study showed that metabolic response assessed by ^{18}F-FDG PET-CT may complement RECIST criteria in the identification of responders and non-responders thus providing an additional guide for adaptation of therapy in patients with advanced or recurrent thymic epithelial tumors.

Abbreviations
^{18}F-FDG PET-CT: ^{18}F-Fluorodeoxyglucose Positron Emission Tomography-Computed Tomography; CE-CT: Contrast-Enhanced Computed Tomography; CR: Complete Response; EORTC: European Organization for Research and Treatment of Cancer; MDCT: Multidetector Computed Tomography; MTV: Metabolic Tumor Volume; PD: Progressive Disease; PERCIST: PET Response Criteria in Solid Tumors; PR: Partial Response; RECIST: Response Evaluation Criteria in Solid Tumor; ROC: Receiver Operating Characteristic; SD: Stable Disease; SUV$_{max}$: Maximum Standardized Uptake Value; TETs: Thymic Epithelial Tumors; TLG: Total Lesion Glycolysis; WHO: World Health Organization; ΔSUV$_{max}$: percentage change of SUV$_{max}$ in pre- and post-treatment scans.

Acknowledgements
The authors would like to acknowledge AIRC, Associazione Italiana per la Ricerca sul Cancro (project No. IG-17249) and POR (Programma Operativo Regionale) Campania FESR (Fondo Europeo Sviluppo Regionale) 2007/2013, Rete delle Biotecnologie Campane.
The authors would like to thank Dr Viviana De Rosa for her help in the preparation of this manuscript and the Rare Tumors Reference Center of University of Naples Federico II for patient's care.

Funding
This work was partly supported by AIRC, Associazione Italiana per la Ricerca sul Cancro (project No. IG-17249) and POR (Programma Operativo Regionale) Campania FESR (Fondo Europeo Sviluppo Regionale) 2007/2013, Rete delle Biotecnologie Campane.

Authors' contributions
SS, SDV, GP and MO were responsible for study design and conception; data collection was performed by MO, SP and VD; SS, SDV, RF and LP were responsible for data analysis and interpretation; RF and SP carried out image processing; manuscript was drafted by SS and SDV. All authors read and approved the final manuscript.

Competing interests
The authors declare that they have no competing interests.

Author details
[1]Department of Advanced Biomedical Sciences, University of Naples Federico II, Via Pansini 5, Edificio 10, 80131 Naples, Italy. [2]Institute of Biostructures and Bioimaging, National Research Council, Via T. De Amicis 95, 80145 Naples, Italy. [3]Rare Tumors Reference Center, University of Naples Federico II, Via S. Pansini 5, 80131 Naples, Italy. [4]Department of Medicine and Surgery, University of Salerno, Via S. Allende, 84081 Baronissi, Salerno, Italy.

References
1. Srirajaskanthan R, Toubanakis C, Dusmet M, Caplin ME. A review of thymic tumours. Lung Cancer. 2008;60:4–13.
2. Priola AM, Priola SM. Imaging of thymus in myasthenia gravis: from thymic hyperplasia to thymic tumor. Clin Radiol. 2014;69:e230–45.
3. Masaoka A. Staging system of thymoma. J Thorac Oncol. 2010;5:S304⁻12.
4. Detterbeck FC, Nicholson AG, Kondo K, Van Schil P, Moran C. The Masaoka-Koga stage classification for thymic malignancies: clarification and definition of terms. J Thorac Oncol. 2011;6:S1710–6.
5. Rena O, Papalia E, Maggi G, Oliaro A, Ruffini E, Filosso P, et al. World Health Organization histologic classification: an independent prognostic factor in resected thymomas. Lung Cancer. 2005;50:59–66.
6. Strobel P, Bauer A, Puppe B, Kraushaar T, Krein A, Toyka K, et al. Tumor recurrence and survival in patients treated for thymomas and thymic squamous cell carcinomas: a retrospective analysis. J Clin Oncol. 2004;22:1501–9.
7. Benveniste MF, Rosado-de-Christenson ML, Sabloff BS, Moran CA, Swisher SG, Marom EM. Role of imaging in the diagnosis, staging, and treatment of thymoma. Radiographics. 2011;31:1847–61. discussion 61-3.
8. Girard N, Ruffini E, Marx A, Faivre-Finn C, Peters S, Committee EG. Thymic epithelial tumours: ESMO Clinical Practice Guidelines for diagnosis, treatment and follow-up. Ann Oncol. 2015;26 Suppl 5:v40–55.
9. Falkson CB, Bezjak A, Darling G, Gregg R, Malthaner R, Maziak DE, et al. The management of thymoma: a systematic review and practice guideline. J Thorac Oncol. 2009;4:911–9.
10. Girard N, Mornex F, Van Houtte P, Cordier JF, van Schil P. Thymoma: a focus on current therapeutic management. J Thorac Oncol. 2009;4:119–26.
11. Loehrer Sr PJ, Jiroutek M, Aisner S, Aisner J, Green M, Thomas Jr CR, et al. Combined etoposide, ifosfamide, and cisplatin in the treatment of patients with advanced thymoma and thymic carcinoma: an intergroup trial. Cancer. 2001;91:2010–5.
12. Lemma GL, Lee JW, Aisner SC, Langer CJ, Tester WJ, Johnson DH, et al. Phase II study of carboplatin and paclitaxel in advanced thymoma and thymic carcinoma. J Clin Oncol. 2011;29:2060–5.
13. Hirai F, Yamanaka T, Taguchi K, Daga H, Ono A, Tanaka K, et al. A multicenter phase II study of carboplatin and paclitaxel for advanced thymic carcinoma: WJOG4207L. Ann Oncol. 2015;26:363–8.
14. Palmieri G, Merola G, Federico P, Petillo L, Marino M, Lalle M, et al. Preliminary results of phase II study of capecitabine and gemcitabine (CAP-GEM) in patients with metastatic pretreated thymic epithelial tumors (TETs). Ann Oncol. 2010;21:1168–72.
15. Marom EM, Milito MA, Moran CA, Liu P, Correa AM, Kim ES, et al. Computed tomography findings predicting invasiveness of thymoma. J Thorac Oncol. 2011;6:1274–81.
16. Zhao Y, Chen H, Shi J, Fan L, Hu D, Zhao H. The correlation of morphological features of chest computed tomographic scans with clinical characteristics of thymoma. Eur J Cardiothorac Surg. 2015;48:698–704.
15. Marom EM, Milito MA, Moran CA, Liu P, Correa AM, Kim ES, et al. Computed tomography findings predicting invasiveness of thymoma. J Thorac Oncol. 2011;6:1274–81.
16. Zhao Y, Chen H, Shi J, Fan L, Hu D, Zhao H. The correlation of morphological features of chest computed tomographic scans with clinical characteristics of thymoma. Eur J Cardiothorac Surg. 2015;48:698–704.
17. Tomiyama N, Honda O, Tsubamoto M, Inoue A, Sumikawa H, Kuriyama K, et al. Anterior mediastinal tumors: diagnostic accuracy of CT and MRI. Eur J Radiol. 2009;69:280–8.
18. Marom EM. Advances in thymoma imaging. J Thorac Imaging. 2013;28:69–80. quiz 1-3.
19. Qu YJ, Liu GB, Shi HS, Liao MY, Yang GF, Tian ZX. Preoperative CT findings of thymoma are correlated with postoperative Masaoka clinical stage. Acad Radiol. 2013;20:66–72.
20. Therasse P, Arbuck SG, Eisenhauer EA, Wanders J, Kaplan RS, Rubinstein L, et al. New guidelines to evaluate the response to treatment in solid tumors. European Organization for Research and Treatment of Cancer, National Cancer Institute of the United States, National Cancer Institute of Canada. J Natl Cancer Inst. 2000;92:205–16.
21. Eisenhauer EA, Therasse P, Bogaerts J, Schwartz LH, Sargent D, Ford R, et al. New response evaluation criteria in solid tumours: revised RECIST guideline (version 1.1). Eur J Cancer. 2009;45:228–47.
22. De Luca S, Fonti R, Palmieri G, Federico P, Del Prete G, Pacelli R, et al. Combined imaging with 18F-FDG-PET/CT and 111In-labeled octreotide SPECT for evaluation of thymic epithelial tumors. Clin Nucl Med. 2013;38:354–8.
23. Sung YM, Lee KS, Kim BT, Choi JY, Shim YM, Yi CA. 18F-FDG PET/CT of thymic epithelial tumors: usefulness for distinguishing and staging tumor subgroups. J Nucl Med. 2006;47:1628–34.
24. Endo M, Nakagawa K, Ohde Y, Okumura T, Kondo H, Igawa S, et al. Utility of 18FDG-PET for differentiating the grade of malignancy in thymic epithelial tumors. Lung Cancer. 2008;61:350–5.
25. Nakajo M, Kajiya Y, Tani A, Yoneda S, Shirahama H, Higashi M, et al. (1)(8)FDG PET for grading malignancy in thymic epithelial tumors: significant differences in (1)(8)FDG uptake and expression of glucose transporter-1 and hexokinase II between low and high-risk tumors: preliminary study. Eur J Radiol. 2012;81:146–51.
26. Park SY, Cho A, Bae MK, Lee CY, Kim DJ, Chung KY. Value of 18F-FDG PET/CT for Predicting the World Health Organization Malignant Grade of Thymic Epithelial Tumors: Focused in Volume-Dependent Parameters. Clin Nucl Med. 2016;41:15–20.
27. Benveniste MF, Moran CA, Mawlawi O, Fox PS, Swisher SG, Munden RF, et al. FDG PET-CT aids in the preoperative assessment of patients with newly diagnosed thymic epithelial malignancies. J Thorac Oncol. 2013;8:502–10.
28. Terzi A, Bertolaccini L, Rizzardi G, Luzzi L, Bianchi A, Campione A, et al. Usefulness of 18-F FDG PET/CT in the pre-treatment evaluation of thymic epithelial neoplasms. Lung Cancer. 2011;74:239–43.
29. Viti A, Terzi A, Bianchi A, Bertolaccini L. Is a positron emission tomography-computed tomography scan useful in the staging of thymic epithelial neoplasms? Interact Cardiovasc Thorac Surg. 2014;19:129–34.
30. Thomas A, Mena E, Kurdziel K, Venzon D, Khozin S, Berman AW, et al. 18F-fluorodeoxyglucose positron emission tomography in the management of patients with thymic epithelial tumors. Clin Cancer Res. 2013;19:1487–93.
31. Wahl RL, Jacene H, Kasamon Y, Lodge MA. From RECIST to PERCIST: Evolving Considerations for PET response criteria in solid tumors. J Nucl Med. 2009;50 Suppl 1:122S–50S.
32. Juweid ME, Cheson BD. Positron-emission tomography and assessment of cancer therapy. N Engl J Med. 2006;354:496–507.
33. Kaira K, Murakami H, Miura S, Kaira R, Akamatsu H, Kimura M, et al. 18F-FDG uptake on PET helps predict outcome and response after treatment in unresectable thymic epithelial tumors. Ann Nucl Med. 2011;25:247–53.
34. Kaira K, Endo M, Abe M, Nakagawa K, Ohde Y, Okumura T, et al. Biologic correlation of 2-[18F]-fluoro-2-deoxy-D-glucose uptake on positron emission tomography in thymic epithelial tumors. J Clin Oncol. 2010;28:3746–53.
35. Korst RJ, Bezjak A, Blackmon S, Choi N, Fidias P, Liu G, et al. Neoadjuvant chemoradiotherapy for locally advanced thymic tumors: a phase II, multi-institutional clinical trial. J Thorac Cardiovasc Surg. 2014;147:36–44. 6 e1.
36. Kim HS, Lee JY, Lim SH, Sun JM, Lee SH, Ahn JS, et al. A Prospective Phase II Study of Cisplatin and Cremophor EL-Free Paclitaxel (Genexol-PM) in

Patients with Unresectable Thymic Epithelial Tumors. J Thorac Oncol. 2015;10:1800–6.

37. Wahl RL, Zasadny K, Helvie M, Hutchins GD, Weber B, Cody R. Metabolic monitoring of breast cancer chemohormonotherapy using positron emission tomography: initial evaluation. J Clin Oncol. 1993;11:2101–11.

38. Weber WA, Wieder H. Monitoring chemotherapy and radiotherapy of solid tumors. Eur J Nucl Med Mol Imaging. 2006;33 Suppl 1:27–37.

39. Fonti R, Salvatore B, Quarantelli M, Sirignano C, Segreto S, Petruzziello F, et al. 18F-FDG PET/CT, 99mTc-MIBI, and MRI in evaluation of patients with multiple myeloma. J Nucl Med. 2008;49:195–200.

40. Marom EM, Detterbeck FC. Overview. J Thorac Oncol. 2014;9:S63–4.

41. Detterbeck FC, Stratton K, Giroux D, Asamura H, Crowley J, Falkson C, et al. The IASLC/ITMIG Thymic Epithelial Tumors Staging Project: proposal for an evidence-based stage classification system for the forthcoming (8th) edition of the TNM classification of malignant tumors. J Thorac Oncol. 2014;9:S65–72.

42. Nicholson AG, Detterbeck FC, Marino M, Kim J, Stratton K, Giroux D, et al. The IASLC/ITMIG Thymic Epithelial Tumors Staging Project: proposals for the T Component for the forthcoming (8th) edition of the TNM classification of malignant tumors. J Thorac Oncol. 2014;9:S73–80.

43. Kondo K, Van Schil P, Detterbeck FC, Okumura M, Stratton K, Giroux D, et al. The IASLC/ITMIG Thymic Epithelial Tumors Staging Project: proposals for the N and M components for the forthcoming (8th) edition of the TNM classification of malignant tumors. J Thorac Oncol. 2014;9:S81–7.

44. Benveniste MF, Korst RJ, Rajan A, Detterbeck FC, Marom EM, International Thymic Malignancy Interest G. A practical guide from the International Thymic Malignancy Interest Group (ITMIG) regarding the radiographic assessment of treatment response of thymic epithelial tumors using modified RECIST criteria. J Thorac Oncol. 2014;9:S119–24.

45. Kasamon YL, Wahl RL. FDG PET and risk-adapted therapy in Hodgkin's and non-Hodgkin's lymphoma. Curr Opin Oncol. 2008;20:206–19.

46. Kasamon YL, Jones RJ, Wahl RL. Integrating PET and PET/CT into the risk-adapted therapy of lymphoma. J Nucl Med. 2007;48 Suppl 1:19S–27S.

47. Young H, Baum R, Cremerius U, Herholz K, Hoekstra O, Lammertsma AA, et al. Measurement of clinical and subclinical tumour response using [18F]-fluorodeoxyglucose and positron emission tomography: review and 1999 EORTC recommendations. European Organization for Research and Treatment of Cancer (EORTC) PET Study Group. Eur J Cancer. 1999;35:1773–82.

48. Lin C, Itti E, Haioun C, Petegnief Y, Luciani A, Dupuis J, et al. Early 18F-FDG PET for prediction of prognosis in patients with diffuse large B-cell lymphoma: SUV-based assessment versus visual analysis. J Nucl Med. 2007;48:1626–32.

49. Ott K, Herrmann K, Lordick F, Wieder H, Weber WA, Becker K, et al. Early metabolic response evaluation by fluorine-18 fluorodeoxyglucose positron emission tomography allows in vivo testing of chemosensitivity in gastric cancer: long-term results of a prospective study. Clin Cancer Res. 2008;14:2012–8.

50. Avril N, Sassen S, Schmalfeldt B, Naehrig J, Rutke S, Weber WA, et al. Prediction of response to neoadjuvant chemotherapy by sequential F-18-fluorodeoxyglucose positron emission tomography in patients with advanced-stage ovarian cancer. J Clin Oncol. 2005;23:7445–53.

51. Moon SH, Kim HS, Cho YS, Sun JM, Ahn JS, Park K, et al. Value of volume-based early metabolic response in patients with unresectable thymic epithelial tumor. Lung Cancer. 2016;100:24–9.

4

Lymphomatosis cerebri: a rare variant of primary central nervous system lymphoma and MR imaging features

Hui Yu[1†], Bo Gao[2†], Jing Liu[1], Yong-Cheng Yu[3], Mark S. Shiroishi[4], Ming-Ming Huang[1], Wen-Xiu Yang[5] and Zhi-Zhong Guan[5*] (iD)

Abstract

Background: Lymphomatosis cerebri (LC) is a rare variant of primary central nervous system lymphoma (PCNSL), characterized by diffuse infiltration without the formation of a discrete mass. The diagnosis of LC is a challenge because the imaging findings are atypical for lymphoma. The purpose of present study is to investigate MRI characteristics and clinical features of LC and potentially facilitate an early and accurate diagnosis of this often-missed disease.

Methods: Seven patients (average 44 years, 19–58 years) with LC proved basing on MRI and histology were retrospectively reviewed the clinical data and cerebral MR imaging findings.

Results: The common presenting symptoms were cognitive decline, behavioral disturbance, gait disturbance. All patients had both deep and lobar lesion distribution, and two of them had infratentorial involvement. Lack of contrast enhancement and subtle patchy enhanced pattern were observed in two and three patients, respectively. The remaining two patients presented multiple patchy enhancement. Most of the lesions were slightly hyperintense to normal brain on DWI as well as hyperintense on ADC maps. Three patients presented a pattern of marked decrease of NAA/Cr, increase of Cho/Cr, and two of the three cases showed increased Lip/Cr and Lac/Cr on MRS.

Conclusions: We conclude that diffuse bilateral lesions especially in deep and lobar region including white and gray matter, without enhancement or with patchy enhancement, marked decrease of NAA/Cr and increase of Cho/Cr, and increased Lip/Cr and Lac/Cr are suggestive of LC. Prompt recognition of these imaging patterns may lead to early diagnosis of LC and brain biopsy with improved prognosis.

Keywords: Lymphomatosis cerebri, Primary central nervous system lymphoma, Magnetic resonance imaging, Diffusion weighted imaging, Magnetic resonance spectroscopy

Background

Lymphomatosis cerebri (LC) is a rare variant of primary central nervous system lymphoma (PCNSL), characterized by diffuse infiltration without the formation of a discrete mass and with little contrast enhancement [1], appearing similar to gliomatosis cerebri [2]. This uncommon entity is a diagnostic challenge because the clinical presentation is subacute and the imaging findings are very different from other PCNSLs which typically presents as single or multiple T2-hyperintense, nodular contrast-enhancing mass lesions on MRI [1]. Central nervous system infections, inflammatory, toxic, and metabolic disorders can also mimic the radiologic features of LC [3, 4]. Therefore, early and accurate diagnosis of LC could be crucial for its appropriate treatment choices [5]. Besides traditional MRI, diffusion weighted imaging (DWI) and magnetic resonance spectroscopy (MRS) can also be informative and useful for diagnosis of this rare disease. Neuroimaging studies of LC are rare, and the characteristics of MRI findings remain to be fully

* Correspondence: zhizhongguan@yahoo.com
†Equal contributors
5Department of Pathology, Affiliated Hospital of Guizhou Medical University, Guiyang 550004, People's Republic of China
Full list of author information is available at the end of the article

elucidated. This study was designed to retrospectively analyze the MRI and clinical manifestations of 7 patients with histopathologically confirmed LC. This summary of the MRI features of LC may facilitate early diagnosis and intervention of this often-missed disease.

Case presentation

Patients and methods

We retrospectively reviewed the clinical data and cerebral MR imaging of 7 patients (from January 2012 to December 2016)who were diagnosed basing on the following criteria: (i) presence of diffuse lesions in the brain MRI without contrast enhancement or with patchy contrast enhancement and (ii) histology revealing lymphoma. Patients with concurrent systemic lymphoma and intravascular lymphoma were excluded. All the patients underwent stereotactic brain biopsy and were diagnosed with lymphoma by two experienced neuropathologists (each with 7 and 15 years of experience, respectively) according to hematoxylin-eosin (H&E) staining and immunohisto-chemical examinations. All patients provided informed consent for MRI examination and for the use of personal data.

MRIs of three patients were performed on 3.0 Tesla Philips Achieva(Netherlands) scanner, three other cases were imaged on a 1.5 Tesla Siemens Magnetom Avanto(Germany), one patient was imaged on 1.5 Tesla GE(America). All patients had T2-weighted fluid attenuated inversion recovery(FLAIR), T2- and T1-weighted images. Post-contrast T1-weighted images were available for all patients after intravenous administration of 0.1 mmol/kg gadopentetate dimeglu-mine(Beilu Inc.). DWI was available in 5 patients, while MRS was available in 3 patients. The DWI was obtained using B-values of 0, 1000 s/mm^2. The mean ADC values in the lesions and in normal-appearing white matter were measured by two experienced neuroradiologists (each with 7 and 15 years of experi-ence, respectively). MR spectroscopy was performed with a intermediate echo time (135 ms or 40 ms) as multi-voxel or single-voxel 2D exam encompassing the lesion. For MRS, the major metabolites(Choline (Cho), N-acetylaspartate (NAA) and Creatine (Cr)) were determined. Also, the presence of lipids(Lip) and lactate(Lac) peaks was determined. For each spectrum, the peak height of total creatine (Cr) was used as the internal reference to quantify other metabolites.

The two neuroradiologists, who were blinded to patient data, reviewed and analyzed the cerebral MRI in consensus. All scans were reviewed noting lesions loca-tion in the brain, patterns of contrast enhancement, the signal of DWI and corresponding ADC map, and MRS

metabolic patterns. The lesions distribution were classi-fied into deep, lobar, and infratentorial categories(Type I,II and III respectively). Deep regions included the basal ganglia, thalamus, internal capsule, external capsule, corpus callosum, and deep and periventricular white matter (DPWM); lobar regions included cortical gray matter and subcortical regions(including lateral white matter adjacent to DPWM); infratentorial regions in-cluded the brainstem and cerebellum. DPWM was de-fined as white matter adjacent to or within approximately 10 mm of the lateral ventricular margin. Contrast enhancement was defined as patchy when a minimally or moderately heterogeneous, not well-defined area of contrast enhancement was present, re-gardless of size. The criterion for diffusion restriction le-sions was hyperintense areas on DWI with corresponding hypointensity on the ADC map. Disagree-ments were resolved by consensus.

Results

Our case series was composed of 3 men and 4 women, ranging from 19 to 58 years of age (average year is 44 and medium year is 49). Presenting symptoms were cognitive decline in 4, behavioral disturbance in 2, gait disturbance in 2, coma in 1 and altered level of consciousness in 1 patient. Five patients were diagnosed with diffuse large B-cell lymphoma and two patients had T-cell lymphoma. One patient was treated with corticosteroids and died 1 month after the biopsy. After courses of chemotherapy in remaining 6 patients, there was some neurological and radiological improvement in four cases, but one patient died 9 months after the bi-opsy and another one patient appeared a mass lesion in parietal lobe after six courses of chemotherapy.

Patient demographics, cerebral MRI findings and pathological types are summarized in Table 1. Repre-sentative FLAIR, pre-contrast T1WI and post-contrast T1WI, available DWI and ADC maps, available MRS are shown in Figs. 1, 2, 3, 4 and 5. All patients had both deep and lobar lesion distribution, and two of them had infratentorial involvement. Lack of contrast enhancement and subtle patchy enhanced pattern were observed in two and three patients, respectively. The remaining two patients presented multiple patchy enhancement. Most of the lesions were slightly hyper-intense to normal brain on DWI as well as hyperin-tense on ADC maps, which were consistent with the increasing diffusivity. Two cases showed increased peak of Lip and Lac on MRS. The pathology was characterized by dispersed round neoplastic cells spreading along the white matter tracts without caus-ing tissue destruction or mass formation and was oc-casionally clustered around blood vessels (Fig. 6 A). Five cases were strongly labeled CD20, a B cell

Table 1 MRI features of the LC cases and histological diagnosis

Case	Sex/ Age (years)	Types of lesions distribution			Enhancement	DWI	1H–MRS	Pathological type
		I	II	III				
1	M/55	"+"	"+"	"+"	Multiple patchy	Slightly hyperintense		B
2	F/49	"+"	"+"		Partial patchy	NE		B
3	F/45	"+"	"+"		Partial patchy	Slightly hyperintense	Cho/Cr ↑ NAA/Cr↓ Lac/Cr ↑	B
4	F/57	"+"	"+"		Partial patchy	Slightly hyperintense		B
5	M/27	"+"	"+"		Multiple patchy	Slightly hyperintense	Cho/Cr ↑ NAA/Cr↓ Lip/Cr ↑	T
6	M/19	"+"	"+"	"+"	No	Slightly hyperintense	Cho/Cr ↑ NAA/Cr↓	T
7	F/58	"+"	"+"		No	NE		B

LC lymphomatosis cerebri, *NE* not evaluated, *DWI* diffusion-weighted imaging, *MRS* magnetic resonance spectroscopy, *Cho* choline, *Lip* Lipid, *Lac* lactate, *NAA* N-acetylaspartate, *Cr* creatine, *B* diffuse large B-cell lymphoma, *T*, T-cell lymphoma

marker (Fig. 6 B) and two cases were positive for CD3, consistent with T-cell lymphoma.

Discussion

About 90% of PCNSL's are diffuse large B-cell lymphomas and only 5% constitute low-grade B-cell type lymphoma, including mucosa-associated lymphoid tissue type and T-cell type lymphoma [6]. LC is a rare type of CNS lymphoma characterized by lymphoma cells diffusely infiltrating the brain parenchyma without forming a mass or distorting the cerebral architecture [2]. MR imaging typically reveals diffuse white matter disease variably involving bilateral cerebral hemispheres, periventricular region, basal ganglia, thalami, or the brainstem [1]. With the aim

of improving knowledge of this entity, we documented the clinical features and brain MR imaging findings from 7 patients with LC and analyzed the abnormal findings of multiparametric MRI focusing on: 1) distribution of lesions on conventional MRI, 2) patterns of contrast enhancement, 3) signal of DWI, and 4) metabolite changes on MRS.

Clinical features

Patients with LC may have variable clinical symptoms such as gait disturbance, focal weakness, decline of cognitive function, memory disturbance, personality changes, dementia, anorexia, orthostatic hypotension, paraparesis and weight loss [3]. Of these, the most common presenting symptoms are cognitive

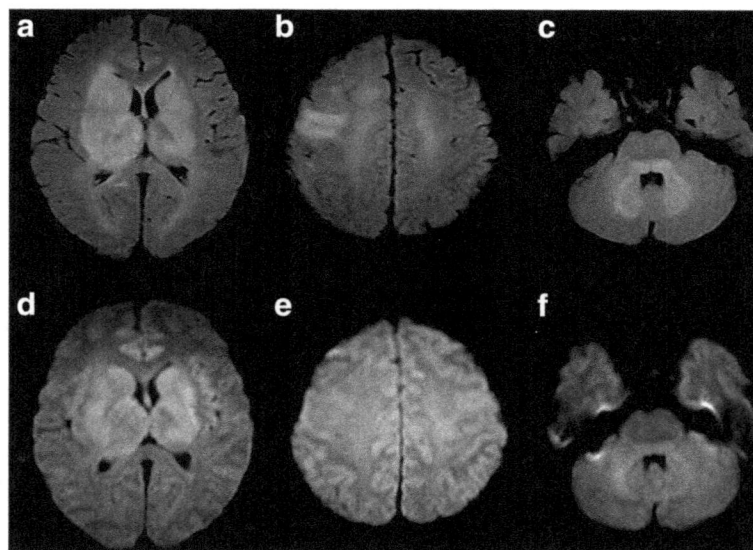

Fig. 1 Nineteen-year-old man with lymphomatosis cerebri. **a**, **b** and **c**, Axial T2-weighted-FLAIR with STIR show the lesions distribution of type I, II and III respectively, which involved bilateral superior cerebellar peduncles, dentate nucleus of cerebellum, basal ganglia, internal capsule, thalamus and right frontal lobes. **d**, **e** and **f**, DWI images show slight hyperintensity in the lesions, but corresponding ADC maps (not shown) indicate no water of restriction

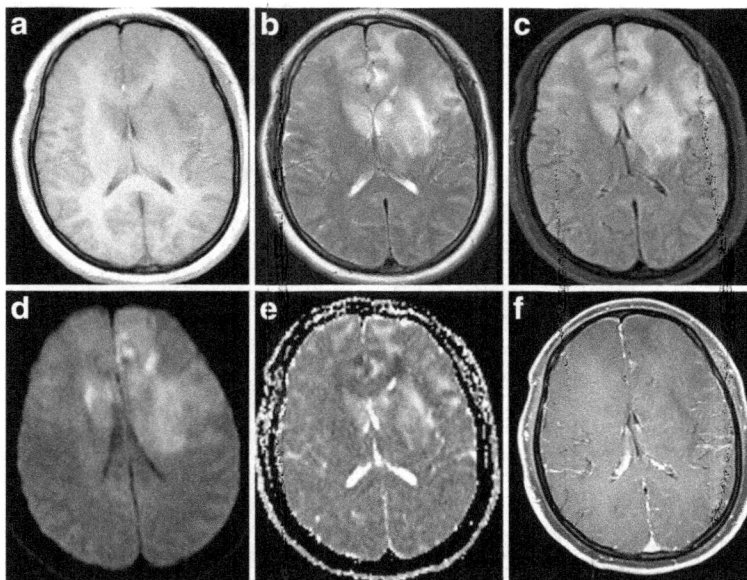

Fig. 2 Forty five-year-old woman with lymphomatosis cerebri. **a**, **b** and **c**, Axial T1WI, T2WI and T2-weighted-FLAIR show the distribution of type I and II lesions, which involved bilateral frontal lobes and basal ganglia, left thalamus, and genu of corpus callosum. **d** and **e**, DWI shows slight hyperintensityand corresponding low ADC in portions of the genu of corpus callosum and left frontal lobe. **f**, Post-contrast T1WI shows subtle patchy contrast enhancement in the left frontal lobe

decline(59.5%), gait disturbances(54.8%) and behavioral changes(50%) [5]. Similar to most reported cases presented with rapidly progressing dementia accompanied by extensive leukoencephalopathy on MRI [2, 7, 8], four of our cases were typical of previously described LC cases. But the clinical presentation of these patients were easily mistaken for other, more common, conditions such as infectious, inflammatory, vascular, toxic, or neurodegenerative etiologies that can cause white-matter injury. Our cases suggested that it is

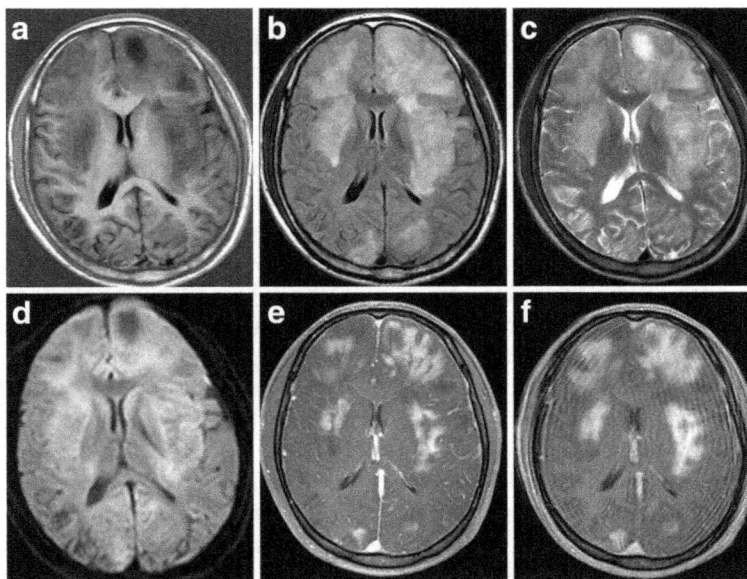

Fig. 3 Twenty one-year-old man with lymphomatosis cerebri. **a**, **b** and **c**, Axial T1WI,T2-weighted FLAIR and T2WI show the distribution of type I and II lesions, which involved bilateral frontal lobes, occipital lobes, basal ganglia and insula. **d** DWI shows slight hyperintensity in the lesions, which were also slightly hyperintense on ADC map(not shown). **e** Post-contrast T1WI shows multiple patchy contrast enhancement in the lesions. **f**, Delayed scanning of post-contrast T1WI shows extended enhancement range of the lesions

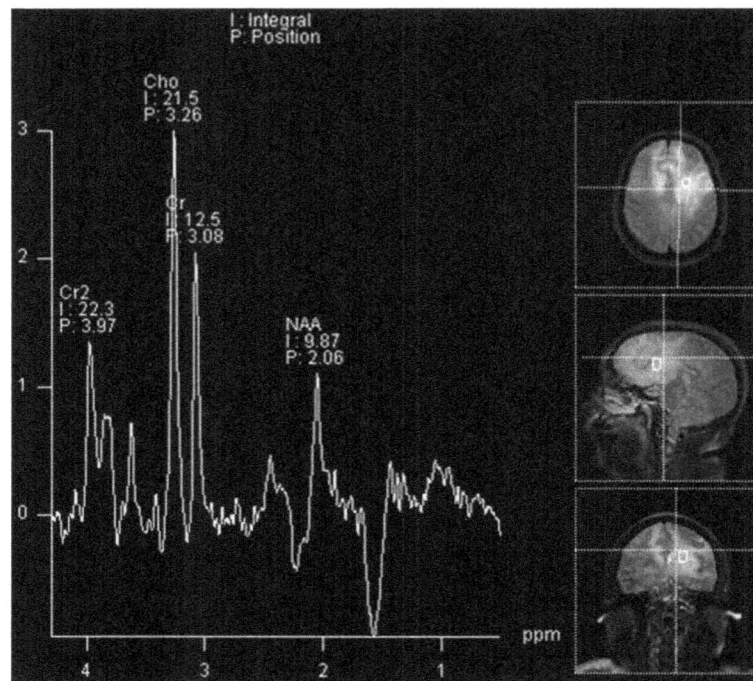

Fig. 4 The same case shown in Fig.2. Multiple-voxel spectra are acquired with a point-resolved spectroscopy (PRESS) sequence, TR 1500 ms, TE 135 ms, NSA 128. MRS shows elevation of Cho/Cr and marked reduction of NAA/Cr in the lesion. In addition, there is an inverted Lac peak

important for clinicians to be aware of this LC form of PCNSL and LC should be added to the differential diagnosis of cognitive decline.

Distribution of lesions

It is noteworthy that all the patients had bilateral hemispheric lesions on MRI. Conventional MRI without contrast enhancement showed extensive, diffuse hyperintense lesions involving bilateral cerebral hemispheres on both T2-weighted FLAIR sequences. Case 1 and 6 of our series had concurrent infratentorial and supratentorial infiltration. The remaining patients presented with isolated supratentorial infiltration. The most common regions involved were the white matter of both hemispheres, in the frontal and deep periventricular regions including corpus callosum, and the lesions extended into the gray matter such as basal ganglia,thalamus and cortex. We classified these lesions by distribution into deep, lobar, and infratentorial categories as TypeI,II and III, respectively. The two most common lesion distribution in LC included those in the deep and lobar categories regardless if the lesions involved gray or white matter. The lesions of deep brain regions type were always bilateral and incompletely symmetrical distribution in LC, but the lesions of lobar type were always unilateral. Lymphomatous cells have a tendency to traffic in rows between white matter fibers rather than expanding diffusely [9]. The diffuse findings can be explained by the theory that lymphoma has to be

considered as a whole brain disease even when it presents with a cohesive mass [10].

Given the multifocal distribution of the lesions in white matter, the main differential considerations were Binswanger's disease(subcortical ischemic vascular dementia), infectious leukoencephalitis, toxic encephalopathy, or neoplasms such as gliomatosis cerebri [2, 11–13]. However, diffuse involvement of both hemispheres and incompletely symmetrical distribution, including involved white matter and deep gray matter simultaneously, distinguish LC from other entities considered in the differential diagnosis.

Patterns of contrast enhancement

Most patients of our series showed patchy contrast enhancement. Bakshi et al. [2] defined cases of LC as diffuse white matter infiltration without the formation of discrete mass lesions and with little contrast enhancement. Rollinset al. [12]reviewed the pathological findings of LC. In LC, there is a diffuse pattern of brain infiltration coupled with the associated perivascular cuffing by both lymphoma cells and non-neoplastic lymphocytes that can mimic an encephalitic pattern [2]. The common reason for a lack of contrast enhancement on MRI is assumed to be an intact blood-brain barrier (BBB), or that significant BBB disruption by lymphoma cells is not yet produced [14]. However, subtle or patchy contrast enhancement has been described in some cases [6, 7]. In

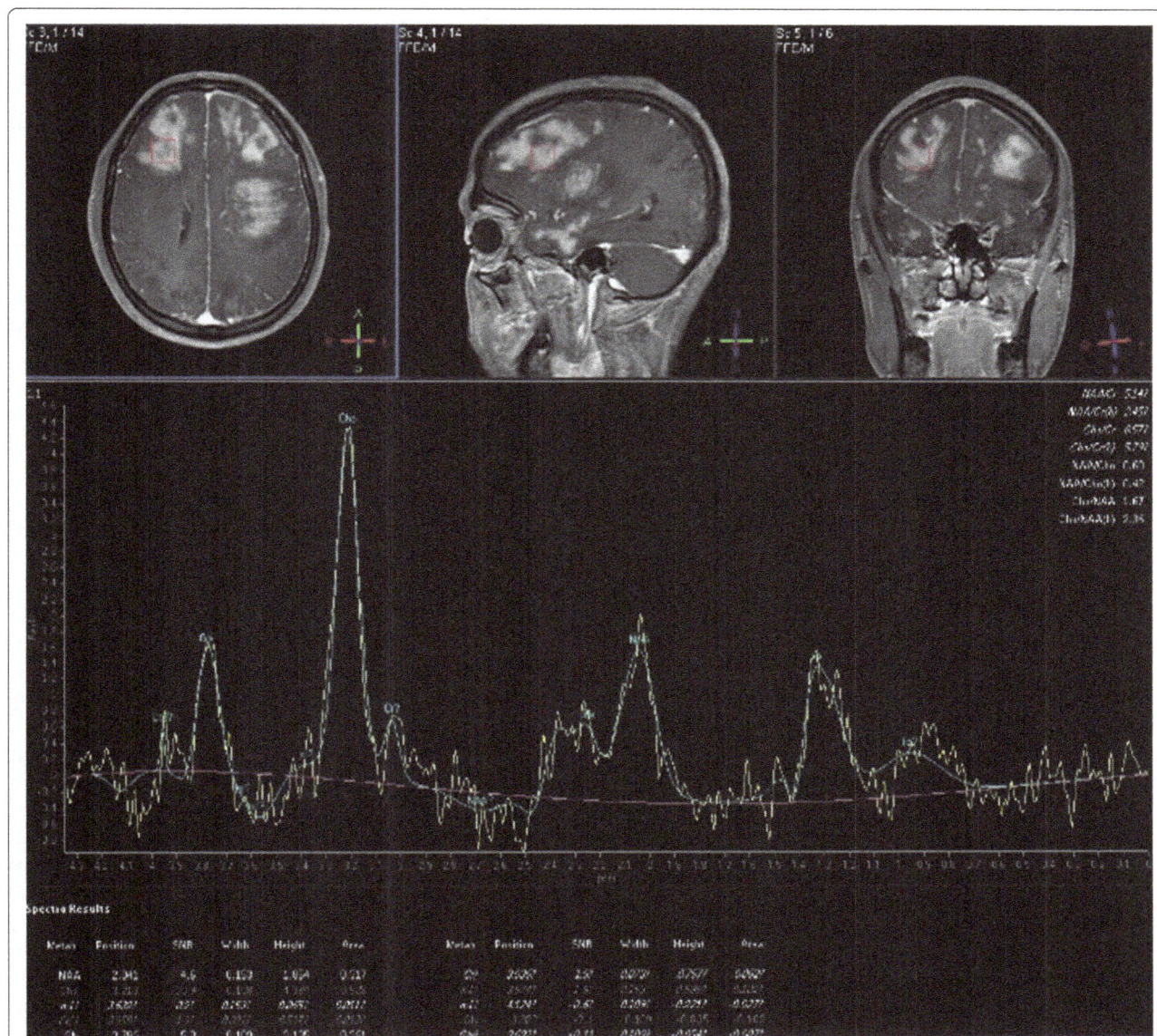

Fig. 5 The same case shown in Fig.3. Single-voxel spectra are acquired with a point-resolved spectroscopy (PRESS) sequence, TR 2000 ms, TE 40 ms, NSA 128. MRS shows elevation of Cho/Cr and marked reduction of NAA/Cr in the lesion. In addition, there is a large Lip peak

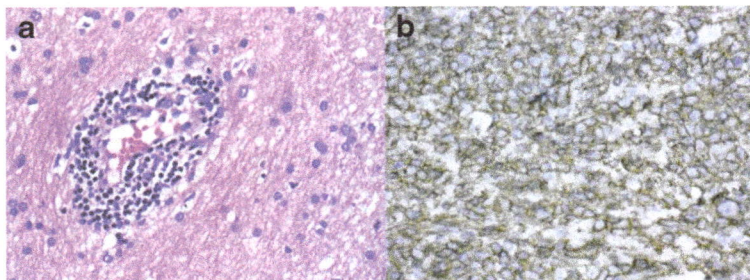

Fig. 6 a Brain biopsy specimen from the case 1 shows dispersed round neoplastic cells spreading along the white matter tracts without causing tissue destruction or mass formation and are occasionally clustered around blood vessels (H&E × 400). **b** Immunohistochemistry shows that the atypical cells were positive for CD20, a marker for **b** cells

these cases, biopsy revealed tumor cells that induced subtle contrast enhancement distributed throughout the white matter; the atypical cells were neither cohesive nor did they form a mass [3]. Subtle patchy contrast enhancement was found in 3 of our 7 patients and 2 patients showed multiple patchy. Our Case 5 showed more substantial contrast enhancement in both cerebral hemispheres, which was misdiagnosed with encephalitis based on the initial MRI and improved after steroid treatment. Histopathological analysis of this patient revealed severe tumor cell infiltration with small round lymphatic cells cuffing and destroying microvasculature, which is consistent with the imaging finding of multifocal patchy contrast enhancement due to BBB disruption. Delayed scanning post-contrast T1WI was 20 min after the initial scan and showed marked contrast enhancement (Figure 3). Other reports [4, 15] have reported that contrast enhancement patterns can change in LC patients on follow-up MRI. A systematic review LC patients found that 26.6% of those without contrast enhancement on the initial MRI and 16.6% of those who showed patchy contrast enhancement eventually developed nodular contrast enhancing lesions at follow-up imaging [5]. The transformation from a non-enhancing to enhancing lesion reflects the eventual disruption of the BBB [16]; this is likely a late event that is due to factors at the cellular level [17]. Although the reason for this transformation remains unclear, we speculate that LC without contrast enhancement might be an early-stage appearance of this specific type of PCNSL with diffuse infiltrating neoplastic cells.

Diffusion weighted imaging

DWI reflects the motion of intra- and extra-cellular water. It is helpful in distinguishing between PCNSL and other tumors and tumor-mimicking lesions [18]. Highly cellular tumors, like central nervous system(CNS) lymphoma, generally present as single or multiple contrast-enhancing mass lesions on MRI scans, with hyperintensity on DWI and hypointensity on ADC maps [19]. Decreased ADC value suggests increased cellularity [20].We observed subjective diffusion restriction in portions of the lesions in two cases, suggesting high cellularity in these portions of the lesions. But most of the lesions were slightly hyperintense to normal brain on DWI and hyperintense on ADC maps, consistent with increased diffusivity. The hyperintensity on DWI and hyperintensity on ADC map may have reflect diffuse cerebral infiltration of non-cohesive malignant lymphoid cells and T2 shine-through effect. Histopathological analysis revealed blastic lymphocytic cells with large pleomorphic nuclei and distinct nucleoli diffusely infiltrating the parenchyma. These lymphocytes showed the typical angiocentric infiltration pattern, and tumor cells invaded

the neural parenchyma with a diffuse growth pattern from these perivascular cuffs. Although DWI was not suggestive of LC in our cases, the variation of DWI signal intensity may be a reflection of the variation of tumor cellular density. However, the slight DWI hyperintensity is difficult to differentiate from gliomatosis cerebri, infectious leukoencephalitis, and toxic encephalopathy.

MR spectroscopy(MRS)

MRS allows for the semiquantitative in-vivo evaluation of metabolites, such as NAA, Cho, Cr, Lac, and Lip. In PCNSL,MRS has demonstrated elevated Lip and Lac peaks, high Cho/Cr ratios, decreased NAA levels and high Cho/NAA ratios [21, 22]. PCNSL grows rapidly and behaves similar to other high-grade brain tumors with evidence of high cell membrane turnover on MRS(high Cho peak), neuronal damage (decreased NAA levels), and anaerobiosis (high lactate levels) [18, 19, 22].These findings are similar to those for high-grade gliomas and metastases; however, MRS is useful to suggest PCNSL because lipids were found to be useful to discriminate between PCNSL and glioblastoma/metastasis at short TE [23].In our three LC patients, MRS (at TE 135 ms or 40 ms) consistently presented a pattern of marked decrease of NAA/Cr, increase of Cho/Cr, which is suggestive of malignant neoplastic disease. Two patients showed increased Lip/Cr and Lac/Cr. The presence of this MRS pattern may help in the differential diagnosis of brain non-neoplastic diseases [20]. We determined that MRS is potentially useful to reinforce the suspicion of LC when bilateral hemispheric lesions were found on an MRI exam. Although LC is a relatively rare type of PCNSL, establishing suspicion of LC by imaging could be a pivotal step in determining management strategies for patients, as it would result in a consideration of biopsy before initiation of treatment with steroids [23].

Limitations

There are several limitations in this study. First, LC is rare and the cases came from multiple institutions. As a result, we had a small sample size and heterogeneity of the dataset where DWI and MRS were not available in all cases; variable imaging sequences were performed in each case. Other advanced imaging techniques were also not available for these challenging cases, including MR perfusion and diffusion tensor imaging (DTI). Perfusion MRI can improve the diagnostic accuracy of PCNSL, particularly when the brain parenchyma is affected [24]. DTI takes advantage of highly ordered white matter fibers, and the FA values for PCNSL can help in the differentiation of glioblastoma [25].

Conclusion

In conclusion, it is important for clinicians and radiologists to be aware of the LC form of PCNSL. Diffuse bilateral lesions especially in deep and lobar region including white and gray matter, without enhancement or with patchy enhancement, marked decrease of NAA/Cr and increase of Cho/Cr, and increased Lip/Cr and Lac/Cr are suggestive of LC. Prompt recognition of these imaging patterns may lead to early diagnosis of LC and brain biopsy with improved prognosis.

Abbreviations
ADC: Apparent diffusion coefficient; BBB: Blood-brain barrier; Cho: Choline; CNS: Central nervous system; Cr: Creatine; DPWM: Deep and periventricular white matter; DTI: Diffusion tensor imaging; DWI: Diffusion-weighted imaging; FLAIR: Fluid attenuated inversion recovery; HE: Hematoxylin-eosin staining; Lac: Lactate; LC: Lymphomatosis cerebri; Lip: Lipid; MRS: Magnetic resonance spectroscopy; NAA: N-acetylaspartate; PCNSL: Primary central nervous system lymphoma

Acknowledgements
We thank all surgeons and neurologists who contributed to patients' management.

Funding
Collection, interpretation of data and writing manuscript were supported by Chinese National Natural Science Foundation GR-81260173,Guizhou Provincial Education Department KY[2016]012, SC CTSI (NIH/NCRR/NCATS) GR-KL2TR000131 and NIH 1 L30 CA209248-01.

Authors' contributions
The manuscript has been seen and approved by all authors, whose individual contributions were as follows: HY, BG, JL contributed to patients'selection, reviewed the MRI findings, conceptualized and wrote the paper; YCY interpreted the patients clinical data. MMH performed the analysis for the DWI and MRS part. MSS wrote part of the paper and polished the manuscript. ZZG conceptualized and reviewed the manuscript. WXY interpreted the histological examination of the specimen.

Competing interests
The authors declare that they have no competing interests.   .

Author details
[1]Department of Radiology, Affiliated Hospital of Guizhou Medical University, Guiyang 550004, People's Republic of China. [2]Department of Radiology, Yantai Yuhuangding Hospital, Yantai 264000, Shandong, People's Republic of China. [3]Department of Neurology, the second affiliated Hospital of Guizhou Medical University, Kaili 556000, People's Republic of China. [4]Department of Radiology,Keck School of Medicine, University of Southern California, Los Angeles, CA, USA. [5]Department of Pathology, Affiliated Hospital of Guizhou Medical University, Guiyang 550004, People's Republic of China.

References
1. Hatanpaa KJ, Fuda F, Koduru P, Young K, Lega B, Chen W. Lymphomatosis Cerebri: A Diagnostic Challenge. JAMA Neurol. 2015;72:1066–7.
2. Bakshi R, Mazziotta JC, Mischel PS, Jahan R, Seligson DB, Vinters HV. Lymphomatosis cerebri presenting as a rapidly progressive dementia: clinical, neuroimaging and pathologic findings. Dement Geriatr Cogn Disord. 1999;10:152–7.
3. Kitai R, Hashimoto N, Yamate K, Ikawa M, Yoneda M, Nakajima T, Arishima H, Takeuchi H, Sato K, Kikuta K. Lymphomatosis cerebri: clinical characteristics, neuroimaging, and pathological findings. Brain Tumor Pathol. 2012;29:47–53.
4. Lewerenz J, Ding XQ, Matschke J, Schnabel C, Emami P, von Borczyskowski D, Buchert R, Krieger T, de Wit M, Munchau A. Dementia and leukoencephalopathy due to lymphomatosis cerebri. BMJ Case Rep. 2009; 2009 10.1136/bcr.08.2008.0752.
5. Izquierdo C, Velasco R, Vidal N, Sanchez JJ, Argyriou AA, Besora S, Graus F, Bruna J. Lymphomatosis cerebri: a rare form of primary central nervous system lymphoma. Analysis of 7 cases and systematic review of the literature. Neuro-Oncology. 2016;18:707–15.
6. Sugino T, Mikami T, Akiyama Y, Wanibuchi M, Hasegawa T, Mikuni N. Primary central nervous system anaplastic large-cell lymphoma mimicking lymphomatosis cerebri. Brain Tumor Pathol. 2013;30:61–5.
7. Raz E, Tinelli E, Antonelli M, Canevelli M, Fiorelli M, Bozzao L, Di Piero V, Caramia F. MRI findings in lymphomatosis cerebri: description of a case and revision of the literature. J Neuroimaging. 2011;21:e183–6.
8. Weaver JD, Vinters HV, Koretz B, Xiong Z, Mischel P, Kado D. Lymphomatosis cerebri presenting as rapidly progressive dementia. Neurologist. 2007;13:150–3.
9. Vital A, Sibon I. A 64-year-old woman with progressive dementia and leukoencephalopathy. Brain Pathol. 2007;17:117–8. 121
10. Lai R, Rosenblum MK, DeAngelis LM. Primary CNS lymphoma: a whole-brain disease? Neurology. 2002;59:1557–62.
11. Filley CM, Kleinschmidt-DeMasters BK. Toxic leukoencephalopathy. N Engl J Med. 2001;345:425–32.
12. Rollins KE, Kleinschmidt-DeMasters BK, Corboy JR, Damek DM, Filley CM. Lymphomatosis cerebri as a cause of white matter dementia. Hum Pathol. 2005;36:282–90.
13. Lewerenz J, Ding X, Matschke J, Schnabel C, Emami P, von Borczyskowski D, Buchert R, Krieger T, de Wit M, Munchau A. Dementia and leukoencephalopathy due to lymphomatosis cerebri. J Neurol Neurosurg Psychiatry. 2007;78:777–8.
14. Terae S, Ogata A. Nonenhancing primary central nervous system lymphoma. Neuroradiology. 1996;38:34–7.
15. Courtois F, Gille M, Haven F, Hantson P. Lymphomatosis cerebri Presenting as a Recurrent Leukoencephalopathy. Case Rep Neurol. 2012; 4:181–6.
16. Samani A, Davagnanam I, Cockerell OC, Ramsay A, Patani R, Chataway J. Lymphomatosis cerebri: a treatable cause of rapidly progressive dementia. J Neurol Neurosurg Psychiatry. 2015;86:238–40.
17. Phan TG, O'Neill BP, Kurtin PJ. Posttransplant primary CNS lymphoma. Neuro-Oncology. 2000;2:229–38.
18. da Rocha AJ, Sobreira Guedes BV, da Silveira da Rocha TM, Maia Junior AC, Chiattone CS. Modern techniques of magnetic resonance in the evaluation of primary central nervous system lymphoma: contributions to the diagnosis and differential diagnosis. Rev Bras Hematol Hemoter. 2016; 38:44–54.
19. Zacharia TT, Law M, Naidich TP, Leeds NE. Central nervous system lymphoma characterization by diffusion-weighted imaging and MR spectroscopy. J Neuroimaging. 2008;18:411–7.
20. Haldorsen IS, Espeland A, Larsson EM. Central nervous system lymphoma: characteristic findings on traditional and advanced imaging. AJNR Am J Neuroradiol. 2011;32:984–92.
21. Taillibert S, Guillevin R, Menuel C, Sanson M, Hoang-Xuan K, Chiras J, Duffau H. Brain lymphoma: usefulness of the magnetic resonance spectroscopy. J Neuro-Oncol. 2008;86:225–9.
22. Raizer JJ, Koutcher JA, Abrey LE, Panageas KS, DeAngelis LM, Lis E, Xu S, Zakian KL. Proton magnetic resonance spectroscopy in immunocompetent patients with primary central nervous system lymphoma. J Neuro-Oncol. 2005;71:173–80.
23. Mora P, Majos C, Castaner S, Sanchez JJ, Gabarros A, Muntane A, Aguilera C, Arus C. (1)H-MRS is useful to reinforce the suspicion of primary central nervous system lymphoma prior to surgery. Eur Radiol. 2014;24:2895–905.

5

How we read pediatric PET/CT: indications and strategies for image acquisition, interpretation and reporting

Gabrielle C. Colleran, Neha Kwatra, Leah Oberg, Frederick D. Grant, Laura Drubach, Michael J. Callahan, Robert D. MacDougall, Frederic H. Fahey and Stephan D. Voss*

Abstract: PET/CT plays an important role in the diagnosis, staging and management of many pediatric malignancies. The techniques for performing PET/CT examinations in children have evolved, with increasing attention focused on reducing patient exposure to ionizing radiation dose whenever possible and minimizing scan duration and sedation times, with a goal toward optimizing the overall patient experience.

This review outlines our approach to performing PET/CT, including a discussion of the indications for a PET/CT exam, approaches for optimizing the exam protocol, and a review of different approaches for acquiring the CT portion of the PET/CT exam. Strategies for PACS integration, image display, interpretation and reporting are also provided.

Most practices will develop a strategy for performing PET/CT that best meets their respective needs. The purpose of this article is to provide a comprehensive overview for radiologists who are new to pediatric PET/CT, and also to provide experienced PET/CT practitioners with an update on state-of-the art CT techniques that we have incorporated into our protocols and that have enabled us to make considerable improvements to our PET/CT practice.

Keywords: PET/CT, Diagnostic CT, Pediatric oncology, Hybrid imaging, Dose reduction, Attenuation correction, Multidisciplinary interpretation

Introduction

Positron Emission Tomography/Computed Tomography (PET/CT) plays an important role in the diagnosis, staging and management of a wide range of pediatric malignancies including Hodgkin and non-Hodgkin lymphoma, malignant soft tissue and bone sarcomas, head and neck tumors, Langerhans cell histiocytosis (LCH) and neuroblastoma [1–4]. PET/CT is the most common hybrid imaging technique currently in use, owing to the increased sensitivity and specificity of PET/CT for detecting metabolically active malignancies. ^{18}Fluorine-2-fluoro-2-deoxy-d-glucose (FDG) is still the most commonly used radiopharmaceutical in routine clinical use, but a number of new PET tracers are being developed with potential for use in imaging children with cancer.

In addition to the discovery and development of novel radiopharmaceuticals for detection of malignant disease, the techniques used to acquire PET images have also

evolved. PET imaging was initially confined to review of emission imaging data. Non-diagnostic quality transmission scans were obtained only for soft tissue attenuation correction of the PET raw data, but provided no additional anatomic information. With the development of integrated hybrid PET/CT scanners, many new opportunities emerged for obtaining high quality co-registered CT images [5]. Because we now have numerous options for obtaining CT images as part of the PET/CT acquisition there is an increasing need for awareness and selection of appropriate CT imaging techniques. These CT techniques may vary substantially, and are largely dependent on whether the CT images are intended for attenuation correction only, anatomic co-localization, or diagnostic interpretation [6].

This review will outline our approach to performing PET/CT in children with a variety of pediatric cancers. We will review current indications and common practices for using PET/CT and the evidence supporting these practices, and discuss the practical aspects of performing and interpreting PET/CT examinations in children.

* Correspondence: stephan.voss@childrens.harvard.edu
Department of Radiology, Boston Children's Hospital, Harvard Medical School, 300 Longwood Avenue, Boston, MA 02115, USA

Indications

Indications for performing (and reimbursing) PET/CT differ between countries and healthcare systems. In the US, reimbursement programs also differ between states and between insurance companies. While private insurers may exercise more latitude in considering payment for imaging pediatric cancers, most third party payers initially rely on the national coverage determinations provided by the Centers for Medicare and Medicaid Services (CMS) for guidance. CMS has expanded the reimbursable indications for use of PET/CT to include the majority of adult cancers [7]. In some cases there is overlap with pediatric cancers, such as lymphoma and melanoma, although for the majority of pediatric malignancies CMS does not provide explicit guidance or approval. As such, in most pediatric cancer centers such as ours, insurance pre-authorization is sought for nearly all new cancer diagnoses prior to obtaining a PET/CT, whether for initial staging or for interim response assessment. CMS approved indications, for which specific reimbursement codes exist, include both Hodgkin and non-Hodgkin lymphoma, melanoma, neuroendocrine tumors, and Langerhans Cell Histiocytosis, as well as other malignancies more commonly seen in adults but occasionally occurring in children (e.g. colorectal and esophageal cancer). In the case of Hodgkin lymphoma, the use of FDG PET/CT to evaluate early metabolic response to therapy has led to new response-based treatment algorithms and completely changed the approach therapy (Fig. 1) [3, 8].

In many other pediatric cancers, including Ewing sarcoma, rhabdomyosarcoma, synovial cell sarcoma, osteosarcoma, gastrointestinal stromal tumor (GIST) and MPNST, there is accumulating data showing the importance of PET/CT in staging, and in some cases response

assessment. For the staging of osteosarcoma, Ewing sarcoma and rhabdomyosaroma there is consistent evidence of improved sensitivity of PET/CT for detecting skeletal metastases when compared to conventional techniques such as bone scintigraphy [2]. The data is less clear regarding the utility of PET/CT for assessing response and predicting outcome in the malignant sarcomas, although several small studies have shown a correlation between changes in FDG uptake (standardized uptake value, SUV) and response to therapy and outcome [9–11]. Pediatric malignancies are comparatively rare, making it difficult to design large clinical trials to demonstrate the utility of FDG PET/CT in the management of most pediatric cancers. As of yet no prospective trials have incorporated response-based treatment decisions into algorithms that rely solely on changes in FDG uptake to dictate course of therapy, which limits our assessment of the prognostic value of PET in these malignancies.

In neurofibromatosis type-1, FDG uptake is an effective biomarker for predicting evolution of benign neurofibromas into either premalignant atypical neurofibromas or malignant peripheral nerve sheath tumors (MPNST) [12]. Many other pediatric cancers have been shown to be FDG-avid and a staging PET/CT has been shown in many small studies to have improved sensitivity over existing techniques [4, 13, 14]. In contrast, neuroblastoma, despite being the most common non-CNS solid tumor occurring in children, is not routinely imaged by FDG PET/CT, owing mostly to the large body of evidence showing the value of ^{123}I-MIBG for staging and predicting outcome after response to induction therapy, in addition to establishing the extent of disease prior to beginning treatment with ^{131}I-MIBG [15, 16]. In addition, in many cases neuroblastoma is

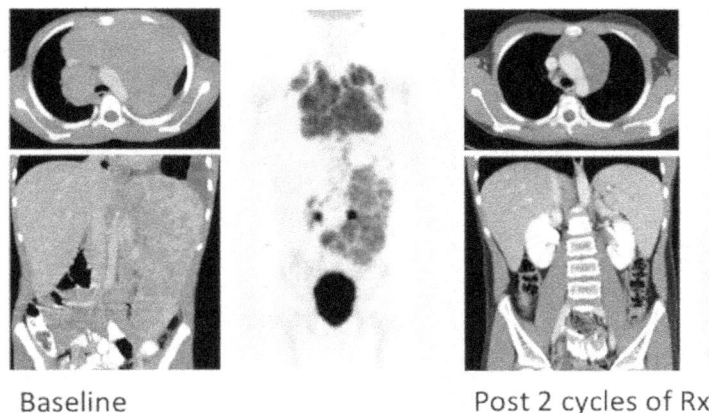

Baseline   Post 2 cycles of Rx

Fig. 1 PET/CT in Hodgkin Lymphoma. Baseline PET/CT shows bulky mediastinal, extensive splenic and intra-abdominal nodal disease. Following 2 cycles of chemotherapy the ^{18}F-FDG PET/CT shows a complete metabolic response to therapy, whereas residual mediastinal soft tissue mass and splenic lesions remain. Following a response-based treatment algorithm, subsequent therapeutic decisions are made based on the metabolic complete response (CR) shown by PET/CT

FDG-negative and as such the routine use of FDG PET in staging and response assessment in neuroblastoma has been largely restricted to those few patients with MIBG-negative disease [17]. Wilms tumor is the most common renal tumor occurring in childhood, although physiologic excretion of FDG from the kidneys has limited the routine use of PET/CT for management of Wilms tumor [18]. In our experience, however, PET imaging may still be useful for staging, particularly for characterizing extrarenal sites of disease, and for restaging at the time of relapse.

Unique molecular targets are also being identified for many pediatric malignancies. Tumors such as inflammatory myofibroblastic tumor (IMFT), as well as other uncommon pediatric neoplasms, are receiving renewed attention based on the identification of molecular markers against which targeted therapies can be directed. The use of FDG PET/CT to monitor changes in tumor metabolic activity in response to treatment with molecularly targeted agents, may be an important surrogate for establishing pharmacologic activity of new drugs being evaluated in early phase clinical trials [19]. In particular, alterations in tumor metabolic activity can play an important role in guiding therapy, even in when significant measureable changes in lesion size and/or number are not observed (Fig. 2).

Practical aspects of PET/CT: ordering, protocoling, acquiring, and interpreting the PET/CT examination

Ordering a PET/CT

PET/CT is typically performed as either an examination of the whole body or the torso (eyes-to-thighs), although more focused limited examinations may be specified by the ordering physician. In general, lymphoma patients undergo examinations of the torso, which assures coverage of the majority of the lymphoid tissue, extending from Waldeyer's ring through the inguinal lymph nodes. Because of the potential for metastatic disease occurring anywhere in the body, sarcoma patients usually undergo a whole-body PET/CT. For other patients the extent of coverage should be determined in conjunction with the ordering clinician to ensure adequate coverage of specific

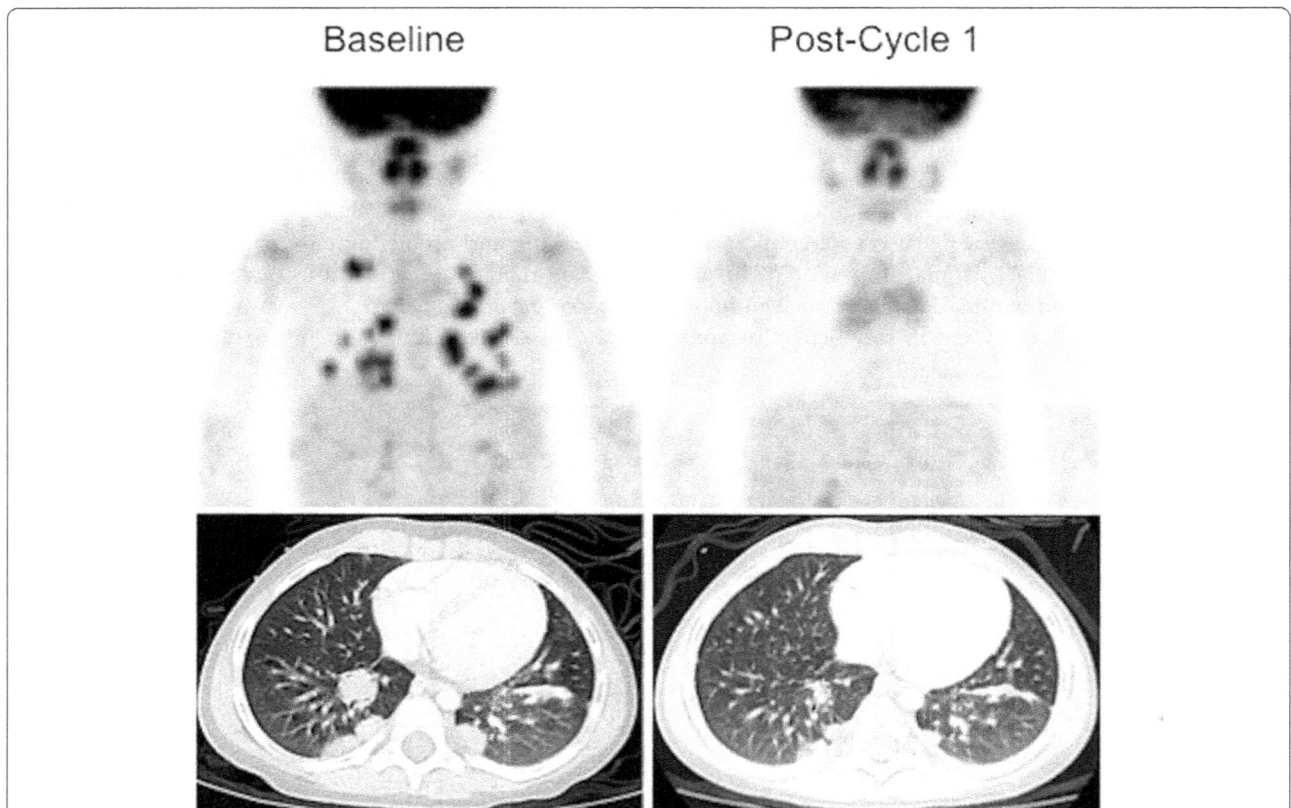

Fig. 2 PET response to targeted experimental Phase 1 therapy: Crizotinib in ALK[+] IMFT. ^{18}F-FDG-PET and CT imaging of Crizotinib response in IMFT: Baseline whole body ^{18}F-FDG-PET and Chest CT show multiple FDG-avid pulmonary nodules, confirmed by biopsy to be IMFT. Following 1 cycle of therapy, no residual abnormal FDG accumulation is seen (metabolic CR). The lesions have decreased significantly in size by CT, meeting criteria for partial reponse (PR), but not CR. This patient has remained free of disease for >36 months [32].

regions of interest based on the patient's disease, and to be in compliance with coverage determined at the time of insurance pre-authorization. Some third party payers will approve a PET/CT of the torso, but deny coverage for a whole-body exam.

At the time a PET/CT study is ordered, the referring clinician should determine if a diagnostic quality CT (Dx CT) is required or whether a low-dose CT for anatomical correlation will suffice [20]. To aid clinicians in ordering the correct examination, an algorithmic approach is useful (Fig. 3). If a diagnostic study is required, the necessary extent of body coverage must be clearly stated by the referring physician. Exam techniques and parameters must then be clearly delineated by the protocolling radiologist. For example, if a diagnostic abdomen and pelvis examination is required, the Dx CT should be protocoled with intravenous and oral contrast media, using established departmental guidelines. The same is true for a Dx CT of the entire torso (Neck/Chest/Abdomen and Pelvis). If only a diagnostic chest CT is required, a determination must be made whether the CT chest is for the purpose of characterizing mediastinal adenopathy and soft tissue disease, in which case IV contrast media is required, or for the identification and characterization of pulmonary nodules. In this latter instance, a non-contrast protocol is typically used and the examination is performed at end-inspiration to optimize visualization of small lung nodules.

If a Dx CT is not required, the CT portion of the PET/CT examination is protocoled using the lower dose attenuation correction CT (AC CT, lowest dose) protocol. Many departments distinguish between an AC CT and an anatomic co-localization CT (slightly higher CT dose, but not as high as a diagnostic CT), and a diagnostic quality CT. We only have a single AC CT protocol, with slighter higher tube current for patients > 55 kg, as compared to smaller patients < 55 kg (see later), and routinely utilize IV contrast for the AC CT, to improve anatomic localization and image quality despite the lower CT dose. Importantly, referring clinicians should understand that the low dose AC CT, while not considered to be of diagnostic quality, nonetheless contains images that in many instances are comparable to diagnostic scans (Fig. 4). As such, it is our practice to routinely issue a separate report summarizing any pertinent findings detected on the AC CT. This assures a rigorous review of all the patient's imaging data, and in some instances, may identify an unexpected finding that alters patient management (Fig. 5), which is consistent with reported rates of 3-5% for clinically significant incidental findings identified on AC CT images [21].

Patient preparation

Patients being sedated for the PET/CT have nothing by mouth (NPO) after midnight the night before the study. For studies being performed without sedation, patients should be NPO at least 4 h before the exam. In all cases the patients remain fasting during the 1-h FDG uptake

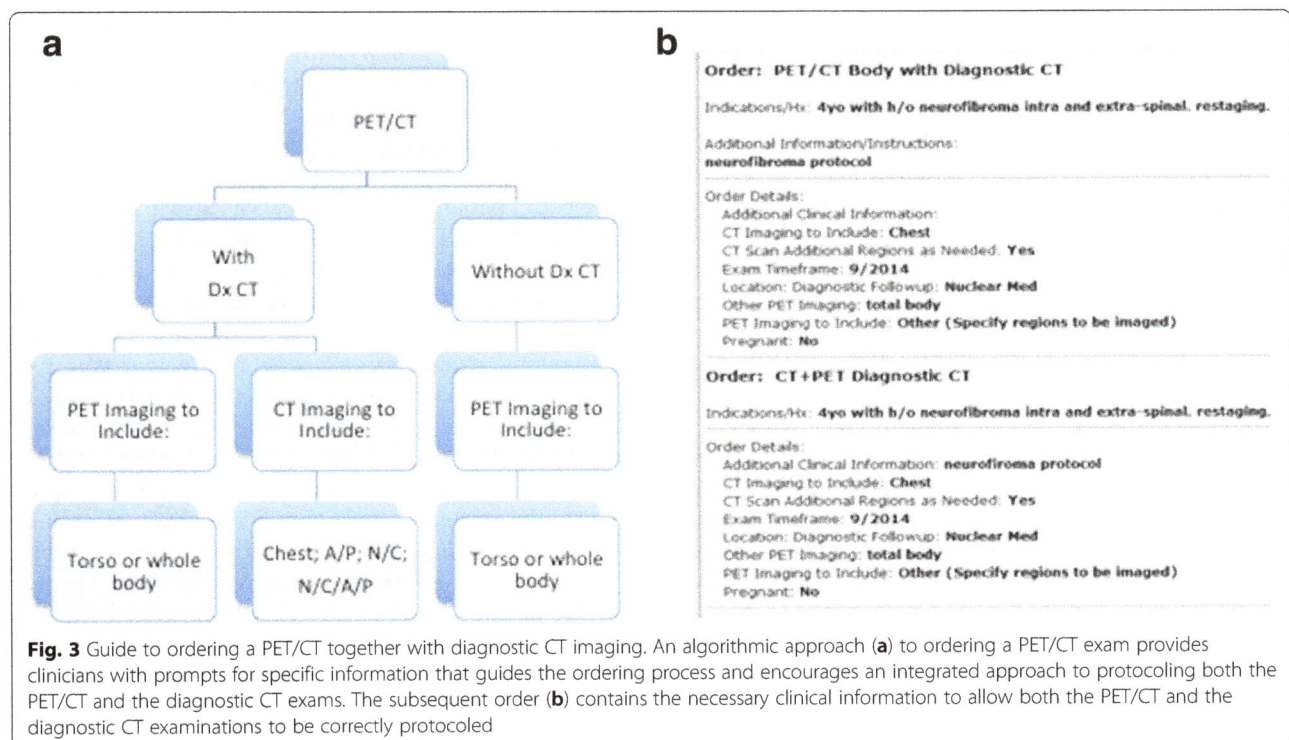

Fig. 3 Guide to ordering a PET/CT together with diagnostic CT imaging. An algorithmic approach (a) to ordering a PET/CT exam provides clinicians with prompts for specific information that guides the ordering process and encourages an integrated approach to protocoling both the PET/CT and the diagnostic CT exams. The subsequent order (b) contains the necessary clinical information to allow both the PET/CT and the diagnostic CT examinations to be correctly protocoled

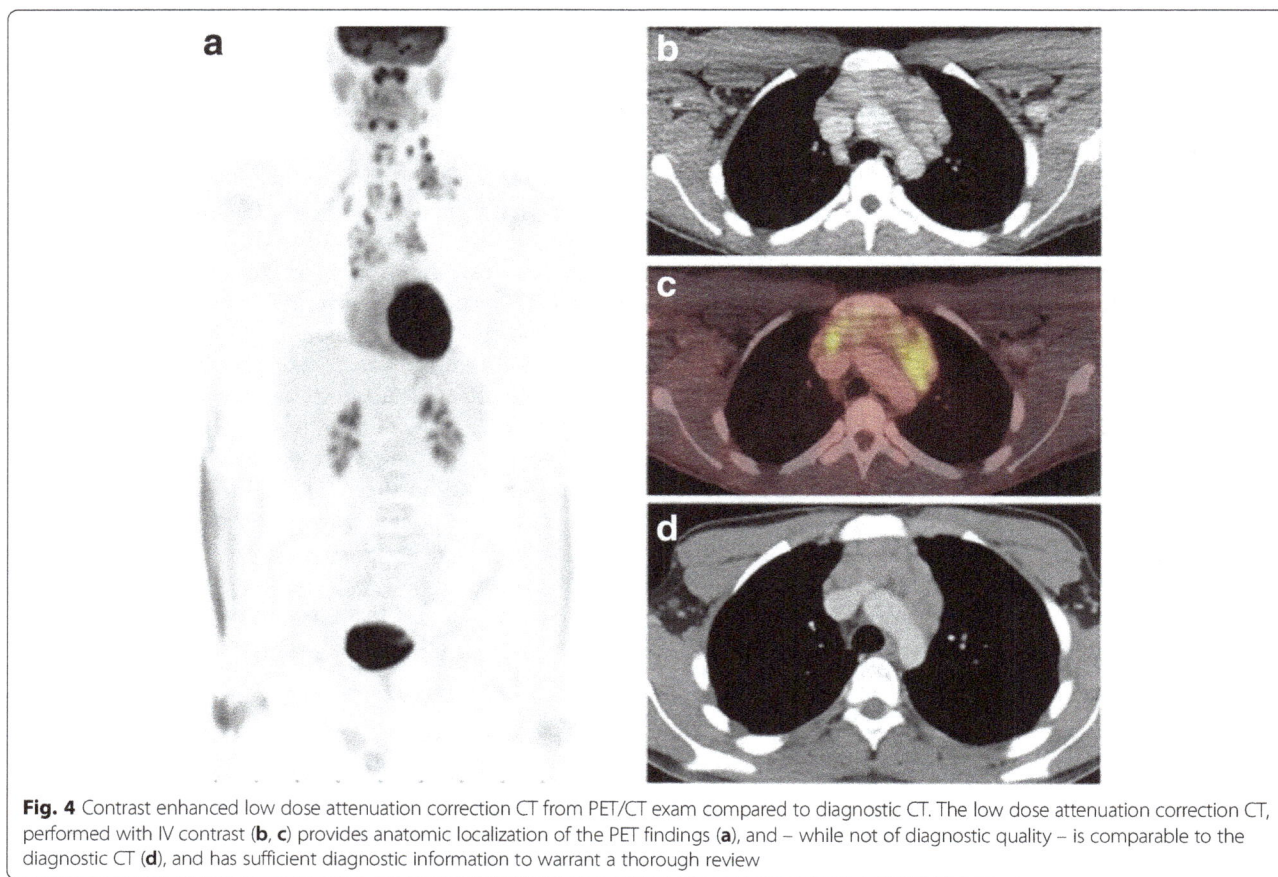

Fig. 4 Contrast enhanced low dose attenuation correction CT from PET/CT exam compared to diagnostic CT. The low dose attenuation correction CT, performed with IV contrast (**b**, **c**) provides anatomic localization of the PET findings (**a**), and – while not of diagnostic quality – is comparable to the diagnostic CT (**d**), and has sufficient diagnostic information to warrant a thorough review

period. Because insulin secretion is stimulated by caloric intake, high levels of FDG uptake can occur in both skeletal and cardiac muscle, limiting the interpretability of the PET scan. NG tube feeds, parenteral nutrition, and all dextrose-containing IV solutions should also be discontinued. If IV hydration is required a simple isotonic solution of normal saline is preferred. Note that even non-caloric artificial sweeteners such as Nutrasweet® can stimulate insulin secretion and are contraindicated prior to performing FDG PET/CT [22]. Strenuous exercise is also avoided for 24 h prior to the examination to minimize background uptake in skeletal muscle.

The possibility of pregnancy must be considered in all post-pubertal females. Even though the likelihood of pregnancy is very small in oncology patients due to on-going chemotherapy and the underlying oncologic illness, most institutions have a policy that requires anyone undergoing a CT examination (and by extension a PET/CT examination) to have a negative pregnancy test prior to the procedure. In our institution, all post-menarcheal female patients age 12 and older undergo urine pregnancy testing prior to the PET/CT exam only if they are also having a diagnostic CT of the abdomen or pelvis; pregnancy tests are not obtained for routine

PET/CT studies. The practical and ethical considerations that attend this policy, particularly regarding patient confidentiality for older teenage patients and procedures for responding to a positive pregnancy test, are beyond the scope of this review and must be individualized for each institution.

Diabetic patients require special instructions when preparing for an FDG PET/CT examination [22]. Having a skilled nursing team available to communicate with the patient and family several days prior to arrival will help to avoid either a cancelled examination or an un-interpretable study. Diabetic patients (whether type 1 or 2) can have high circulating glucose levels, either due to absence of insulin production (type 1) or insulin resistance (type 2). Ideally diabetic patients should be scheduled early in the morning. Type 1 patients require exogenous insulin to maintain basal levels of insulin, even while fasting. The long acting form of insulin (NPH), when given around bedtime the prior evening, should be sufficient to maintain appropriate insulin levels until the examination is complete. Blood glucose levels must be checked prior to tracer injection. If higher than 200 mg/dl the examination should probably not be performed as high serum glucose levels can compete

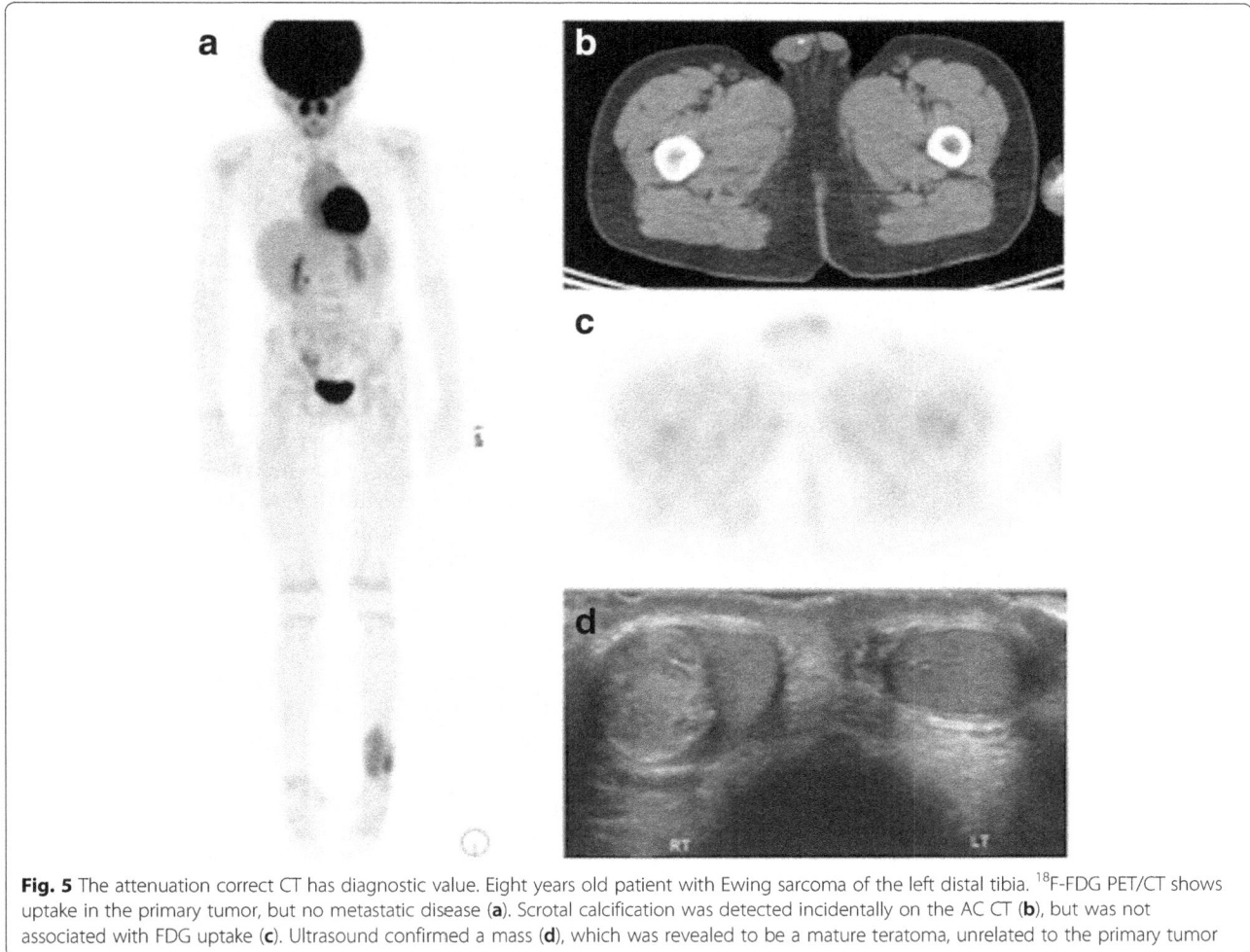

Fig. 5 The attenuation correct CT has diagnostic value. Eight years old patient with Ewing sarcoma of the left distal tibia. ^{18}F-FDG PET/CT shows uptake in the primary tumor, but no metastatic disease (**a**). Scrotal calcification was detected incidentally on the AC CT (**b**), but was not associated with FDG uptake (**c**). Ultrasound confirmed a mass (**d**), which was revealed to be a mature teratoma, unrelated to the primary tumor

with the trace amounts of FDG being administered, thereby reducing the sensitivity of the PET/CT examination.

Short acting insulin should not be administered prior to, or during the PET examination as insulin-mediated muscle uptake will occur, and may limit interpretability of the scan. Many patients with type 1 diabetes mellitus use an insulin pump, and any alteration in the insulin-pump regimen should be made in consultation with the clinician who routinely helps the patient and family manage the insulin pump. Although type 2 diabetes is less common in children, its prevalence is increasing in pediatric populations. Patients with type 2 diabetes mellitus may be treated with metformin, which is associated with undesirable colonic, hepatic and muscle uptake of FDG. Ideally, metformin is discontinued for at least 2-3 days prior to the FDG PET examination, although this may not be possible if it will result in unacceptable hyperglycemia. In rare instances it may be necessary to suppress myocardial FDG uptake (e.g. cardiac and pericardial tumors). This can be accomplished by restricting the patient to a high-fat ketogenic diet, although in practice

we use this technique primarily for non-oncologic cardiac imaging applications.

For patients who are having a Dx CT as part of their PET/CT examination, special care must be taken when administering IV and oral contrast agents, to ensure the high diagnostic quality of the CT examination. To the interpreting radiologist, a Dx CT that is obtained on the PET/CT scanner as part of the PET examination should be equivalent in quality to a CT performed on a comparably equipped standalone CT scanner. For oral contrast media, we routinely use between 90 and 300 ml (adjusted by patient age) of contrast, prepared as a 1:30 solution of non-ionic iodinated contrast (Optiray 320, Ioversol, Liebel-Flarsheim Company LLC, Raleigh, NC) diluted into water: for example a 10 yo child will receive 180 ml of contrast, prepared as 6 ml of Optiray 320 diluted into 180 ml water. Although many children may prefer contrast diluted in juice, most juices contain sweeteners and should be avoided. In practice, the non-ionic contrast, when diluted into water, is tasteless and generally well-tolerated. Most dilute barium preparations

(BaroCAT) and other palatable oral contrast media contain sweeteners and should be avoided.

Sedation

For patients requiring sedation, additional direct communication with the sedation or anesthesia team should take place prior to performing the PET/CT examination. This will ensure that any fasting or feeding requirements, and the administration of enteric contrast, is in accordance with anesthesia guidelines. We generally wait approximately 60 min after the last administration of enteric contrast before sedating a patient, thereby reducing the risk of an aspiration event that can occur in a patient with a full stomach. The sedation team also should be aware of the need for all IV fluids, including IV medications in saline solutions, to be glucose/dextrose-free.

Sedated patients typically receive continuous IV fluids both prior to and during the examination. As a result, the bladder may become quite full and in small children, as well as in children with pelvic neoplasms, excreted FDG in a very full bladder can obscure areas of interest and concern, and thereby compromise the examination. Placement of a bladder catheter is ideally done after consultation with the referring oncology team, although in practice catheter placement can be accomplished quickly and without incident. In neutropenic patients, who are at increased risk for development of infection, and in patients with hemorrhagic cystitis, placement of a bladder catheter may be contraindicated, and the decision to place a catheter should be made only after conferring with the ordering oncologist.

PET/CT acquisition

Although this review is focused on PET/CT, it should be noted that PET/MR has been shown to result in substantial reductions in radiation dose to the patient, primarily due to the elimination of the CT component of the PET/CT [23, 24]. Increased sensitivity of newer generation solid state PET detectors and longer PET acquisition times during the PET/MR exam can further contribute to dose reduction by allowing for lower administered activities of PET radiopharmaceutical. In some instances PET/MR may be preferable, particularly when anatomic co-localization of disease evident on MRI cannot be accomplished by CT [25]. In almost all cases, assuming a portion of the MRI is being performed for diagnostic purposes and not simply for attenuation correction, the combined PET/MR examination will require considerably more time (up to three times longer, depending on the protocol) than a PET/CT providing comparable coverage.

We have recently published a survey of 19 North American institutions where a large volume of pediatric

PET/CT examinations are performed [5]. There was surprising variability in practice between institutions, particularly when the PET/CT was ordered together with a diagnostic CT. What follows is a description of the approach developed at Boston Children's Hospital for performance of PET/CT, with an aim toward optimizing the scanning technique to avoid duplicate CT scanning over the same coverage area and to provide improved anatomic detail when needed to correlate with findings on the accompanying FDG PET scan.

Attenuation correction CT

The attenuation correction CT portion of the PET/CT exam is usually obtained prior to the PET acquisition. Attenuation correction accounts for differences in the location of positron annihilation events and the degree to which tissues "attenuate" the PET annihilation photons (Fig. 6). Photons emitted from the center of the patient must pass through more attenuating tissue, and thus are less likely to be detected than those from the periphery. Furthermore, photons emitted from tissues with minimal attenuation (i.e. air/lung) are more likely to reach the detector than photons emitted from locations within or near dense structures like bone. A more extensive discussion of the physics underlying the use of CT for PET attenuation correction is beyond the scope of this review and can be found in the recent review by Fahey et al., and references therein [5].

Traditionally, the CT component of a torso PET/CT exam had been performed at our institution as a low-dose non-diagnostic scan using one of two weight-based low dose CT protocols. When a Dx CT was also requested, this frequently resulted in duplicate imaging of the same coverage area, with as much as 25-50% additional CT dose (Fig. 7). By integrating the non-Dx and the Dx CT data there was an opportunity to eliminate duplicate scanning over regions where both CT's were being acquired. The Dx CT provides diagnostic quality data for anatomic correlation and can also be used for attenuation correction [20]. However, two concerns were frequently expressed: 1) IV contrast media used for diagnostic CT changes tissue attenuation and thereby might affect the attenuation corrected PET data and SUV calculations, and 2) existing software only allowed for a single series CT acquisition during the PET/CT. If just a Dx Abdomen/Pelvis CT was required, there was no means of merging the Dx CT and low dose AC CT data in a single reconstructed data set.

To address these concerns, others have shown [26, 27], and we have verified (Fig. 8) that IV contrast does not significantly impact either SUV max or SUV mean calculations. We then worked with our PET/CT manufacturer (Siemens Healthineers, Hoffman Estates,

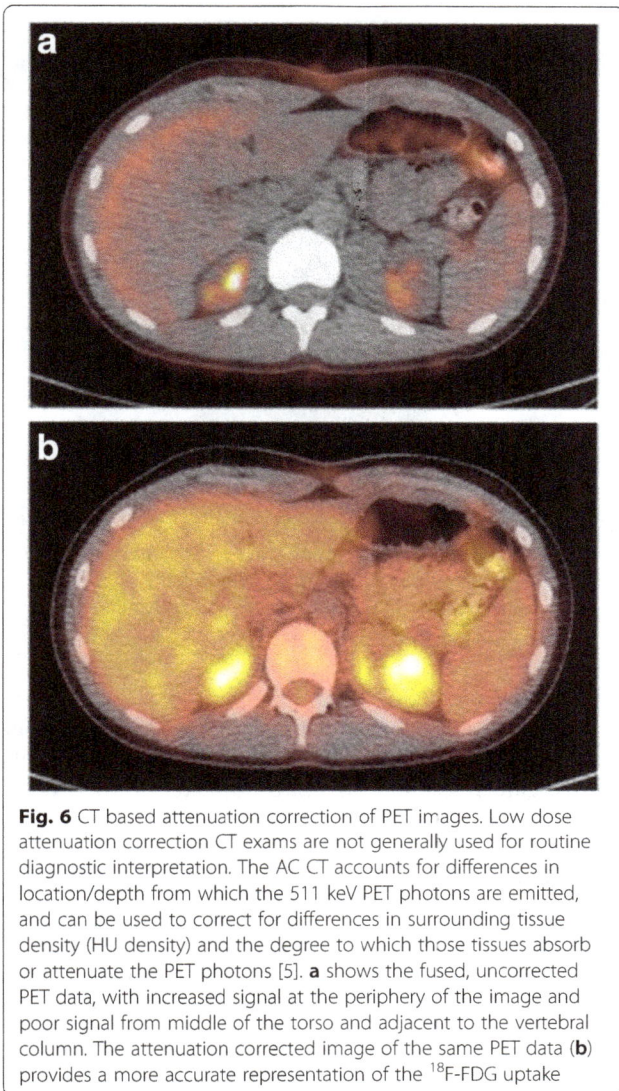

Fig. 6 CT based attenuation correction of PET images. Low dose attenuation correction CT exams are not generally used for routine diagnostic interpretation. The AC CT accounts for differences in location/depth from which the 511 keV PET photons are emitted, and can be used to correct for differences in surrounding tissue density (HU density) and the degree to which those tissues absorb or attenuate the PET photons [5]. **a** shows the fused, uncorrected PET data, with increased signal at the periphery of the image and poor signal from middle of the torso and adjacent to the vertebral column. The attenuation corrected image of the same PET data (**b**) provides a more accurate representation of the ^{18}F-FDG uptake

Tables 1 and 2 provide details for the attenuation correction and diagnostic CT parameters used during PET/CT exams.

As described earlier in the "Ordering the Examination" section, and shown diagrammatically in Fig. 3, the following imaging algorithm is now routinely used:

1) Determine whether the PET/CT examination is to be done with or without a diagnostic CT
2) Determine what the PET coverage will be (Torso, whole body, or limited).
3) For PET/CT without a Dx CT, follow the approach outlined in Table 1, with weight based tube current modulation. We routinely use IV contrast for the attenuation correction CT, with a dose of 2 cc/kg and a rate of 2 cc/sec. Axial, sagittal and coronal reconstructions are generated, in addition to axial reconstructions using a lung algorithm.
4) For a PET/CT with a Dx CT, the ordering clinician must specify the CT coverage. Regardless of the Dx CT coverage, the patient preparation (IV, oral contrast), weight-based reference mAs, pitch and reconstruction techniques should match the standard Dx CT protocols in use on other CT scanners in the department. These are summarized in Table 2.

Based on the Dx CT coverage, one of three acquisition techniques are used:

a) PET/CT with a separate Dx CT (for example, an non-contrast Chest CT to evaluate for lung nodules is performed separately from – usually before – the PET/CT exam given the need for end-inspiration CT imaging and no need for IV contrast for the diagnostic CT exam).
b) PET/CT with a Dx CT of the same coverage (Torso CT is used both for diagnostic interpretation and PET attenuation correction). This scenario is common for lymphoma patients.
c) PET/CT with a Dx CT limited to a specific region of interest that can be readily incorporated into the PET examination. This scenario is common for lymphoma patients who may have had a Dx neck and chest CT at the time of initial presentation. Once the diagnosis is confirmed, an Abdomen/Pelvis CT is required for completion of staging, together with a torso PET. In this scenario, the examination is performed in 3 series: a low dose Neck/Chest series, a diagnostic Abdomen/Pelvis series, and a small low dose series of the extremities to match the PET bed positions. As described earlier, these 3 series are merged into a single data set and used for attenuation correction, fusion/anatomic co-localization with the PET, and diagnostic interpretation (Fig. 10).

IL, USA) to develop and validate the acquisition software to allow for obtaining a multi-series CT acquisition as part of the PET/CT exam, such that the patient receives only the dose required for each area, with minimal overlap. For example, as shown in Fig. 9, a non-diagnostic attenuation correction scan can be acquired from the skull base through the thorax, followed by a diagnostic scan of the abdomen and pelvis, finishing with a non-diagnostic low dose scan to the mid-thighs to match the remaining PET bed position. These separate series are then merged into a single data set, which can be used for attenuation correction, anatomical correlation and diagnostic interpretation. This multi-series PET/CT approach is now routine for the majority of our PET/CT acquisitions that require both diagnostic and non-diagnostic CT exams.

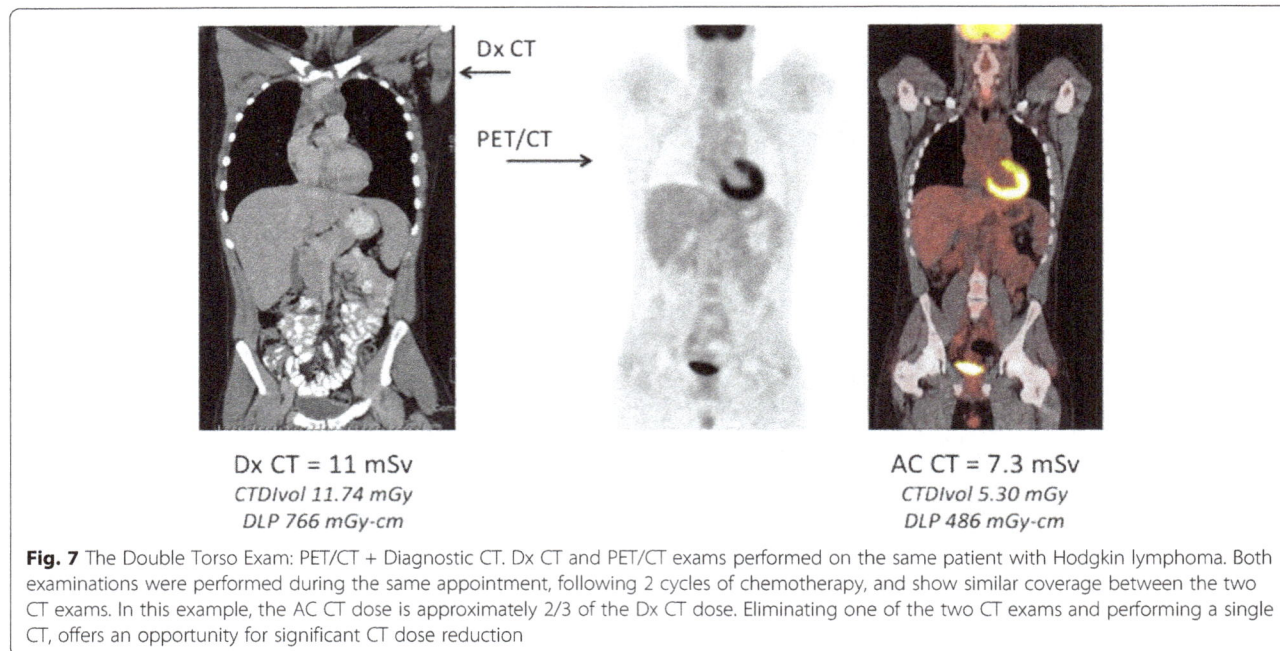

Dx CT = 11 mSv
CTDIvol 11.74 mGy
DLP 766 mGy-cm

AC CT = 7.3 mSv
CTDIvol 5.30 mGy
DLP 486 mGy-cm

Fig. 7 The Double Torso Exam: PET/CT + Diagnostic CT. Dx CT and PET/CT exams performed on the same patient with Hodgkin lymphoma. Both examinations were performed during the same appointment, following 2 cycles of chemotherapy, and show similar coverage between the two CT exams. In this example, the AC CT dose is approximately 2/3 of the Dx CT dose. Eliminating one of the two CT exams and performing a single CT, offers an opportunity for significant CT dose reduction

PET/CT acquisition techniques vary considerably between institutions [5]. One result of implementing our multi-series acquisition technique has been a reduction in radiation dose at our institution. In phantom experiments, Fahey et al. showed that dose reductions of as much as 44% can be achieved using an integrated multi-series PET/CT acquisition technique, as compared to 2 separately acquired examinations [5]. In addition to reducing unnecessary radiation dose, having diagnostic quality CT data for image co-registration and fusion can also improve the diagnostic accuracy of the PET examination and provide anatomic correlation for lesions that would have been difficult to discern on a low dose attenuation correction CT.

In all cases, the CT used for attenuation correction, whether low dose or of diagnostic quality, should be acquired with the same patient positioning and the same quiet breathing used for the PET acquisition. This is particularly important for lesions in the chest and upper abdomen, where large differences in patterns of breathing (e.g. end-inspiration vs quiet breathing) can lead to mis-registration artifacts [22]. If an end-inspiratory diagnostic quality chest CT is required as part of diagnostic CT torso exam, we will often obtain this separately at the end of the PET/CT examination. Sedated patients will have similar quiet breathing patterns for both the CT and PET acquisitions and co-registered images can usually be accurately generated without difficulty. We do not routinely intubate patients for the purposes of breath-holding during PET/CT.

PET acquisition

PET imaging is performed using standard techniques in accordance with the North American and EANM consensus guidelines and the 2016 update of the North American guidelines [28, 29], using administered activities of 3.7-5.2 MBq/kg (0.10-0.14 mCi/kg) for ^{18}F-FDG, resulting in effective doses ranging from 5.2-7.4 mSv per examination. Lower administered activities have also been used in an effort to generate sub-mSv PET examinations [30], however these usually require longer acquisition times and have not been rigorously validated to ensure sensitivities and specificities that are comparable with the existing techniques.

Patients are placed in a warm injection room (~24 °C/75 ° F) for at least 30 min prior to FDG injection to reduce FDG uptake in brown adipose tissue. Others have reported using β-blockers, such as propranolol, low dose benzodiazepine (diazepam), or short-acting opiates such as intravenous fentanyl in an effort to reduce brown fat uptake [22]. In our experience, proper patient preparation, with instructions to avoid cold exposure and dress warmly (even during warm summer months, ambient temperatures in air conditioned cars and hospitals may be quite cold for a lightly dressed child), followed by warming of the patient prior to, and during the uptake period, can substantially eliminate brown fat uptake in most patients. We do not routinely administer benzodiazepines, opiates, or other pharmaceuticals during the PET/CT examination, and in many institutions use of these agents is considered procedural sedation and requires prior consultation with anesthesia and/or sedation services. During the uptake period patients are also

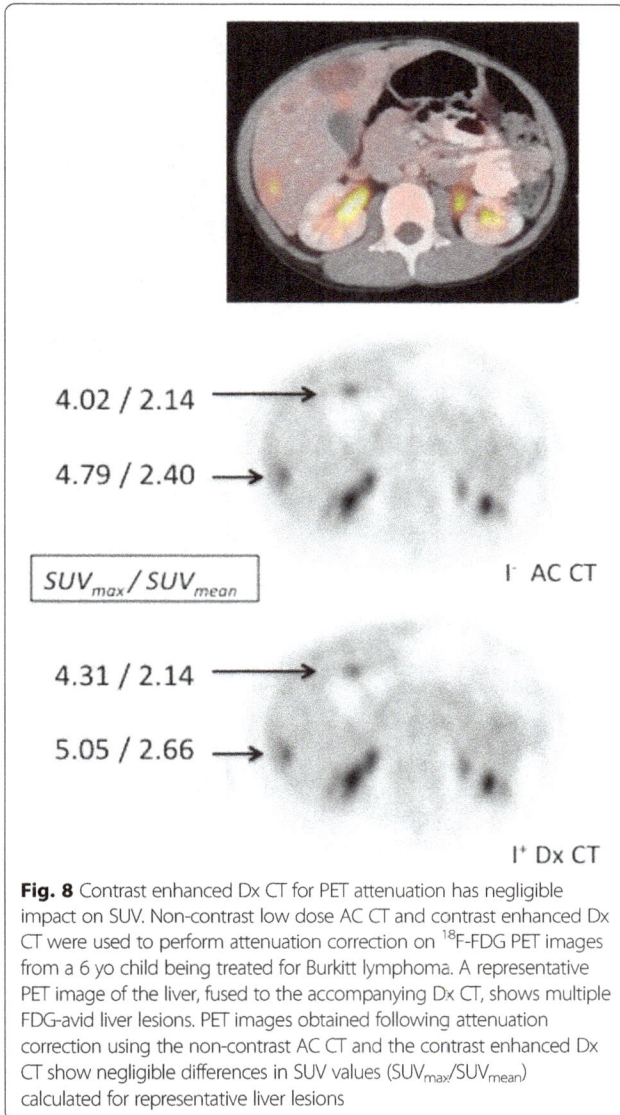

Fig. 8 Contrast enhanced Dx CT for PET attenuation has negligible impact on SUV. Non-contrast low dose AC CT and contrast enhanced Dx CT were used to perform attenuation correction on ^{18}F-FDG PET images from a 6 yo child being treated for Burkitt lymphoma. A representative PET image of the liver, fused to the accompanying Dx CT, shows multiple FDG-avid liver lesions. PET images obtained following attenuation correction using the non-contrast AC CT and the contrast enhanced Dx CT show negligible differences in SUV values (SUV_{max}/SUV_{mean}) calculated for representative liver lesions

is generally accepted that absolute SUV values are prone to 10-15% variability, related both to unavoidable differences in uptake time and variability in tissue biodistribution between examinations [31].

The PET/CT acquisition and reconstruction parameters will depend on the equipment available. On our Siemens mCT 40 PET/CT with a 20-cm axial field of view, PET images are acquired in 3D mode using an acquisition time of 3 min per bed position (Table 3), with the acquisition proceeding from head to toe. Reversing the direction of the PET acquisition, moving from feet to head, may be indicated, particularly for bladder and pelvic neoplasms where excreted tracer in the bladder can obscure tumor uptake, although as noted earlier, placement of a bladder catheter could be considered in such circumstances. Arms may be positioned above the head or be placed at the patient's side, depending on the indication for the exam. Head and neck tumors are best imaged with the arms down to minimize CT beam-hardening artifacts in the neck. Similarly, tumors in the thorax and upper abdomen may benefit from having the arms up, although young children often find it difficult to hold their arms above the head for the ~20 min PET acquisition without some additional support (handles or the head holders supplied by most manufacturers). In practice, having the arms at the patient's side, slightly elevated off the bed to reduce the beam hardening that can occur when upper arms and the vertebral column are in alignment, is adequate for most pediatric indications, and preferred for sedated patients in whom having the arms above the head may compromise the airway and IV access.

Iterative reconstruction of the PET data has been standard for more than 15 years. However, the reconstruction of the 3D PET data will require either a 3D reconstruction algorithm or rebinning of the data into a 2D set prior to reconstruction. Many sites utilize ordered subset expectation maximization (OSEM) iterative reconstruction leading to a reduction in reconstruction time. Lastly, we routinely use iterative reconstruction with resolution recovery which has improved the imaging of small structures, particularly in our younger patients.

PACS integration

Once the PET/CT examination is complete, attenuation correction of the PET imaging data and co-registration with the previously determined CT dataset is performed at the acquisition workstation. For routine examinations done without a diagnostic CT, the PET and attenuation correction CT exams are automatically processed and sent to the Picture Archiving and Communication System (PACS). When a diagnostic CT is being integrated into the PET/CT exam, the respective low dose and

instructed to minimize repetitive muscle activity in an effort to reduce background muscle uptake, although in practice the patterns of muscle uptake in children related to, for example, inconsolable crying, use of a pacifier, or use of electronic devices such as cell phones, can usually be readily recognized and interpreted.

Following FDG injection, an uptake period of 60 min is standard for most body imaging and oncologic applications. For brain tumor imaging, a shorter uptake period can be utilized (30 min) but should be standardized for all such studies. The PET/CT acquisition is ideally started as soon as possible after the 60 min tracer uptake period. Wide variability in uptake times can affect the reproducibility and comparability of SUV values between studies, although in practice it is challenging – particularly for sedated patients – to adhere rigorously to the 60 min uptake period guideline, and it

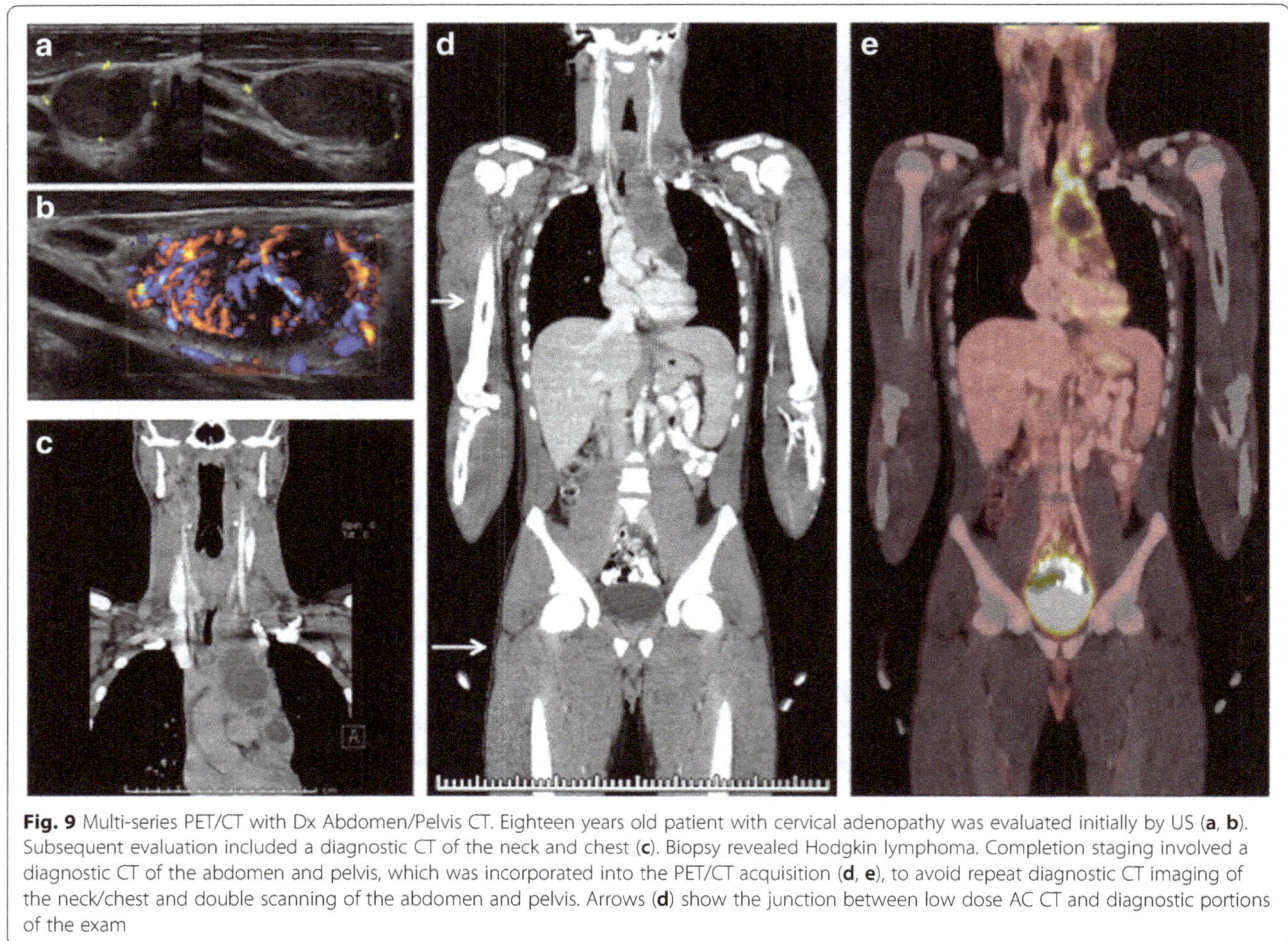

Fig. 9 Multi-series PET/CT with Dx Abdomen/Pelvis CT. Eighteen years old patient with cervical adenopathy was evaluated initially by US (**a**, **b**). Subsequent evaluation included a diagnostic CT of the neck and chest (**c**). Biopsy revealed Hodgkin lymphoma. Completion staging involved a diagnostic CT of the abdomen and pelvis, which was incorporated into the PET/CT acquisition (**d**, **e**), to avoid repeat diagnostic CT imaging of the neck/chest and double scanning of the abdomen and pelvis. Arrows (**d**) show the junction between low dose AC CT and diagnostic portions of the exam

diagnostic CT series are first merged, followed by attenuation correction of, and co-registration to, the PET data.

When sending the PET/CT data to the PACS system, at a minimum the following series should be sent with every examination: 1) the attenuation-corrected PET exam, 2) the non-attenuation corrected PET data, and 3) the co-registered CT images used for attenuation correction. Inclusion of the uncorrected PET data is important to allow apparent focal areas of FDG uptake that are related to attenuation correction artifacts, rather than disease, to be evaluated. Additional series that we routinely include with all PET/CT examinations include a maximum-intensity-projection (MIP) image of the PET examination, axial, sagittal, and coronal fused PET/CT images, axial, sagittal, and coronal CT images reconstructed using a soft-tissue

Table 1 Protocol Details – I+ low dose AC CT

• Low dose I+ enhanced optimized AC CT

  - 2 cc/kg IV contrast (Optiray320); 1 cc/kg if <10 kg; 22 G
  - 2 cc/s injection, 10–20 cc saline flush, scan
  - No oral contrast routinely used
  - Arms down, elevated off table with blanket
    • (arms up possible, depending on pt)

• CT scan top - > down (eyes - > thighs, vertex-toes)

    • Thickness: 1.2 mm, Pitch: 1.3
    • Tube current modulation (reference mAs, weight-based): 20 mAs (< 55 kg); 35 mAs (> 55 kg)
  - Reconstructions:
    • Sag, Cor: standard algorithm
    • Axial: lung algorithm
    • Iterative Reconstructions: 2 iterations

Table 2 Protocol Details – Dx CT for Attenuation Correction

• Standard dose po/I+ contrast enhanced Dx CT

  - 2 cc/kg IV contrast (Optiray320); 1 cc/kg if <10 kg
  - 2 cc/s injection, 10-20 cc saline flush
  - Oral contrast (1 cc Opti 320/30 cc water, max 300 cc)
    • Adjustment for sedation (60 min delay after last cup)
  - Arms down, elevated off table with blanket
    • (arms up is possible, depending on pt)

• CT scan top - > down (eyes - > thighs, vertex-toes)

    • Thickness: 0.5 mm
    • Pitch: 1.3
  - Tube current modulation/reconstructions: standard Dx CT
  - Dedication lung CT, end-inspiration, as dedicated

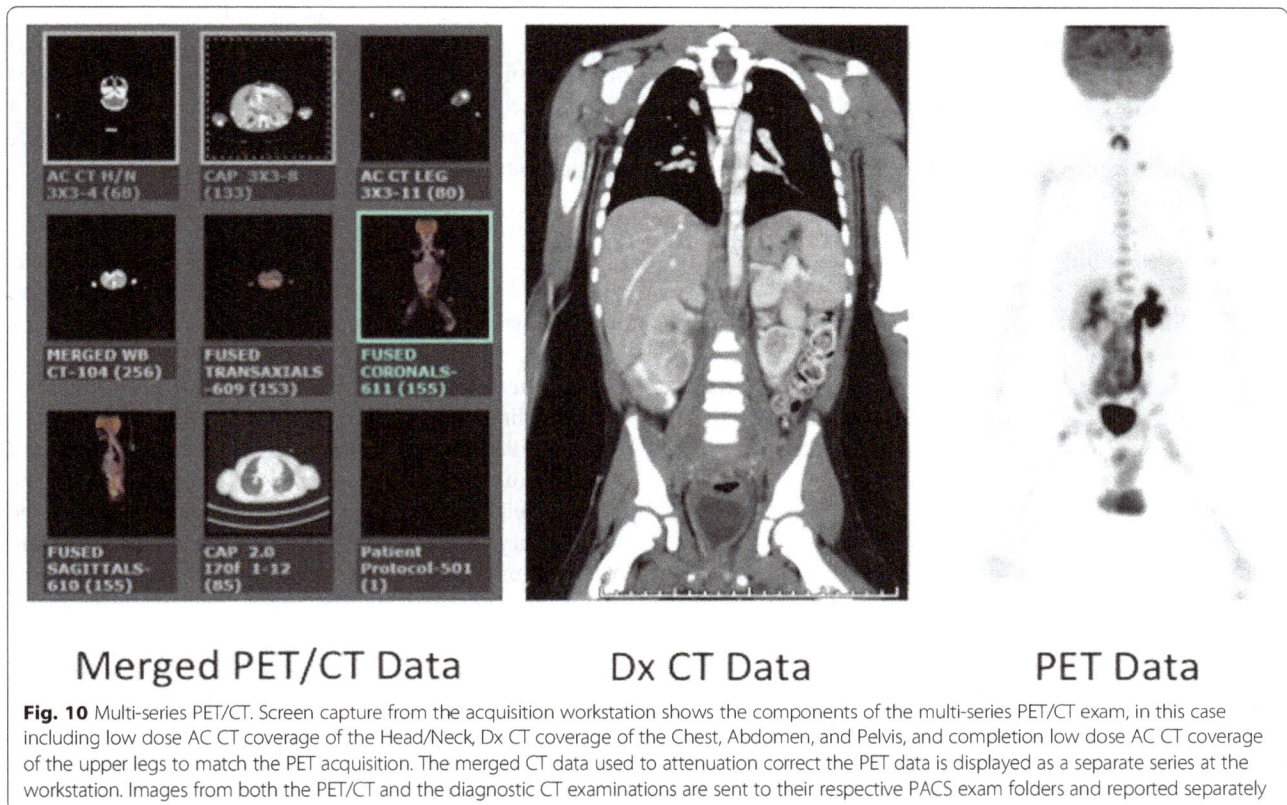

Merged PET/CT Data   Dx CT Data   PET Data

Fig. 10 Multi-series PET/CT. Screen capture from the acquisition workstation shows the components of the multi-series PET/CT exam, in this case including low dose AC CT coverage of the Head/Neck, Dx CT coverage of the Chest, Abdomen, and Pelvis, and completion low dose AC CT coverage of the upper legs to match the PET acquisition. The merged CT data used to attenuation correct the PET data is displayed as a separate series at the workstation. Images from both the PET/CT and the diagnostic CT examinations are sent to their respective PACS exam folders and reported separately

reconstruction kernel, and axial images of the thorax processed using a lung technique.

When a Dx CT has been integrated into the PET/CT examination, special considerations are needed to allow the diagnostic CT images to reside simultaneously in the PACS system within both the PET/CT folder and the Dx CT folder. Most PACS systems prevent the same imaging data from being sent to two different destinations within a given patient's examination folder by assigning each acquisition series a unique ID or UID. This is to prevent the inadvertent placement of duplicate exams in the patient's image archive, which can result in confusion and potentially lead to erroneous image interpretation. Depending on both the PET/CT platform and the PACS vendor, a protocol must be developed to allow the diagnostic CT data to co-exist within the PET/CT exam

Table 3 Protocol Details – ^{18}F-FDG PET

• Either I⁻ or I⁺ low dose-optimized AC CT or Dx CT is obtained prior to PET imaging

• PET – ^{18}F-FDG

  – 150 uCi/kg (5.55 MBq)
    • min: 500uCi (18.5 MBq)
    • max: 10 mCi (370 MBq)
  – Arms down, elevated off table with blanket
    • (arms up is possible, depending on pt)
  – PET imaging top - > bottom (eyes- > thighs, vertex-toes)
  – 3 min/bed position (20-30 min), depending on size

folder, either separately or as part of a merged CT dataset, and within the diagnostic CT folder.

For example, using the scenario described previously, in which a patient undergoes a torso PET with a Dx CT of the Abdomen/Pelvis, the following workflow is used:

1) Both the PET/CT Torso and the Abdomen/Pelvis Dx CT exam orders are activated, which assigns PACS acquisition numbers to each of the orders.
2) Once the PET/CT is complete, the PET examination is processed using the merged CT data, as detailed above. When the processing of the PET/CT exam is complete and the images have been sent to PACS, the Dx CT portion of the PET/CT examination is transferred into the Dx CT folder on the acquisition workstation (this folder will only be available if the both the diagnostic CT and PET/CT orders have been activated prior to the exam) and then sent to PACS. Other strategies are possible, but we have found this to be an efficient workflow that minimizes procedural errors during the image transfer process.

It is also the practice in many nuclear medicine departments to send PET/CT images to a dedicated nuclear medicine viewing workstation to afford a more comprehensive review of the PET/CT data. At our institution, images are reviewed using the Hermes GOLD™ (Hermes Medical Solutions) viewing platform, although other vendors such as MIM Software, Inc. provide similar functionality. Most PACS vendors also include some type of PET/CT viewing capability within the PACS environment (e.g. Synapse 3-D, GE Centricity Universal Viewer, etc.), which may be adequate, depending on the clinical environment.

3) Once the examination has been completely processed and delivered to the appropriate PACS folders, the technologist performing the examination should confirm receipt of the correct images in PACS and assure that both the diagnostic CT and PET/CT folders have the appropriate images needed for interpretation. Separate dictations are then issued for each of the respective examinations.

PET/CT interpretation

Interpretation

Each department will have its own preferred workflow for interpreting PET/CT examinations, although in practice most radiologists and nuclear medicine physicians review these complex examinations similarly.

All PET images should be reviewed in the transverse/axial, coronal and sagittal planes, reviewing both the fused and un-fused data. This is best accomplished using either a dedicated nuclear medicine processing and viewing workstation or a PACS-integrated nuclear medicine viewing functionality. Regardless of the viewing environment chosen, it is essential that PET image thresholds be scalable and adjustable. The fusion workstation should have the capability of displaying fused images with different percentages of PET and CT blending, and should have the capability of measuring SUV, including use of volumetric ROI.

We generally review the PET component of the exam first, using the greyscale images on an appropriately calibrated monitor. Beneath the PET images, the fused images are displayed, which allows for convenient anatomic co-localization of any PET abnormalities. The fused images are then separately reviewed in all three planes, followed by a dedicated review of the CT images in all three planes (whether low dose attenuation correction CT, diagnostic CT or merged hybrid CT images).

The CT images are also reviewed at a diagnostic PACS workstation in all three planes, using soft tissue, bone and lung windows, to evaluate for incidental/unexpected findings. If a Dx CT scan was requested and performed as part of the PET/CT examination, then the Dx CT should be reported separately to remain compliant with regulatory and reimbursement requirements. The physicians interpreting the PET/CT or the Dx CT must satisfy institutional credentialing requirements, and in our practice the radiologist interpreting the diagnostic CT is usually separate from the physician interpreting the PET/CT. Although is it not standard practice in most institutions, we issue a separate report for the attenuation correction CT portion of the exam, making reference to any pertinent findings on the accompanying PET examination, and ensuring a thorough and comprehensive review of all the available imaging data.

Report generation

In general, three reports are provided for each examination: the PET report, the attenuation correction CT report and, when applicable, a diagnostic CT report.

PET report In accordance with ACR and SNMMI practice guidelines, the PET report should contain a description of the radiopharmaceutical used, the administered activity and route of administration, serum glucose level, patient weight and time of injection. Since this will be the primary report reviewed by the referring clinician, any additional information, such as need for sedation or contrast reactions, should be noted.

Description of any areas of abnormal FDG uptake should be noted, with relation made to any correlative findings on the CT images and with provision of any quantitative or semi-quantitative measures of FDG accumulation (SUV). Any image artifacts or technical problems that could lead to image misinterpretation should also be noted.

Attenuation correction CT Although not standard practice or required by the guidelines, it is our practice to review the attenuation correction CT images with the same rigor used for reviewing a diagnostic CT. A standardized reporting template is used, with brief descriptions of any CT findings that correlate with PET abnormalities, and note made of any pertinent incidental or unexpected findings (e.g. spondylolysis, vertebral compression, malpositioned support lines or catheters, etc).

Diagnostic CT This is reported by the covering body radiologist using standard dictation templates, in a similar fashion to a Dx CT being obtained without an accompanying PET examination. In most cases the radiologist reviews the Dx CT together with the individual interpreting the PET examination, which insures a comprehensive review and allows both the PET and Dx CT reports to convey uniform information.

Artifacts

A discussion of the numerous artifacts that one may encounter during PET/CT examinations is beyond the scope of this review and has been described previously [22]. Where indicated strategies for minimizing specific artifacts or physiologic variants (i.e. muscle and brown fat uptake) have been noted elsewhere throughout this review.

Conclusions

PET/CT plays an important role in the management of many pediatric malignancies. This review provides an overview of our approach to determining when and how a PET/CT examination is performed, with attention to optimizing the CT component of the PET/CT exam. A multi-disciplinary approach is needed to ensure that the indications for PET/CT are appropriate, that the correct examination is performed, and the appropriate imaging techniques are used. As hybrid imaging technologies such as PET/CT have evolved, new strategies for image acquisition and interpretation have emerged, leading to many exciting opportunities for improving the overall quality of the PET/CT experience.

Acknowledgements
Richard Powers, Ph.D., Siemens Healthcare, for his contribution to the development of the multi-series PET/CT software described in this review.

Funding
No external sources of funding were used.

Authors' contributions
All authors contributed to preparation, editing, and final approval of the submitted manuscript.

Competing interests
The authors declare that they have no competing interests.

References

1. Freebody J, Wegner EA, Rossleigh MA. 2-deoxy-2-((18)F)fluoro-D-glucose positron emission tomography/computed tomography imaging in paediatric oncology. World J Radiol. 2014;6(10):741–55

2. Harrison DJ, Parisi MT, Shulkin BL. The role of 18F-FDG-PET/CT in pediatric sarcoma. Semin Nucl Med. 2017;47(3):229–41.

3. Kluge R, Kurch L, Georgi T, Metzger M. Current role of FDG-PET in pediatric Hodgkin's lymphoma. Semin Nucl Med. 2017;47(3):242–57.

4. Uslu L, Donig J, Link M, Rosenberg J, Quon A, Daldrup-Link HE. Value of 18F-FDG PET and PET/CT for evaluation of pediatric malignancies. J Nucl Med. 2015;56(2):274–86.

5. Fahey FH, Goodkind A, MacDougall RD, Oberg L, Ziniel SI, Cappock R, Callahan MJ, Kwatra N, Treves ST, Voss SD. Operational and Dosimetric aspects of pediatric PET/CT. J Nucl Med. 2017;58(9):1360–366.

6. Parisi MT, Bermo MS, Alessio AM, Sharp SE, Gelfand MJ, Shulkin BL. Optimization of pediatric PET/CT. Semin Nucl Med. 2017;47(3):258–74.

7. Jacques L, Jensen TS, Rollins J, Caplan S, Roche JC: Decision memo for positron emission tomography (FDG) for solid tumors (CAG-00181R4). Edited by Services CfMaM; 2013.

8. Flerlage JE, Kelly KM, Beishuizen A, Cho S, De Alarcon PA, Dieckmann U, Drachtman RA, Hoppe BS, Howard SC, Kaste SC, et al. Staging evaluation and response criteria harmonization (SEARCH) for childhood, adolescent and young adult Hodgkin lymphoma (CAYAHL): methodology statement. Pediatr Blood Cancer. 2017;64(7):e26421/1-10.

9. Hawkins DS, Conrad EU 3rd, Butrynski JE, Schuetze SM, Eary JF. [F-18]-fluorodeoxy-D-glucose-positron emission tomography response is associated with outcome for extremity osteosarcoma in children and young adults. Cancer. 2009;115(15):3519–25.

10. Hawkins DS, Schuetze SM, Butrynski JE, Rajendran JG, Vernon CB, Conrad EU 3rd, Eary JF. [18F]Fluorodeoxyglucose positron emission tomography predicts outcome for Ewing sarcoma family of tumors. J Clin Oncol. 2005; 23(34):8828–34.

11. Raciborska A, Bilska K, Drabko K, Michalak E, Chaber R, Pogorzala M, Polczynska K, Sobol G, Wieczorek M, Muszynska-Roslan K, et al. Response to chemotherapy estimates by FDG PET is an important prognostic factor in patients with Ewing sarcoma. Clin Transl Oncol. 2016;18(2):189–95.

12. Tsai LL, Drubach L, Fahey F, Irons M, Voss S, Ullrich NJ. [18F]-Fluorodeoxyglucose positron emission tomography in children with neurofibromatosis type 1 and plexiform neurofibromas: correlation with malignant transformation. J Neuro-Oncol. 2012;108(3):469–75.

13. Kiratli PO, Tuncel M, Bar-Sever Z. Nuclear medicine in pediatric and adolescent tumors. Semin Nucl Med. 2016;46(4):308–23.

14. Franzius C. FDG-PET/CT in pediatric solid tumors. Q J Nucl Med Mol Imaging. 2010;54(4):401–10.

15. Dumba M, Jawad N, McHugh K. Neuroblastoma and nephroblastoma: a radiological review. Cancer Imaging. 2015;15(5):1–14.

16. Sharp SE, Trout AT, Weiss BD, Gelfand MJ. MIBG in Neuroblastoma diagnostic imaging and therapy. Radiographics. 2016;36(1):258–78.

17. Sharp SE, Shulkin BL, Gelfand MJ, Salisbury S, Furman WL. 123I-MIBG scintigraphy and 18F-FDG PET in neuroblastoma. J Nucl Med. 2009;50(8):1237–43.

18. Moinul Hossain AK, Shulkin BL, Gelfand MJ, Bashir H, Daw NC, Sharp SE, Nadel HR, Dome JS. FDG positron emission tomography/computed tomography studies of Wilms' tumor. Eur J Nucl Med Mol Imaging. 2010; 37(7):1300–8.

19. Weiser DA, Kaste SC, Siegel MJ, Adamson PC. Imaging in childhood cancer: a Society for Pediatric Radiology and Children's oncology group joint task force report. Pediatr Blood Cancer. 2013;60(8):1253–60.

20. Wong TZ, Paulson EK, Nelson RC, Patz EF Jr, Coleman RE. Practical approach to diagnostic CT combined with PET. AJR Am J Roentgenol. 2007;188(3):622–9.

21. Osman MM, Cohade C, Fishman EK, Wahl RL. Clinically significant incidental findings on the unenhanced CT portion of PET/CT studies: frequency in 250 patients. J Nucl Med. 2005;46(8):1352–5.

22. Grant FD. Normal variations and benign findings in pediatric 18F-FDG-PET/CT. PET Clin. 2014;9(2):195–208.

23. Schafer JF, Gatidis S, Schmidt H, Guckel B, Bezrukov I, Pfannenberg CA, Reimold M, Ebinger M, Fuchs J, Claussen CD, et al. Simultaneous whole-body PET/MR imaging in comparison to PET/CT in pediatric oncology: initial results. Radiology. 2014;273(1):220–31.

24. Gatidis S, Schmidt H, Gucke B, Bezrukov I, Seitz G, Ebinger M, Reimold M, Pfannenberg CA, Nikolaou K, Schwenzer NF, et al. Comprehensive oncologic imaging in infants and preschool children with substantially reduced radiation exposure using combined simultaneous (1)(8)F-Fluorodeoxyglucose positron emission tomography/magnetic resonance imaging: a direct comparison to (1)(8)F-Fluorodeoxyglucose positron emission tomography/computed tomography. Investig Radiol. 2016; 51(1):7–14.

25. Gatidis S, Bender B, Reimold M, Schafer JF. PET/MRI in children. Eur J Radiol. 2017;94:A64–A70.

26. Aschoff P, Plathow C, Beyer T, Lichy MP, Erb G, Oksuz MO, Claussen CD, Pfannenberg C. Multiphase contrast-enhanced CT with highly concentrated contrast agent can be used for PET attenuation correction in integrated PET/CT imaging. Eur J Nucl Med Mol Imaging. 2012;39(2):316–25.

27. Berthelsen AK, Holm S, Loft A, Klausen TL, Andersen F, Hojgaard L. PET/CT with intravenous contrast can be used for PET attenuation correction in cancer patients. Eur J Nucl Med Mol Imaging. 2005;32(10):1167–75.

28. Treves ST, Gelfand MJ, Fahey FH, Parisi MT. 2016 update of the north American consensus guidelines for pediatric administered radiopharmaceutical activities. J Nucl Med. 2016;57(12):15N–8N.

29. Lassmann M, Treves ST, Group ESPDHW. Paediatric radiopharmaceutical administration: harmonization of the 2007 EANM paediatric dosage card (version 1.5.2008) and the 2010 north American consensus guidelines. Eur J Nucl Med Mol Imaging. 2014;41(5):1036–41.

30. Hope T, Phelps A, Behr S, Seo Y, Corbin K, MacKenzie J. Sub-mSv whole body PET/MRI in pediatric patients. Pediatr Radiol. 2017;47(Suppl 1):163.

31. Lodge MA. Repeatability of SUV in oncologic 18F-FDG PET. J Nucl Med. 2017;58(4):523–32.

32. Mossé YP, Voss SD, Lim MS, Rolland D, Minard CG, Fox E, Adamson P, Wilner K, Blaney SM, Weigel BJ. Targeting ALK With Crizotinib in Pediatric Anaplastic Large Cell Lymphoma and Inflammatory Myofibroblastic Tumor: A Children's Oncology Group Study. J Clin Oncol. 2017; 35(28):3215–21.

3D analysis of apparent diffusion coefficient histograms in hepatocellular carcinoma: correlation with histological grade

Tomohisa Moriya[1], Kazuhiro Saito[1*], Yu Tajima[1], Taiyo L. Harada[1], Yoichi Araki[1], Katsutoshi Sugimoto[2] and Koichi Tokuuye[1]

Abstract

Background: To evaluate the usefulness of differentiation of histological grade in hepatocellular carcinoma (HCC) using three-dimensional (3D) analysis of apparent diffusion coefficient (ADC) histograms retrospectively.

Methods: The subjects consisted of 53 patients with 56 HCCs. The subjects included 12 well-differentiated, 35 moderately differentiated, and nine poorly differentiated HCCs. Diffusion-weighted imaging (b-values of 100 and 800 s/mm^2) were obtained within 3 months before surgery. Regions of interest (ROIs) covered the entire tumor. The data acquired from each slice were summated to derive voxel-by-voxel ADCs for the entire tumor. The following parameters were derived from the ADC histogram: mean, standard deviation, minimum, maximum, mode, percentiles (5th, 10th, 25th, 50th, 75th, and 90th), skew, and kurtosis. These parameters were analyzed according to histological grade. After eliminating steatosis lesions, these parameters were re-analyzed.

Results: A weak correlation was observed in minimum ADC and 5th percentile for each histological grade ($r = -0.340$ and $r = -0.268$, respectively). The minimum ADCs of well, moderately, and poorly differentiated HCC were 585 ± 388, 411 ± 278, and $235 \pm 102 \times 10^{-6}$ mm^2/s, respectively. Minimum ADC showed significant differences among tumor histological grades ($P = 0.009$). The minimum ADC of poorly differentiated HCC and that of combined well and moderately differentiated HCC were 236 ± 102 and $437 \pm 299 \times 10^{-6}$ mm^2/s. The minimum ADC of poorly differentiated HCC was significantly lower than that of combined well and moderately differentiated HCC ($P = 0.001$). The sensitivity and specificity, when a minimum ADC of 400×10^{-6} mm^2/s or lower was considered to be poorly differentiated HCC, were 100 and 54%, respectively. After exclusion of the effect of steatosis, the sensitivity and specificity did not change, although the statistical differences became strong ($P < 0.0001$).

Conclusion: Minimum ADC was most useful to differentiate poorly differentiated HCC in 3D analysis of ADC histograms.

Keywords: Hepatocellular carcinoma, Diffusion-weighted imaging, ADC histogram, Histological differentiation

Background

The histological grade of hepatocellular carcinoma (HCC) is a major contributing factor to recurrence after surgery, and poorly differentiated HCC tends to have higher recurrence rates than well and moderately differentiated HCC [1, 2]. Therefore, distinguishing the histological grade of HCC before therapy can be effective to create a therapeutic strategy and estimate the prognosis. It has been previously reported that poorly differentiated HCC showed decreasing arterial blood flow using CT hepatic arteriography [3]. However, the decreased arterial blood supply is observed in not only poorly differentiated HCC but also in well differentiated HCC [4], and this makes the discrimination of these two entities difficult. To clearly distinguish tumor histological grade, diffusion-weighted imaging (DWI) that is independent of vascularity has been proposed. Some papers have already reported about the diagnosis of tumor histological grade using the apparent diffusion coefficient

* Correspondence: saito-k@tokyo-med.ac.jp
[1]Department of Radiology, Tokyo Medical University, 6-7-1 Nishishinjuku, Shinjuku-ku, Tokyo 160-0023, Japan
Full list of author information is available at the end of the article

(ADC). However, the methodology and results were variable and inconsistent [5–9]. The region of interest (ROI) setting is significant to eliminate bias, for example, if the ROI is set in the tumor avoiding areas of necrosis, this measurement involves arbitrariness of the researchers. Furthermore, when the ROI is set at the entire tumor on a slice, the measured ADC is represented only on the selected slice. Some different histological grade components are often included in an HCC nodule; therefore, the ROI set through the entire lesion three-dimensionally may lead to a more accurate diagnosis. The usefulness of differentiation of brain glioma grade using ADC histogram analysis in which ROI is set to the entire lesion three-dimensionally has already been reported [10]. We evaluated the usefulness of differentiating the histological grade of HCC using 3D analysis of ADC histograms derived from the ROI set at the entire tumor.

Methods

This retrospective study was approved by an institutional review board and informed consent was waived.

Subjects

The researchers referred to medical records and a radiological database and the eligibility criteria were determined as follows: (a) the same parameter of DWI, (b) resected and pathologically confirmed HCC, (c) patients previously not receiving radiofrequency ablation and trans-arterial chemoembolization, (d) MRI was performed within 3 months prior to surgery. Exclusion criteria were as follows: (a) patients with artifacts associated with body metal and/or body movement, (b) patients whose tumors are present at the left lobe lateral segment, (c) boundary of the tumor is unclear due to an infiltrative feature. Finally, 52 patients with 56 nodules were enrolled in this study, which included 41 men and 11 women with a mean age of 68 years and a median age of 66 years. Underlying liver diseases were hepatitis B ($n = 6$), hepatitis C ($n = 13$), non-B non-C hepatitis ($n = 1$), alcoholic liver ($n = 12$), non-alcoholic steatohepatitis ($n = 1$), fatty liver ($n = 1$), primary sclerosing cholangitis ($n = 2$), idiopathic portal hypertension ($n = 1$), and absence of underling liver disease ($n = 15$). Partial hepatectomy, liver subsegmentectomy, segmentectomy, and lobectomy were performed in 30, 7, 11, and 4 patients, respectively. All patients were classified into Child-Pugh "A". Makuuchi criteria were used to select the surgical indication [11]. The indocyanine green test (ICG15) and technetium-99 m diethylenetriamine pentaacetic acid galactosyl human serum albumin single photon emission computed tomography were also performed to evaluate liver functional reserve. Four patients had two tumors in a resected liver. Histological grade of HCC was classified into well, moderately, and poorly differentiated

HCC [12]. When multiple components of histological grade were contained within a lesion, the major component was regarded as the tumor grade. Finally, this study included 12 well, 35 moderately, and nine poorly differentiated HCCs.

MRI protocols

All magnetic resonance imaging examinations were performed with a 1.5 T superconductive MRI system (Avanto, Siemens, Erlangen, Germany) with a 32-channel body phased-array coil. The maximum gradient strength of the system was 45 mT/m and the maximum slew rate was 200 T/m/s. The non-contrast T1-weighted imaging (T1WI) was performed using a breath-hold two-dimensional gradient-echo sequence with the following parameters: repetition time/echo time, (TR/TE), 125 ms/2.38 ms for opposed phase and 4.76 ms for in-phase; flip angle, 75°; slice thickness, 5 mm; intersection gap, 1 mm; matrix, 320×154; field of view (FOV), 400 mm × 446 mm; average, 1; bandwidth, 470 Hz/pixel. The T2-weighted imaging (T2WI) was performed using the navigator-assisted technique for respiratory gating (2D-PACE). The T2WI parameters were as follows: TR/TE, 1600 ms/81 ms; flip angle, 150°; matrix, 512×176; FOV, 400 mm × 447 mm; slice thickness, 5 mm; intersection gap, 1 mm; average, 1; bandwidth, 260 Hz/pixel; fat suppression, chemical shift selective (CHESS). DWI was performed using a spin-echo-based echo-planar imaging sequence. The parameters were as follows: TR/TE, 1600 ms/66 ms; b-values, 100 and 800 s/mm^2; matrix, 128×124; FOV, 400 mm × 447 mm; slice thickness, 5 mm; intersection gap, 1 mm; average, 4; bandwidth, 260 Hz/pixel; fat suppression, CHESS; using the navigator-assisted technique for respiratory gating (2D-PACE). For dynamic and hepatobiliary MRI, gadolinium-ethoxybenzyl-diethylenetriamine pentaacetic acid (Gd-EOB-DTPA) (Primovist, Bayer Schering; 0.025 mmol/kg) was rapidly administered intravenously and immediately followed by 20 mL of sterile saline flush with an injector at 1.0–2.0 mL/s. The hepatobiliary phase images were acquired at 20 min after contrast media injection by three-dimensional volumetric interpolated breath-hold examination (3D-VIBE). The sequence parameters were the following: TR/TE, 3.3 ms/1.2 ms; flip angle, 15.0°; matrix, 320×165; FOV, 400 mm × 446 mm; slice thickness, 2–3 mm; average, 1; intersection gap, 0 mm; fat suppression, CHESS.

Image analysis

Two radiologists (with 4 and 25 years of experience) identified HCC on both images at the hepatobiliary phase and T2WI. Boundary of HCC was defined as a range of low signal intensity at the hepatobiliary phase. In case of revealing both high and low intensity in a lesion at the hepatobiliary phase, the region showing a high intensity in T2WI was defined as HCC. First, the radiologist (4 years of experience) and the radiological technologist (20 years of experience) attempted to match the location on the hepatobiliary phase (or T2WI) with that on the ADC map. They delineated the ROI on hepatobiliary phase or T2-weighted images, because the contour of the tumor was usually blurred on DWI. The hepatobiliary phase (or T2-weighted image) is superimposed on the ADC map automatically at the workstation (Synapse Vincent). However, this fusion imaging has some gap and, therefore, some manual correction is necessary (Fig. 1a, b). Second, the ROIs were set at the entire tumor through all slices on hepatobiliary phase images (Fig. 1c). Third, the information of the ROI setting on the hepatobiliary phase was copied and pasted on the ADC maps (Fig. 1d). Finally, the data acquired from each slice were summated to derive voxel-by-voxel ADC values for the entire tumor and an ADC histogram was generated (Fig. 2). Since the impact of steatosis on ADC has been reported previously, two radiologists (with 4 and 25 years of experience) established a consensus reading and the concomitant fat deposit was classified into the following three categories by chemical shift imaging: "1",

absence of signal decrease; "2", signal decrease in less than half of the tumor; "3", distinct decrease of the signal on more than half of the tumor.

Statistical analysis

The mean, standard deviation, minimum, maximum, mode, skewness, kurtosis, and percentiles (5th, 50th, 75th, and 90th) were derived from the ADC histogram. Correlation between the degree of tumor histological grade and the parameters of ADC histograms were assessed by the Pearson's product moment correlation coefficient. The differences in parameters among tumor histological grades were analyzed by one-way ANOVA with the Tukey-Kramer post hoc test. Poorly differentiated HCC and the group combining well and moderately differentiated HCC were compared using an unpaired Student t-test. In addition, in order to eliminate the interference from steatosis as much as possible, the parameters of the ADC histograms were re-analyzed in the same way as above after excluding the classified cases into "3" on the evaluation of chemical shift imaging. A P value < 0.05 was considered to be significant. ROC curves were created for the parameters found

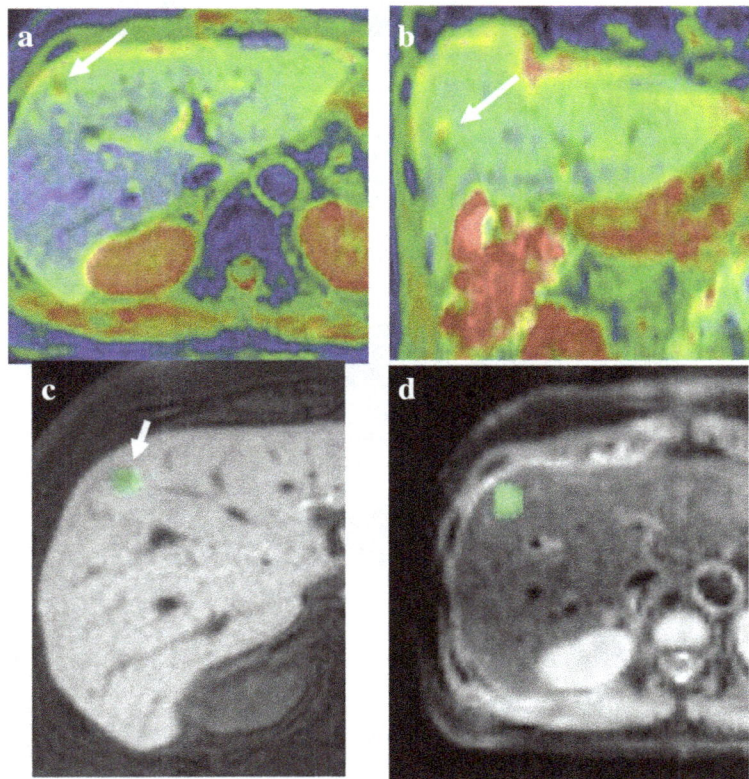

Fig. 1 Process of making the ADC histogram. **a, b** To match the location on the hepatobiliary phase with that on the ADC map, the hepatobiliary phase is superimposed on the ADC map automatically. However, this fusion imaging has some gap and, therefore, some manual correction is necessary. **c, d** The ROIs were set at the entire tumor through all slices on hepatobiliary phase images (**c**). Then, the information of this ROI setting was copied and pasted on ADC maps (**d**)

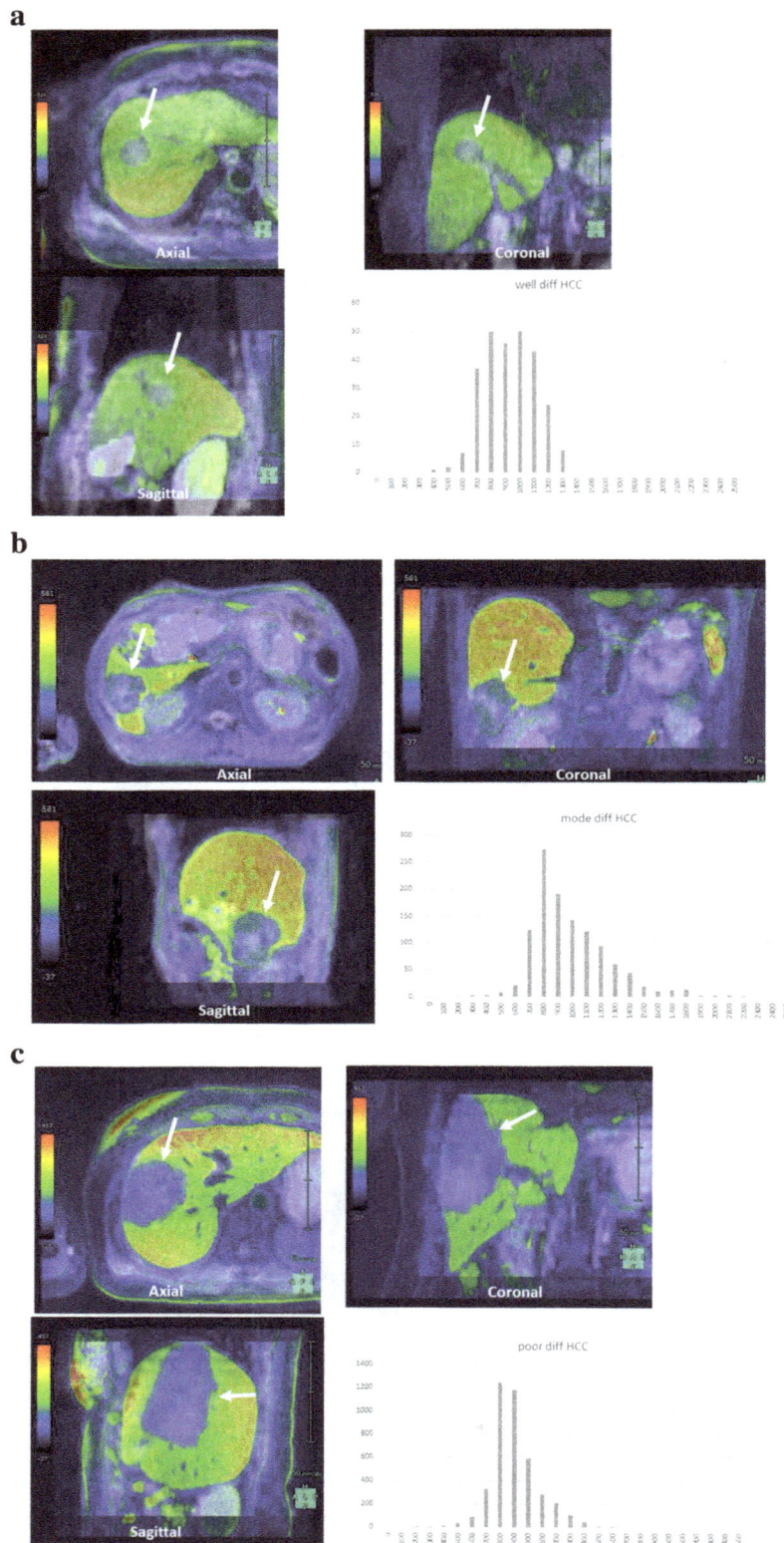

Fig. 2 The representative cases of ADC histogram and 3D ADC map in (**a**) well, (**b**) moderately, and (**c**) poorly differentiated HCC are shown. Smaller minimum ADCs are present in poorly differentiated HCC compared with the other two histological grades. The data acquired from each slice were summated to derive voxel-by-voxel ADC values for the entire tumor and the ADC histogram was generated. Arrows indicates tumor

to be significant from these results, and then the sensitivity and the specificity were calculated by the Youden index. All statistical analyses were performed using SPSS statistics software (version 22, SPSS) for Microsoft Windows.

Results
Overall analysis
Table 1 shows the summary of parameters of ADC histograms associated with each histological grade. Weak correlations were found in minimum ADC and 5th percentile ADC ($r = -0.340$ and $r = -0.268$, respectively).

Minimum ADC showed significant differences among tumor histological grades ($P = 0.009$). The other parameters did not show significant differences. The post hoc test showed significant differences between moderately and poorly differentiated HCC ($P = 0.008$) (Table 1).

The parameters of ADC histograms of poorly differentiated HCC and well and moderately differentiated HCC are shown in Table 2. Minimum ADC showed a significant difference ($P = 0.001$). The sensitivity and specificity, when a minimum ADC of 400×10^{-6} mm^2/s or lower was considered to be poorly differentiated HCC, were 100 and 54%, respectively.

Excluded steatosis lesion
The signal intensity reduction on chemical shift imaging was classified as follows: 1, 41 nodules; 2, 4 nodules; 3, 11 nodules. Of the 11 classified into grade 3, 2 well, 8 moderately, and 1 poorly differentiated HCC were histologically included. The summaries of parameters of ADC histograms, except for grade 3 nodules, are shown in Table 3. Weak correlations were found in minimum

ADC and 5th percentile ADC ($r = -0.469$ and $r = -0.382$, respectively).

Minimum ADC and 5th percentile ADC showed significant differences among three histological grades ($P = 0.006$ and 0.030, respectively). The other parameters did not show significant differences. The post hoc test of minimum ADC showed significant differences between well and poorly differentiated, and between moderately and poorly differentiated HCC ($P = 0.045$ and 0.008, respectively). The 5th percentile ADC of poorly differentiated HCC was significantly lower than that of well differentiated HCC ($P = 0.023$) (Table 3).

Minimum ADC showed significant differences between poorly differentiated HCC and well and moderately differentiated HCC ($P < 0.0001$) (Table 4). The sensitivity and specificity, when a minimum ADC of 400×10^{-6} mm^2/s or lower was considered to be poorly differentiated HCC, were 100 and 54%, respectively.

Discussion
Minimum ADC was useful to distinguish poorly differentiated HCC from well and moderately differentiated HCC because minimum ADC and 5th percentile ADC were weakly correlated with histological grades; furthermore, minimum ADC showed significant differences among tumor histological grades. Nakanishi et al also reported that minimum ADCs in poorly differentiated HCC were significantly lower than those in the other histological grades, although they did not perform ADC histogram analysis [2]. Minimum ADC may reflect the hypercellular component in the tumor. As tumor histological grade increases, the cellularity of the tumor

Table 1 Histological grade of hepatocellular carcinoma, the parameters of ADC histograms, Pearson's product moment correlation coefficient, and one-way ANOVA with the Tukey-Kramer post hoc test

	Well diff HCC	Mod diff HCC	Poor diff HCC	Pearson's correlation coefficient	Pearson's correlation coefficient P value	ANOVA Tukey-Kramer post hoc test
Mean	1051 ± 203	999 ± 163	964 ± 167	−0.141	0.301	n.s.
Standard deviation	180 ± 119	193 ± 86	227 ± 75	0.154	0.257	n.s.
Minimum	585 ± 388	411 ± 278	235 ± 102	−0.340	0.010*	0.009**
Maximum	1641 ± 558	1718 ± 571	1955 ± 704	0.156	0.252	n.s.
Mode	710 ± 517	881 ± 311	829 ± 319	0.074	0.588	n.s.
Skewness	0.58 ± 1.27	0.36 ± 0.88	0.50 ± 1.00	−0.011	0.936	n.s.
Kurtosis	4.75 ± 4.59	4.86 ± 3.14	5.37 ± 3.23	0.056	0.681	n.s.
5th percentile	822 ± 216	718 ± 173	642 ± 147	−0.268	0.046*	n.s.
50th percentile	1034 ± 198	992 ± 160	936 ± 154	−0.170	0.211	n.s.
75th percentile	1149 ± 258	1112 ± 181	1078 ± 187	−0.104	0.448	n.s.
90th percentile	1248 ± 293	1234 ± 223	1244 ± 244	−0.002	0.990	n.s.

Well diff HCC: Well differentiated hepatocellular carcinoma
Mod diff HCC: Moderately differentiated hepatocellular carcinoma
Poor diff HCC: Poorly differentiated hepatocellular carcinoma
*, ** $P < 0.05$
n.s. no significant difference
**Tukey-Kramer post hoc test: Well diff HCC vs Mod diff HCC, $P = 0.521$; Well diff HCC vs Poor diff HCC, $P = 0.121$; Mod diff HCC vs Poor diff HCC, $P = 0.008$

Table 2 Comparison of well differentiated and moderately differentiated hepatocellular carcinoma with poorly differentiated hepatocellular carcinoma using the parameters of ADC histograms

	Well + Mod diff HCC	Poor diff HCC	P value
Mean	1007 ± 168	964 ± 167	0.470
Standard deviation	191 ± 90	227 ± 75	0.251
Minimum	437 ± 299	235 ± 102	0.001*
Maximum	1706 ± 563	1955 ± 704	0.232
Mode	855 ± 348	829 ± 319	0.829
Skewness	0.40 ± 0.94	0.50 ± 1.00	0.752
Kurtosis	4.84 ± 3.34	5.37 ± 3.23	0.648
5th percentile	733 ± 186	642 ± 147	0.151
50th percentile	998 ± 164	936 ± 154	0.276
75th percentile	1118 ± 192	1078 ± 187	0.552
90th percentile	1236 ± 231	1244 ± 244	0.924

Well + Mod diff HCC: Well differentiated and moderately differentiated hepatocellular carcinoma
Poor diff HCC: Poorly differentiated hepatocellular carcinoma
*$P < 0.05$

usually increases. This leads to restricted diffusion. We suppose that the results of the present study support this assumption.

Minimum ADC provided good sensitivity of 100%; however, there was a low specificity of 54% on diagnosis of poorly differentiated HCC. Although several researchers had previously reported the histological grade of the tumor using DWI, the accuracy was relative low. Nishie et al conducted the diagnosis of poorly differentiated HCC using mean ADC and obtained sensitivity of 73.1% and specificity of 72.9% [8]. The ROIs were put on the lowest intensity area in the solid part in the tumor on the ADC map in their report. In contrast, the ROI were set at entire tumors in our examination; therefore, we believe our results are more reproducible. We suppose that the low specificity in the present study was due to the variety of histological structure in well differentiated HCC. Minimum ADC showed significant differences between moderately differentiated HCC and poorly differentiated HCC; however, there were no differences between well differentiated HCC and moderately or poorly differentiated HCC. One of the reasons for this result might be that the minimum ADC of well differentiated HCC had wide variation (actually its standard deviation was large and the skewness was higher, although there was no significant difference). Moreover, the low mode ADC in well differentiated HCC indicates a large amount of histological components that showed restricted diffusion. Well differentiated HCC covers a variable range, from early HCC that is histologically similar to surrounding non-tumorous hepatic tissue [13] to hypervascular well differentiated HCC that often contain steatosis lesions [14, 15]. Steatosis leads to restricted diffusion [16, 17]; therefore, this effect may be present in this study. In the present study, minimum ADC in poorly differentiated HCC was significantly lower than both well and moderately differentiated HCC excluding steatosis-containing lesions. This result supports the concept that steatosis affects minimum ADC.

The effective parameters of ADC histograms for distinguishing histological differentiation are dependent

Table 3 Histological grade of hepatocellular carcinoma (after excluding steatosis lesions), the ADC histogram parameters, Pearson's product moment correlation coefficient, and one-way ANOVA with the Tukey-Kramer post hoc test

	Well diff HCC	Mod diff HCC	Poor diff HCC	Pearson's correlation coefficient	Pearson's correlation coefficient P value	ANOVA Tukey-Kramer post hoc test
Mean	1071 ± 178	1004 ± 157	967 ± 176	−0.164	0.281	n.s.
Standard deviation	147 ± 86	196 ± 89	243 ± 76	0.290	0.053	n.s.
Minimum	738 ± 322	421 ± 271	221 ± 110	−0.469	0.001*	0.006**
Maximum	1588 ± 493	1787 ± 579	1808 ± 606	0.201	0.186	n.s.
Mode	582 ± 531	890 ± 281	799 ± 347	0.122	0.425	n.s.
Skewness	0.91 ± 1.40	0.54 ± 0.84	0.59 ± 0.94	−0.073	0.633	n.s.
Kurtosis	5.39 ± 5.45	5.10 ± 3.38	5.50 ± 3.61	0.017	0.912	n.s.
5th percentile	910 ± 187	734 ± 181	631 ± 158	−0.382	0.010*	0.03***
50th percentile	1042 ± 163	997 ± 154	934 ± 160	−0.192	0.205	n.s.
75th percentile	1139 ± 222	1119 ± 173	1089 ± 199	−0.078	0.610	n.s.
90th percentile	1218 ± 217	1244 ± 219	1271 ± 260	0.065	0.672	n.s.

Well diff HCC: Well differentiated hepatocellular carcinoma
Mod diff HCC: Moderately differentiated hepatocellular carcinoma
Poor diff HCC: Poorly differentiated hepatocellular carcinoma
*, **, *** $P < 0.05$
n.s. no significant difference
**Tukey-Kramer post hoc test: Well diff HCC vs Mod diff HCC, $P = 0.187$; Well diff HCC vs Poor diff HCC, $P = 0.045$; Mod diff HCC vs Poor diff HCC, $P = 0.008$
***Tukey-Kramer post hoc test: Well diff HCC vs Mod diff HCC, $P = 0.110$; Well diff HCC vs Poor diff HCC, $P = 0.023$; Mod diff HCC vs Poor diff HCC, $P = 0.317$

Table 4 Comparison of well differentiated and moderately differentiated hepatocellular carcinoma with poorly differentiated hepatocellular carcinoma using the parameters of ADC histograms (after excluding steatosis lesions)

	Well + Moddiff HCC	Poor diff HCC	P value
Mean	1013 ± 159	967 ± 176	0.474
Standard deviation	189 ± 89	243 ± 76	0.123
Minimum	464 ± 295	221 ± 110	<0.0001*
Maximum	1760 ± 566	2031 ± 769	0.256
Mode	849 ± 333	799 ± 347	0.704
Skewness	0.59 ± 0.92	0.59 ± 1.11	0.999
Kurtosis	5.14 ± 3.63	5.50 ± 3.61	0.799
5th percentile	758 ± 189	631 ± 158	0.085
50th percentile	1003 ± 154	934 ± 160	0.258
75th percentile	1122 ± 177	1089 ± 199	0.640
90th percentile	1241 ± 216	1271 ± 260	0.728

Well + Mod diff HCC: Well differentiated and moderately differentiated hepatocellular carcinoma
Poor diff HCC: Poorly differentiated hepatocellular carcincma
*P < 0.05

on sites originating tumors. Woo et al reported that standard deviation and 75th,90th, and 95th percentiles were useful for differentiating low from high grade in endometrial cancer [18]. The results were reflected by the tissue necrosis in high grade endometrial cancer. On the other hand, high grade HCC usually showing hypercellularity, necrosis, or cystic change was rare. Suo et al. also reported that the mean, minimum, maximum, and 10th, 25th, 50th, 75th, and 90th percentile ADCs were significantly lower, while skewness and entropy ADCs were significantly higher in malignant lesions compared with benign ones in breast tumor [19]. The results reflected hypercellularity and pathological heterogeneity. The present study showed only minimum ADC and skewness showed no significant differences among degrees of tumor differentiation. We supposed these results reflected hypercellularity of HCC and relative pathological homogeneity compared with breast tumors. The pathological homogeneity may lead to making the distinction between tumor differentiation classifications difficult. Therefore, effective parameters of ADC histograms in predicting tumor histological grade were dependent on the characteristics of the tumor. The usefulness of kurtosis was less reported in previous studies of ADC histograms in abdominal and pelvic tumors except for a few reports [18–21], and the present study also showed no significant differences according to tumor differentiation.

The b-values might have affected the results of 3D analysis of ADC histograms. Nasu et al reported the mean ADC values of well, moderately, and poorly differentiated HCC were much higher than those of the present study [6]. They used b-values of 0 and 500 s/mm^2, and used lower b-values than we used. On the other hand, Heo et al reported similar results to the present study, although mean ADC values of poorly differentiated HCC were significantly lower than those of well and moderately differentiated HCC [9]. They used b-values of 0 and 1000 s/mm^2. Therefore, the standardization of b-values is important.

There are several limitations in the present study. First, the sample size of tumor histological differentiation was biased due to many moderately differentiated HCCs. The reason was that operation candidates were collected in the study. Second, some fusion errors from different slice thicknesses might affect the result. This is an important issue for improving this method. Third, we excluded the tumors located in the lateral segment because of cardiac motion. Cardiac motion causes negligible artifact (signal loss). This is a disadvantage of DWI. Recently, some methods have been proposed to reduce the cardiac motion [22–24]. These methods should be tried in the future when performing clinical routines.

Conclusions

In conclusion, minimum ADC was the most promising parameter for distinguishing poorly differentiated HCC from the other histological grades on 3D analysis of ADC histograms.

Abbreviations

3D-VIBE: Three-dimensional volumetric interpolated breath-hold examination; ADC: Apparent diffusion coefficient; CHESS: Chemical shift selective; DWI: Diffusion-weighted imaging; FOV: Field of view; Gd-EOB-DTPA: Gadolinium-ethoxybenzyl-diethylenetriamine pentaacetic acid; HCC: Hepatocellular carcinoma; ROI: Region of interest; T1WI: T1-weighted imaging; T2WI: T2-weighted imaging; TR/TE: Repetition time/Echo time

Acknowledgements

The authors are grateful to the medical editors from the Department of International Medical Communications of Tokyo Medical University for editing and reviewing the English manuscript.

Funding

Not applicable.

Authors' contributions

KS conceived of the study, and participated in its design and coordination. TM, TLH, and YA carried out the image analyses, and KS and YT carried out the statistical analyses. KS and KT carried out the manuscript drafting or revising for important intellectual content. All authors read and approved the final manuscript.

Competing interests

The authors declare that they have no competing interests.

Author details

[1]Department of Radiology, Tokyo Medical University, 6-7-1 Nishishinjuku, Shinjuku-ku, Tokyo 160-0023, Japan. [2]Department of Gastroenterology and Hepatology, Tokyo Medical University, Tokyo, Japan.

References

1. Jonas S, Bechstein WO, Steinmuller T, Herrmann M, Radke C, Berg T, et al. Vascular invasion and histopathologic grading determine outcome after liver transplantation for hepatocellular carcinoma in cirrhosis. Hepatology. 2001;33:1080–6.
2. Nakanishi M, Chuma M, Hige S, Omatsu T, Yokoo H, Nakanishi K, et al. Relationship between diffusion-weighted magnetic resonance imaging and histological tumor grading of hepatocellular carcinoma. Ann Surg Oncol. 2012;19:1302–9.
3. Asayama Y, Yoshimitsu K, Nishihara Y, Irie H, Aishima S, Taketomi A, et al. Arterial blood supply of hepatocellular carcinoma and histologic grading: radiologic-pathologic correlation. Am J Roentgenol. 2008;190:W28–34.
4. Amano S, Ebara M, Yajima T, Fukuda H, Yoshikawa M, Sugiura N, et al. Assessment of cancer cell differentiation in small hepatocellular carcinoma by computed tomography and magnetic resonance imaging. J Gastroenterol Hepatol. 2003;18:273–9.
5. Muhi A, Ichikawa T, Motosugi U, Sano K, Matsuda M, Kitamura T, et al. High-b-value diffusion-weighted MR imaging of hepatocellular lesions: estimation of grade of malignancy of hepatocellular carcinoma. J Magn Reson Imaging. 2009;30:1005–11.
6. Nasu K, Kuroki Y, Tsukamoto T, Nakajima H, Mori K, Minami M. Diffusion-weighted imaging of surgically resected hepatocellular carcinoma: imaging characteristics and relationship among signal intensity, apparent diffusion coefficient, and histopathologic grade. Am J Roentgenol. 2009;193:438–44.
7. Saito K, Moriyasu F, Sugimoto K, Nishio R, Saguchi T, Akata S, et al. Histological grade of differentiation of hepatocellular carcinoma: comparison of the efficacy of diffusion-weighted MRI with T2-weighted imaging and angiography-assisted CT. J Med Imaging Radiat Oncol. 2012;56:261–9.
8. Nishie A, Tajima T, Asayama Y, Ishigami K, Kakihara D, Nakayama T, et al. Diagnostic performance of apparent diffusion coefficient for predicting histological grade of hepatocellular carcinoma. Eur J Radiol. 2011;80:e29–33.
9. Heo SH, Jeong YY, Shin SS, Kim JW, Lim HS, Lee JH, et al. Apparent diffusion coefficient value of diffusion-weighted imaging for hepatocellular carcinoma: correlation with the histologic differentiation and the expression of vascular endothelial growth factor. Korean J Radiol. 2010;11:295–303.
10. Kang Y, Choi SH, Kim YJ, Kim KG, Sohn CH, Kim JH, et al. Gliomas: Histogram analysis of apparent diffusion coefficient maps with standard- or high-b-value diffusion-weighted MR imaging–correlation with tumor grade. Radiology. 2011;261:882–90.
11. Seyama Y, Kokudo N. Assessment of liver function for safe hepatic resection. Hepatol Res. 2009;39:107–16.
12. Liver cancer study group of Japan. The general rules for the clinical and pathological study of primary liver cancer The 5th edition. 2008. p. 40–5.
13. Kojiro M, Roskams T. Early hepatocellular carcinoma and dysplastic nodules. Semin Liver Dis. 2005;25:133–42.
14. Kutami R, Nakashima Y, Nakashima O, Shiota K, Kojiro M. Pathomorphologic study on the mechanism of fatty change in small hepatocellular carcinoma of humans. J Hepatol. 2000;33:282–9.
15. Sano K, Ichikawa T, Motosugi U, Sou H, Muhi AM, Matsuda M, et al. Imaging study of early hepatocellular carcinoma: usefulness of gadoxetic acid-enhanced MR imaging. Radiology. 2011;261:834–44.
16. Poyraz AK, Onur MR, Kocakoc E, Ogur E. Diffusion-weighted MRI of fatty liver. J Magn Reson Imaging. 2012;35:1108–11.
17. Bulow R, Mensel B, Meffert P, Hernando D, Evert M, Kuhn JP. Diffusion-weighted magnetic resonance imaging for staging liver fibrosis is less reliable in the presence of fat and iron. Eur Radiol. 2013;23:1281–7.
18. Woo S, Cho JY, Kim SY, Kim SH. Histogram analysis of apparent diffusion coefficient map of diffusion-weighted MRI in endometrial cancer: a preliminary correlation study with histological grade. Acta Radiol. 2014;55:1270–7.
19. Suo S, Zhang K, Cao M, Suo X, Hua J, Geng X, et al. Characterization of breast masses as benign or malignant at 3.0T MRI with whole-lesion histogram analysis of the apparent diffusion coefficient. J Magn Reson Imaging. 2016;43:894–902.
20. Besa C, Ward S, Cui Y, Jajamovich G, Kim M, Taouli B. Neuroendocrine liver metastases: Value of apparent diffusion coefficient and enhancement ratios for characterization of histopathologic grade. J Magn Reson Imaging. 2016; 44:1432–41.
21. Lin Y, Li H, Chen Z, Ni P, Zhong Q, Huang H, et al. Correlation of histogram analysis of apparent diffusion coefficient with uterine cervical pathologic finding. Am J Roentgenol. 2015;204:1125–31.
22. Liau J, Lee J, Schroeder ME, Sirlin CB, Bydder M. Cardiac motion in diffusion-weighted MRI of the liver: artifact and a method of correction. J Magn Reson Imaging. 2012;35:318–27.
23. Metens T, Absil J, Denolin V, Bali MA, Matos C. Liver apparent diffusion coefficient repeatability with individually predetermined optimal cardiac timing and artifact elimination by signal filtering. J Magn Reson Imaging. 2016;43:1100–10.
24. Murtz P, Flacke S, Traber F, van den Brink JS, Gieseke J, Schild HH. Abdomen: diffusion-weighted MR imaging with pulse-triggered single-shot sequences. Radiology. 2002;224:258–64.

7

^{18}F–FDG-PET/CT and diffusion-weighted MRI for monitoring a BRAF and CDK 4/6 inhibitor combination therapy in a murine model of human melanoma

Ralf S. Eschbach[1*], Philipp M. Kazmierczak[1], Maurice M. Heimer[1], Andrei Todica[2], Heidrun Hirner-Eppeneder[1], Moritz J. Schneider[1,3], Georg Keinrath[1], Olga Solyanik[1], Jessica Olivier[2], Wolfgang G. Kunz[1], Maximilian F. Reiser[1], Peter Bartenstein[2], Jens Ricke[1] and Clemens C. Cyran[1]

Abstract

Background: The purpose of the study was to investigate a novel BRAF and CDK 4/6 inhibitor combination therapy in a murine model of BRAF-V600-mutant human melanoma monitored by ^{18}F–FDG-PET/CT and diffusion-weighted MRI (DW-MRI).

Methods: Human BRAF-V600-mutant melanoma (A375) xenograft-bearing balb/c nude mice ($n = 21$) were imaged by ^{18}F–FDG-PET/CT and DW-MRI before (day 0) and after (day 7) a 1-week BRAF and CDK 4/6 inhibitor combination therapy ($n = 12$; dabrafenib, 20 mg/kg/d; ribociclib, 100 mg/kg/d) or placebo ($n = 9$). Animals were scanned on a small animal PET after intravenous administration of 20 MBq ^{18}F–FDG. Tumor glucose uptake was calculated as the tumor-to-liver-ratio (TTL). Unenhanced CT data sets were subsequently acquired for anatomic coregistration. Tumor diffusivity was assessed by DW-MRI using the apparent diffusion coefficient (ADC). Anti-tumor therapy effects were assessed by *ex vivo* immunohistochemistry for validation purposes (microvascular density – CD31; tumor cell proliferation – Ki-67).

Results: Tumor glucose uptake was significantly suppressed under therapy ($\Delta TTL_{Therapy} - 1.00 \pm 0.53$ vs. $\Delta TTL_{Control}$ 0.85 ± 1.21; $p < 0.001$). In addition, tumor diffusivity was significantly elevated following the BRAF and CDK 4/6 inhibitor combination therapy ($\Delta ADC_{Therapy}$ $0.12 \pm 0.14 \times 10^{-3}$ mm^2/s; $\Delta ADC_{Control} - 0.12 \pm 0.06 \times 10^{-3}$ mm^2/s; $p < 0.001$). Immunohistochemistry revealed a significant suppression of microvascular density (CD31, 147 ± 48 vs. 287 ± 92; $p = 0.001$) and proliferation (Ki-67, 3718 ± 998 vs. 5389 ± 1332; $p = 0.007$) in the therapy compared to the control group.

Conclusion: A novel BRAF and CDK 4/6 inhibitor combination therapy exhibited significant anti-angiogenic and anti-proliferative effects in experimental human melanomas, monitored by ^{18}F–FDG-PET/CT and DW-MRI.

Keywords: Melanoma, BRAF inhibitor, CDK inhibitor, ^{18}F–FDG-PET, Diffusion-weighted MRI, Therapy monitoring

* Correspondence: ralf.eschbach@med.lmu.de
Ralf S. Eschbach and Philipp M. Kazmierczak contributed equally to the project.Ralf S. Eschbach and Philipp M. Kazmierczak share first authorship.
[1]Department of Radiology, Laboratory for Experimental Radiology, University Hospital, Ludwig-Maximilians-University Munich, Marchioninistr. 15, 81377 München, Germany
Full list of author information is available at the enc of the article

Background

The mitogen-activated protein kinase (MAPK) pathway controls cell cycle progression, survival, and proliferation in human cells [1, 2]. B-rapidly accelerated fibrosarcoma (BRAF) gene mutations V600E/K were identified as key drivers of oncogenesis in melanoma, as they lead to overactivation of the MAPK pathway and uncontrolled cell proliferation [2]. Thus, selective inhibition of the BRAF gene emerged as a novel, targeted treatment regimen in advanced or unresectable melanoma [3, 4]. However, tumor response to BRAF inhibitor monotherapy may be limited by intrinsic or acquired resistance [5–7]. Consequently, combination therapies of BRAF inhibitors and additional therapeutics potentially overcoming resistance were investigated in recent years [5, 8]. One possible mechanism of acquired BRAF inhibitor resistance is MAPK pathway activation via the mitogen-activated extracellular signal-regulated kinase (MEK). Co-targeting the MAPK pathway by a BRAF and MEK inhibitor combination therapy yields high response rates as well as prolonged overall and progression-free survival in advanced BRAF-mutant melanoma compared to other available treatment strategies, including BRAF inhibitor monotherapy [9]. A possible mechanism of intrinsic BRAF inhibitor resistance is cyclin D1 overexpression with cyclin-dependent kinase (CDK) 4 mutation/amplification [2, 5]. Cyclin D1 promotes cell cycle progression by binding to CDK 4 and 6, which act as downstream mediators of the MAPK pathway and regulate the cell cycle via the retinoblastoma tumor suppressor protein [2, 5]. Yadav et al. recently demonstrated that the selective inhibition of CDK 4/6 leads to tumor growth regression in a BRAF inhibitor-resistant *in vivo* model of human melanoma (A375) [10]. In 2017, based on the results of the MONALEESA-2 trial, the U.S. Food and Drug Administration approved the CDK 4/6 inhibitor ribociclib combined with an aromatase inhibitor for the treatment of advanced or metastatic, hormone receptor-positive and human epidermal growth factor receptor 2-negative breast cancer in postmenopausal women [11]. The addition of a CDK 4/6 inhibitor to BRAF inhibitor monotherapy represents a novel strategy to overcome cyclin D1-dependent resistance. Dual inhibition of the MAPK pathway by a BRAF and CDK 4/6 inhibitor combination therapy may thus be a promising future therapy regimen in advanced melanoma.

Imaging plays a central role for the non-invasive tumor response assessment in clinical oncology. Morphology-based criteria of tumor response, e. g., RECIST (Response Evaluation Criteria in Solid Tumors), provide a valuable clinical tool to differentiate between partial/complete response, progressive, and stable disease [12]. These criteria are based on the number and size of tumor manifestations, which are commonly assessed by morphological imaging modalities such as computed tomography (CT) or magnetic resonance imaging (MRI). However, in contrast to traditional, primarily cytotoxic therapies, novel targeted therapies exhibit only subtle effects on tumor size [13]. Thus, morphology-based tumor response criteria are of only limited applicability in targeted therapy regimens [14]. Functional and molecular imaging modalities allow for a non-invasive tumor characterization beyond morphology, delivering information on tumor pathophysiology such as tumor glucose metabolism (^{18}F–fluorodeoxyglucose positron emission tomography; ^{18}F–FDG-PET) and tumor cellularity (diffusion-weighted MRI; DW-MRI). Both ^{18}F–FDG-PET and DW-MRI demonstrated their potential to generate non-invasive imaging biomarkers of therapy response in melanoma under targeted therapy [15–18].

As a proof of principle, the present study is a first approach to explore a selective CDK 4/6 inhibitor as novel combination compound for dual inhibition of the MAPK signal pathway in melanoma therapy. The aim of this experimental study was to close this gap of knowledge, evaluating a novel BRAF and CDK 4/6 inhibitor combination therapy in a murine model of human BRAF-V600-mutant melanoma using a multimodal imaging protocol of ^{18}F–FDG-PET/CT and DW-MRI. We hypothesized that a BRAF and CDK 4/6 inhibitor combination therapy exhibits significant anti-angiogenic and anti-proliferative effects in experimental human melanomas in mice and that the according alterations in tumor pathophysiology can be non-invasively monitored by ^{18}F–FDG-PET/CT and DW-MRI *in vivo* validated by *ex vivo* immunohistochemistry.

Methods

The experiments were performed in accordance with the Guidelines for the Care and Use of Laboratory Animals of the National Institutes of Health and with approval by the Government Committee for Animal Research.

Animal model and experimental protocol

After diluting human melanoma cells (A375, ATCC® CRL-1619™, CLS Cell Lines Service GmbH, Eppelheim, Germany) in a total volume of 0.1 mL as a 1:1 solution of phosphate buffered saline (PBS pH 7.4; GIBCO Life Technologies, Darmstadt, Germany) and Matrigel™ (BD Biosciences, San Jose, CA), 3×10^6 cells per mouse were injected subcutaneously into the left abdominal flank of $n = 21$ athymic balb/c nude mice (Charles River, Sulzfeld, Germany). When tumors reached a diameter of 0.5 cm, animals were randomly assigned to either the therapy ($n = 12$) or the control group ($n = 9$). Imaging was performed on day 0 (baseline) and day 7 (follow-up) using a multimodal imaging protocol of ^{18}F–FDG PET/CT and DW-MRI. Imaging was performed under inhalation anesthesia (2.5% in 1.0 L 100% O_2/min for induction, 1.5% in 1.0 L 100% O_2/min for maintenance). Subsequently to the baseline scan, animals were treated daily with either a combination of BRAF inhibitor dabrafenib (20 mg/kg/day; Novartis AG, Basel, Switzerland) and CDK4/6 inhibitor ribociclib (100 mg/kg/day; Novartis AG, Basel, Switzerland) in the therapy group or a volume-equivalent placebo solution (0.5% hydroxymethyl cellulose and 0.2% Tween-80 in dd$H_2$0) in the control group. Immediately after follow-up imaging on day 7, animals were sacrificed and tumors were explanted and fixed in formalin for immunohistochemical analysis with regard to tumor microvascular density (CD31) and tumor cell proliferation (Ki-67). Figure 1 provides an overview of the experimental protocol.

PET imaging

Small-animal PET was performed on a preclinical PET scanner (Inveon µPET, Siemens Healthineers, Erlangen, Germany). For hygienic reasons and allowing regulated anesthesia delivery, mice were placed inside a custom-built acrylic glass-imaging chamber in prone position. 45 min after manual intravenous injection of 20 MBq (~100 µL) ^{18}F–FDG per animal, a transmission scan (15 min) was acquired for scatter and attenuation correction. Subsequently, PET list-mode data acquisition was initiated from 60 to 90 min (30 min emission).

All PET data were post-processed on an Inveon Acquisition Workplace (Siemens Healthineers, Erlangen, Germany). Images were reconstructed as a static image using OSEM 3D (4 iterations) and MAP 3D (32 iterations) algorithm in a 256×256 matrix with a zoom value of 100% as described previously [19]. To calculate the metabolic tumor volume (MTV), a PET/CT-guided volume of interest (VOI) surrounding the tumor was drawn manually and a threshold-value of 30% of the hottest voxels was applied. Background was determined as mean uptake in a 9 mm^3 VOI in the right liver lobe. Tumor-to-liver-ratio (TTL, VOImaxtumor/VOImeanliver) was determined as a semiquantitative measurement of tumor

radiotracer accumulation before (day 0) and after treatment (day 7). Figure 2 demonstrates the process of PET/CT VOI selection.

After PET measurements, additional CT images were acquired on a latest generation clinical CT (SOMATOM Force, Siemens Healthineers, Erlangen, Germany), maintaining the animals in the same position within the acrylic imaging chamber for morphological correlation, as described previously [19].

MRI

MRI measurements were conducted on a clinical 3 Tesla scanner (MAGNETOM Skyra, Siemens Healthineers, Erlangen, Germany) using a 16-channel wrist coil (Siemens Healthineers, Erlangen, Germany). Mice were positioned head-first in prone position. For the assessment of tumor morphology and tumor volume as morphology-based surrogate of tumor response, T2-weighted MR images were acquired using a 2D Turbo Spin Echo sequence (TR = 5470 ms, TE = 91 ms, in-plane resolution 0.3×0.3 mm, matrix size 192×192, slice thickness 1.5 mm). In addition, DW-MRI data sets were acquired using a single shot echo planar imaging sequence (TR = 3200 ms, TE = 50 ms, FOV = 84 mm, acquisition matrix = 64×64, reconstructed matrix = 128×128, slice thickness 2 mm, 8 averages, time to acquisition 180 s; 3 b-values: b = 0 s/mm^2/200 s/mm^2/800 s/mm^2). Apparent diffusion coefficient (ADC) maps were calculated by voxel-wise least-squares fitting of the model

$$S(b) = S_0 \cdot e^{-b \cdot ADC}.$$

MRI data sets were analyzed on an external workstation using a dedicated, in-house written post-processing software (PMI; Platform for Research in Medical Imaging, version 0.4) [20]. For each measurement, a multi-slice VOI was drawn manually over the entire tumor. The median value inside this VOI was used to calculate a representative tumor ADC value for statistical analysis.

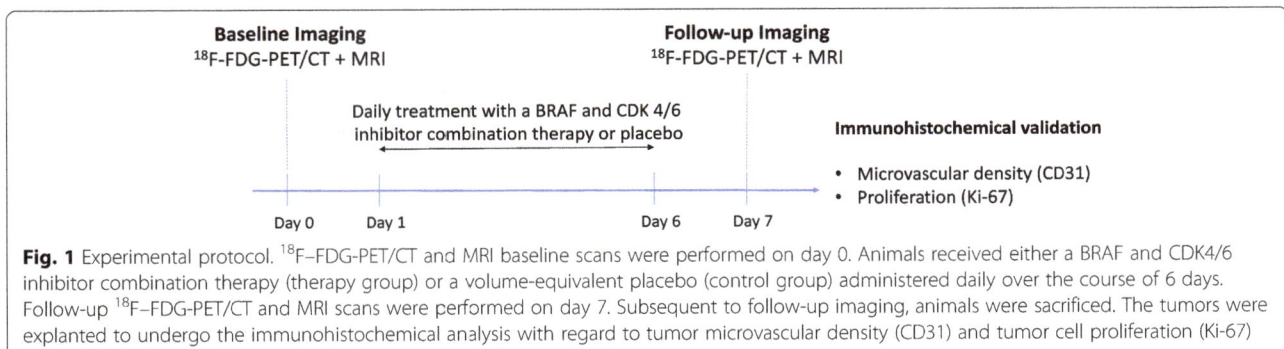

Fig. 1 Experimental protocol. ^{18}F–FDG-PET/CT and MRI baseline scans were performed on day 0. Animals received either a BRAF and CDK4/6 inhibitor combination therapy (therapy group) or a volume-equivalent placebo (control group) administered daily over the course of 6 days. Follow-up ^{18}F–FDG-PET/CT and MRI scans were performed on day 7. Subsequent to follow-up imaging, animals were sacrificed. The tumors were explanted to undergo the immunohistochemical analysis with regard to tumor microvascular density (CD31) and tumor cell proliferation (Ki-67)

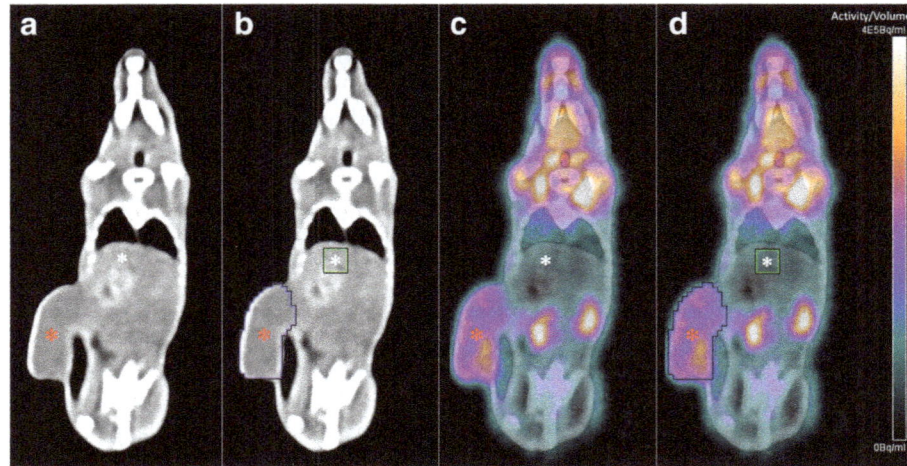

Fig. 2 PET/CT VOI Selection. **a** and **b**: coronal unenhanced CT without (**a**) and with (**b**) VOIs. **c** and **d**: Fused coronal PET/CT data sets without (**c**) and with (**d**) VOIs. Note the tumor in the lateral flank (red asterisk). The liver is indicated by a white asterisk. To calculate the metabolic tumor volume, a PET/CT-guided VOI surrounding the tumor was drawn. Background was determined in a VOI in the right liver lobe and the TTL was calculated accordingly

Immunohistochemistry

Three micrometer tissue sections were cut from the formalin-fixed and paraffin-embedded tumor tissue and stained with regard to microvascular density (CD31) and tumor cell proliferation (Ki-67). After de-waxing and re-hydration following standard procedures (pre-heating at 60 °C, washing in xylene substitute (Neo-Clear, Merck KgaA, Darmstadt, Germany) and rehydration in a graded series of ethanol (100, 95, 80, and 70%, respectively) followed by double distilled water, antigen demasking was performed by microwave irradiation at 600 W in a 0.1 M citrate buffer solution (pH 6.0). Tissue samples were subsequently antibody-incubated at 4 °C over night (antibodies: monoclonal rabbit anti-Ki-67 antibody; SP6, Abcam ab16667 1:100, Cambridge, United Kingdom; polyclonal rabbit anti-CD31 primary antibody; Abcam ab28364 1:50, Cambridge, United Kingdom).

According to the manufacturer's instructions, further work-up of tissue samples was performed using the EnVision + System HRP (DAB or AEC) (DAKO Diagnostika, Hamburg, Germany) kit. Slides were counterstained using Mayer's Haemalaun (Merck KgaA, Darmstadt, Germany) and covered with Kaiser's Glycerin Gelatine (Merck KgaA, Darmstadt, Germany). Results were quantified as the number of positively stained nuclei (Ki-67) or positively stained microvessels (CD31) in ten random fields at 200× magnification.

Statistical analysis

In this randomized placebo-controlled preclinical trial the statistical analyses were performed using commercially available statistics software (SPSS 23, IBM Corp., Armonk, NY). For intergroup comparisons of the imaging and the immunohistochemical parameters, the Mann-Whitney-U-test was applied. For intragroup comparisons between baseline (day 0) and follow-up (day 7), a Wilcoxon signed-rank test was performed. Correlations between the imaging and the immunohistochemical parameters were assessed by Spearman's correlation coefficient. Continuous variables were presented as means with standard deviations. The confirmatory tests were performed against a significance level $\alpha = 0.05$ with Bonferroni corrections.

Results

The experimental protocol was successfully completed in $n = 21$ animals. There were no significant ($p > 0.05$) intergroup differences between therapy and control group in baseline TTL ($TTL_{Baseline}$: 4.19 ± 0.97 vs. 3.70 ± 0.90; $p = 0.193$) and baseline ADC ($ADC_{Baseline}$: $0.78 \pm 0.10 \times 10^{-3}$ mm^2/s vs. $0.79 \pm 0.10 \times 10^{-3}$ mm^2/s; $p = 0.754$) as well as in metabolic (161.1 ± 86.5 mm^3 vs. 217.9 ± 145.8 mm^3; $p = 0.464$) and morphological (94.6 ± 71.4 mm^3 vs. 134.3 ± 89.0 mm^3; $p = 0.219$) tumor volumes.

^{18}F–FDG-PET/CT

We observed a significant reduction of TTL under therapy ($TTL_{Therapy}$ from 4.19 ± 0.97 to 3.19 ± 0.97; $p = 0.002$). In the control group, TTL demonstrated a non-significant increase from baseline to follow-up ($TTL_{Control}$ from 3.70 ± 0.90 to 4.55 ± 0.91; $p = 0.14$). Follow-up TTL values were significantly lower in the therapy group ($TTL_{Follow-up}$: 3.19 ± 0.97 vs. 4.55 ± 0.91; $p = 0.007$). Moreover, ΔTTL ($TTL_{Follow-up} - TTL_{Baseline}$) was negative and significantly lower in the therapy compared to the control group (ΔTTL$_{\text{Therapy}}$ − 1.00 ± 0.53 vs. ΔTTL$_{\text{Control}}$ 0.85 ± 1.21; $p < 0.001$). The metabolic tumor volume increased in the control group (from 217.9 ± 145.8 mm^3 on day 0 to 573.5 ± 294.7 mm^3 on day 7; $p = 0.008$), while no significant change was observed in the therapy group (from 161.1 ± 86.5 mm^3 to 211.6 ± 139.4 mm^3; $p = 0.308$). Metabolic tumor volumes on follow-up were significantly higher in the control than in the therapy group (573.5 ± 294.7 mm^3 vs. 211.6 ± 139.4 mm^3; $p = 0.001$). Figure 3 shows representative ^{18}F–FDG-PET/CT data sets from the therapy and the control group. Individual TTL values and metabolic tumor volumes at baseline and at follow-up are provided in Table 1.

MRI

DW-MRI detected an increase in ADC under therapy with a trend toward significance (ADC$_{\text{Therapy}}$: from $0.78 \pm 0.10 \times 10^{-3}$ mm^2/s to $0.90 \pm 0.13 \times 10^{-3}$ mm^2/s; $p = 0.026$). In the control group, the ADC showed a significant decline (ADC$_{\text{Control}}$: from $0.79 \pm 0.10 \times 10^{-3}$ mm^2/s to $0.68 \pm 0.06 \times 10^{-3}$ mm^2/s; $p = 0.012$). Follow-up ADC values were significantly higher in the therapy group ($0.90 \pm 0.13 \times 10^{-3}$ mm^2/s vs. $0.68 \pm 0.06 \times 10^{-3}$ mm^2/s in the control group; $p < 0.001$). Moreover, ΔADC (ADC$_{\text{Follow-up}}$ − ADC$_{\text{Baseline}}$) was significantly elevated in the therapy group (ΔADC$_{\text{Therapy}}$ $0.12 \pm 0.14 \times 10^{-3}$ mm^2/s; ΔADC$_{\text{Control}}$ − $0.12 \pm 0.06 \times 10^{-3}$ mm^2/s; $p < 0.001$). Analogously to the metabolic tumor volumes, the morphological tumor volumes measured on T2w images significantly increased in the control group (from 134.3 ± 89.0 mm^3 to 381.9 ± 179.4 mm^3; $p = 0.008$). In the therapy group, the morphological tumor volumes showed a non-significant increase between baseline and follow-up (from 94.6 ± 71.4 mm^3 to 130.8 ± 91.3 mm^3; $p = 0.071$). Figure 4 shows representative MRI data sets from the therapy and the control group. Table 2 displays individual ADC values and the morphological tumor volumes for the therapy and the control group. Figure 5 shows boxplot diagrams of ΔTTL and ΔADC for the therapy and the control group.

Immunohistochemistry

Multiparametric immunohistochemistry revealed a significantly lower microvascular density (CD31: 147 ± 48 vs. 287 ± 92; $p = 0.001$) and tumor cell proliferation (Ki-67: 3718 ± 998 vs. 5389 ± 1332; $p = 0.007$) in the therapy compared to the control group. Table 3 summarizes individual immunohistochemical values for both groups. Figure 6 shows representative tumor sections from the therapy and the control group.

Correlations between imaging and immunohistochemical parameters

TTL demonstrated a good, significant correlation to microvascular density (CD31, $\rho = 0.79$; $p < 0.001$) and no significant correlation to the proliferation rate (Ki-67, $\rho = 0.33$; $p = 0.14$). ADC showed a strong and highly significant inverse correlation to microvascular density (CD31, $\rho = -0.80$; $p < 0.001$) but no significant correlation to proliferation (Ki-67, $\rho = -0.42$; $p = 0.061$).

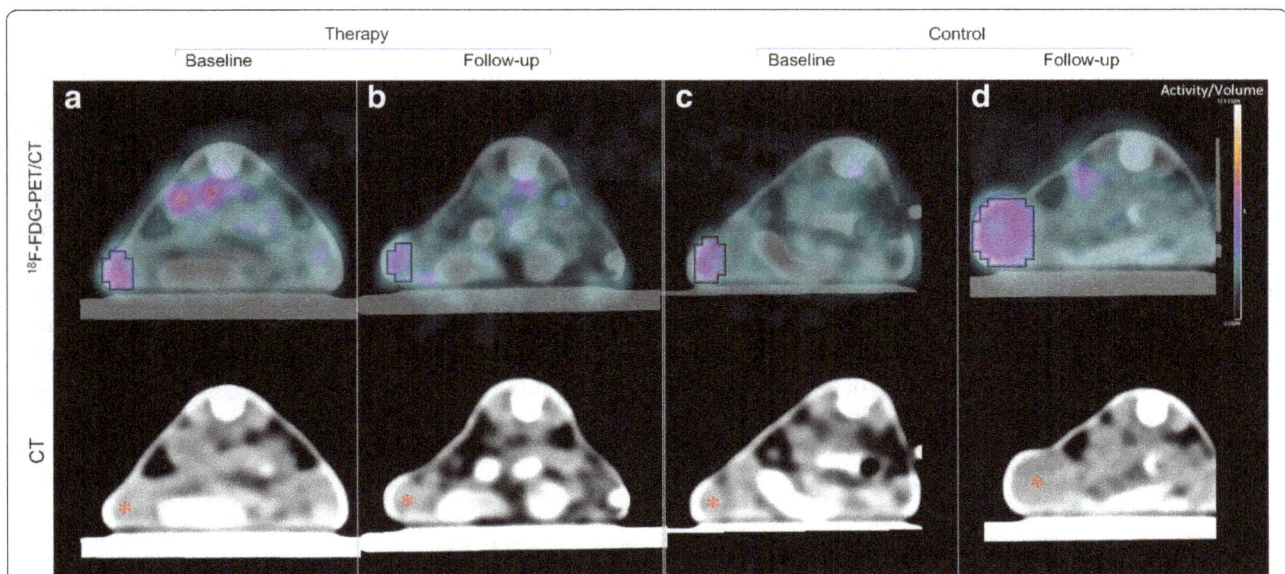

Fig. 3 Axial PET/CT data sets of representative tumors from therapy and control group. Top row: ^{18}F–FDG-PET/CT data sets. Bottom row: CT data sets. **a** therapy group, baseline. **b** therapy group, follow-up. **c** control group, baseline. **d** control group, follow-up. Note the significantly suppressed tumor glucose uptake following the 1-week BRAF and CDK 4/6 inhibitor combination therapy (**b** vs. **a**). Note the significant increase in tumor glucose uptake and tumor volume in the control group (**d** vs. **c**)

Table 1 Individual values for tumor glucose uptake and metabolic tumor volumes at baseline and follow-up

Number	Group[a]	TTL$_{Baseline}$	TTL$_{Follow-Up}$	ΔTTL	Volume$_{Baseline}$ (mm^3)	Volume$_{Follow-up}$ (mm^3)	ΔVolume (mm^3)
1	T	5.63	4.83	−0.79	296.0	311.4	15.4
2	T	4.80	3.13	−1.67	86.8	50.4	−36.4
3	T	5.90	5.26	−0.64	56.1	162.7	106.6
4	T	3.72	2.65	−1.07	155.9	417.9	262.0
5	T	3.94	3.88	0.06	142.5	433.7	291.2
6	T	4.57	3.02	−1.55	230.8	185.2	−45.6
7	T	4.61	2.90	−1.71	112.8	78.2	−34.6
8	T	3.69	2.40	−1.29	162.7	118.0	−44.7
9	T	3.11	2.52	−0.59	332.0	392.0	60.0
10	T	3.59	2.46	−1.13	171.3	161.7	−9.6
11	T	4.14	2.93	−1.21	120.0	80.6	−39.4
12	T	2.57	2.29	−0.28	66.2	147.8	81.6
Mean ± SD[b]	T	4.19 ± 0.97	3.19 ± 0.97	−1.00 ± 0.53	161.1 ± 86.5	211.6 ± 139.4	50.5 ± 117.9
13	C	4.34	4.06	−0.28	96.9	344.0	247.1
14	C	3.07	5.13	2.06	519.1	1192.3	673.2
15	C	5.62	5.50	−0.12	213.0	616.1	403.1
16	C	2.88	3.95	1.07	140.1	329.1	189.0
17	C	4.02	4.13	0.11	222.6	597.8	375.2
18	C	3.31	5.25	1.94	165.1	511.0	345.9
19	C	3.50	5.45	1.95	115.6	421.3	305.7
20	C	2.71	4.73	2.02	392.5	866.5	474.0
21	C	3.81	2.72	−1.09	96.0	283.1	187.1
Mean ± SD[b]	C	3.70 ± 0.90	4.55 ± 0.91	0.85 ± 1.21	217.9 ± 145.8	573.5 ± 294.7	355.6 ± 153.3

[a]T = therapy group; C = control group
[b]SD = standard deviation

ΔTTL and ΔADC showed strong and significant inverse correlations ($ρ = -0.75$; $p = 0.002$).

Discussion

In the present study, we investigated ^{18}F–FDG-PET/CT and DW-MRI for the *in vivo* monitoring of a novel BRAF and CDK4/6 inhibitor combination therapy in human melanoma xenografts in mice. Dual inhibition of the MAPK signal pathway demonstrated significant anti-angiogenic and anti-proliferative effects in the investigated tumor model. The multimodal imaging protocol allowed for the *in vivo* monitoring of tumor glucose metabolism and tumor diffusivity, adding molecular and functional information to the established morphology-based assessments of tumor response.

Our results are in line with previous preclinical and clinical studies investigating tumor response to targeted MAPK signal pathway inhibition. Baudy et al. reported a reduction in tumor glucose metabolism in A375 xenografts in mice following a BRAF (vemurafenib) and MEK inhibitor (GDC-0973) combination therapy over the course of 6 days [21]. However, the authors validated the imaging results by tumor cell glucose transporter 1 and MAPK pathway protein expression but not by immuno-histochemical markers of microvascular density or tumor cell proliferation. Analogously, combined BRAF and MEK targeting (vemurafenib plus cobimetinib or dabrafenib plus trametinib) lead to a significant reduction in tumor maximum standardized uptake value (SUVmax) in patients with advanced melanoma with a mean time to follow-up of 26 days [22]. ^{18}F–FDG-PET even provided predictive imaging biomarkers of therapy response in the investigated patient population, with a significant association of the change in SUVmax and progression-free survival observed for the least responsive tumor focus [22]. These studies underline the applicability and clinical significance of ^{18}F–FDG-based hybrid imaging for therapy monitoring in melanoma under MAPK pathway inhibition. Providing a surrogate of tumor cellularity, DW-MRI confirmed the ^{18}F–FDG-PET results and may thus be a suitable imaging modality to allow for a multi-facetted tumor characterization under targeted therapy. In experimental human BRAF-mutant melanomas, DW-MRI was successfully used for

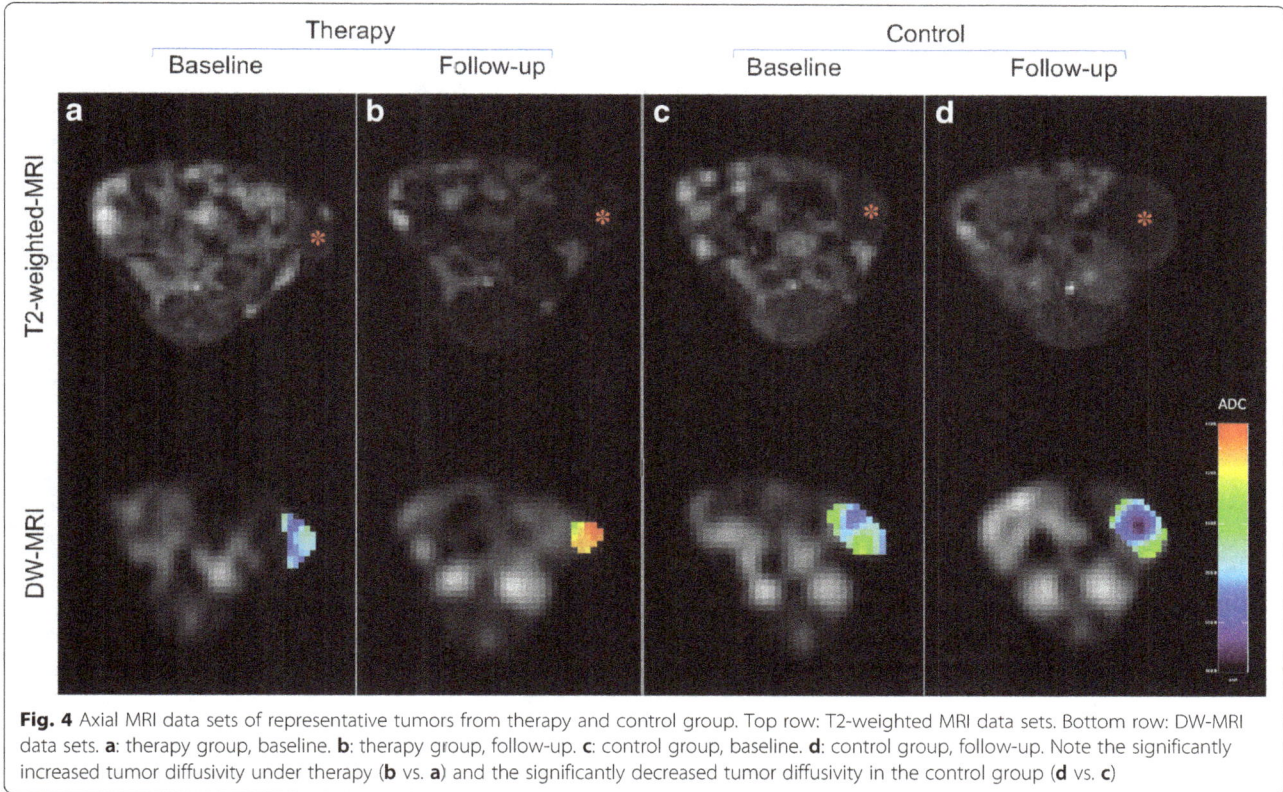

Fig. 4 Axial MRI data sets of representative tumors from therapy and control group. Top row: T2-weighted MRI data sets. Bottom row: DW-MRI data sets. **a**: therapy group, baseline. **b**: therapy group, follow-up. **c**: control group, baseline. **d**: control group, follow-up. Note the significantly increased tumor diffusivity under therapy (**b** vs. **a**) and the significantly decreased tumor diffusivity in the control group (**d** vs. **c**)

the *in vivo* monitoring of a 4-day therapy with the MEK inhibitor selumetinib [17]. Our results confirm the applicability of both ^{18}F–FDG-PET and DW-MRI for therapy monitoring in the same tumors showing a strong, intraindividual correlation between ΔTTL and ΔADC. This correlation may be explained by the fact that a high tumor cell density leads to restricted diffusion with low ADC values and increased tumor glucose metabolism [23].

The addition of a MEK inhibitor to BRAF inhibitor monotherapy proved to be a successful strategy to overcome intrinsic or de novo BRAF inhibitor resistance in BRAF-mutant melanoma [24]. However, resistance was also reported for the BRAF/MEK inhibitor combination therapy [25]. Therefore, novel compounds to be used in combination with BRAF inhibitors are required to address this clinical challenge and need to be investigated in experimental and clinical studies. As a proof of principle, the present study is a first approach to close this gap of knowledge, exploring a selective CDK 4/6 inhibitor as novel combination compound for dual inhibition of the MAPK signal pathway. Our preclinical results add to the literature providing first evidence that a novel BRAF and CDK 4/6 inhibitor combination therapy may be an effective therapeutic regimen in BRAF-mutant melanoma, with significant effects on tumor glucose metabolism, tumor diffusivity, microvascular density, and tumor cell proliferation. However, these

promising preclinical results require further validation in future clinical studies. Selective CDK 4/6 inhibition was shown to significantly improve progression-free survival in patients with advanced breast cancer, but to date there are no clinical data on combined BRAF and CDK 4/6 inhibition [11, 26]. Our results indicate that ^{18}F–FDG-PET/CT and DW-MRI may be applied for non-invasive therapy guidance in clinical trials investigating targeted MAPK pathway inhibition, adding functional and molecular biomarkers of therapy response to morphology-based response criteria. Measurements of tumor radiotracer uptake and ADC can easily be implemented in clinical routine staging reports. Clinically, ^{18}F–FDG-PET/CT is widely applied for staging in advanced melanoma. The current European Society for Medical Oncology guidelines recommend CT or ^{18}F–FDG-PET in advanced cutaneous melanoma (> pT3a) prior to surgical treatment and sentinel lymph node biopsy [27]. The National Comprehensive Cancer Network Clinical Practice Guidelines in Oncology for Melanoma Version 01.2017 recommend CT and/or ^{18}F–FDG-PET for treatment response assessment in patients receiving active non-surgical treatment (www.nccn.org). While ^{18}F–FDG-PET/CT provides a comprehensive whole-body tumor staging at a high spatial resolution, MRI is mainly applied for the local staging of defined body

Table 2 Individual values for tumor diffusivity and morphological tumor volumes at baseline and follow-up

Number	Group[a]	ADC$_{Baseline}$ ($mm^2 \times 10^{-3}/s$)	ADC$_{Follow-up}$ ($mm^2 \times 10^{-3}/s$)	ΔADC ($mm^2 \times 10^{-3}/s$)	Volume$_{Baseline}$ (mm^3)	Volume$_{Follow-up}$ (mm^3)	ΔVolume (mm^3)
1	T	0.84	0.84	0.00	163.0	166.3	3.3
2	T	0.88	1.16	0.28	25.7	33.5	7.8
3	T	0.74	0.72	−0.02	19.1	99.5	80.4
4	T	0.77	0.86	0.09	188.8	255.5	66.7
5	T	0.87	0.82	−0.05	88.5	281.1	192.6
6	T	0.62	0.84	0.22	154.9	107.7	−47.2
7	T	0.79	1.07	0.28	67.2	48.3	−18.9
8	T	0.71	0.87	0.16	38.7	50.8	12.1
9	T	0.66	0.83	0.17	232.5	264.1	31.6
10	T	0.73	0.81	0.08	62.0	123.0	61.0
11	T	0.76	1.07	0.31	48.9	31.9	−17.0
12	T	0.97	0.85	−0.12	45.6	107.9	62.3
Mean ± SD[b]	T	0.78 ± 0.10	0.90 ± 0.13	0.12 ± 0.14	94.6 ± 71.4	130.8 ± 91.3	36.2 ± 63.2
13	C	0.85	0.77	−0.08	119.0	356.0	237.0
14	C	0.70	0.63	−0.07	320.6	777.6	457.0
15	C	0.86	0.69	−0.17	103.1	379.7	276.6
16	C	0.96	0.76	−0.20	81.5	212.9	131.4
17	C	0.78	0.63	−0.15	138.0	371.4	233.4
18	C	0.73	0.61	−0.12	109.0	292.9	183.9
19	C	0.87	0.71	−0.16	72.7	301.7	229.0
20	C	0.61	0.61	0.00	232.7	541.0	308.3
21	C	0.79	0.69	−0.10	31.8	203.5	171.7
Mean ± SD[b]	C	0.79 ± 0.10	0.68 ± 0.06	−0.12 ± 0.06	134.3 ± 89.0	381.9 ± 179.4	247.6 ± 95.1

[a]T = therapy group; C = control group
[b]SD = standard deviation

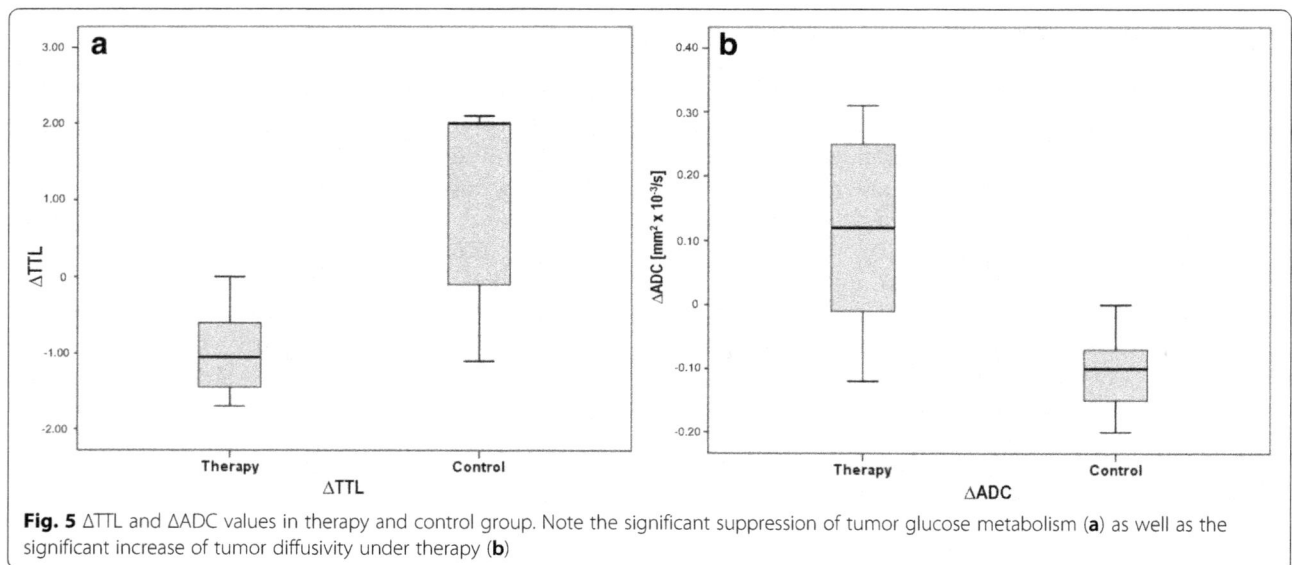

Fig. 5 ΔTTL and ΔADC values in therapy and control group. Note the significant suppression of tumor glucose metabolism (**a**) as well as the significant increase of tumor diffusivity under therapy (**b**)

Table 3 Individual immunohistochemical parameters

Number	Group[a]	CD31	Ki-67
1	T	166	4433
2	T	83	5831
3	T	212	3189
4	T	129	2649
5	T	222	2832
6	T	182	3820
7	T	79	4033
8	T	105	2912
9	T	100	2227
10	T	151	4306
11	T	179	4210
12	T	151	4177
Mean ± SD[b]	T	147 ± 48	3718 ± 998
13	C	271	6801
14	C	336	6349
15	C	447	6489
16	C	191	3799
17	C	307	4562
18	C	358	4582
19	C	261	3379
20	C	284	5718
21	C	132	6824
Mean ± SD[b]	C	287 ± 92	5389 ± 1332

[a]T = therapy group; C = control group
[b]SD = standard deviation

regions, e. g., for the detection of brain and liver metastases, and may therefore complement whole-body imaging protocols for the longitudinal assessment of therapy response [28]. State-of-the-art DW-MRI sequences, e. g., for the brain or abdomen, can be acquired in less than 3 min and may be integrated in standard MRI protocols without significant prolongation of the acquisition time.

Limitations

The study is limited in several aspects. First, although all efforts were made to maintain the same scanning position between PET and MRI as well as between baseline and follow-up, it cannot be fully excluded that the animals were scanned in slightly different planes with potential effects on the semiquantitative parameters. Hybrid imaging on an integrated PET/MRI scanner with simultaneous acquisition of both modalities may improve consistency and concordance of the PET and MRI results due to equalized scanning conditions. Second, *ex vivo* immunohistochemical analysis was performed in selected cross-sections of the tumor and may not necessarily correspond to the whole-tumor VOI. Third, we investigated the BRAF and CDK 4/6 inhibitor combination therapy over the course of 1 week but did not compare the combination therapy to the BRAF inhibitor monotherapy. The comparison of the different therapy regimens in the same tumor model and a longer follow-up interval may provide additional insights in tumor pathophysiology and time course of acquired resistance under MAPK pathway inhibition. Fourth, due to study design, immunohistochemical parameters were only acquired on day 7 after follow-up imaging.

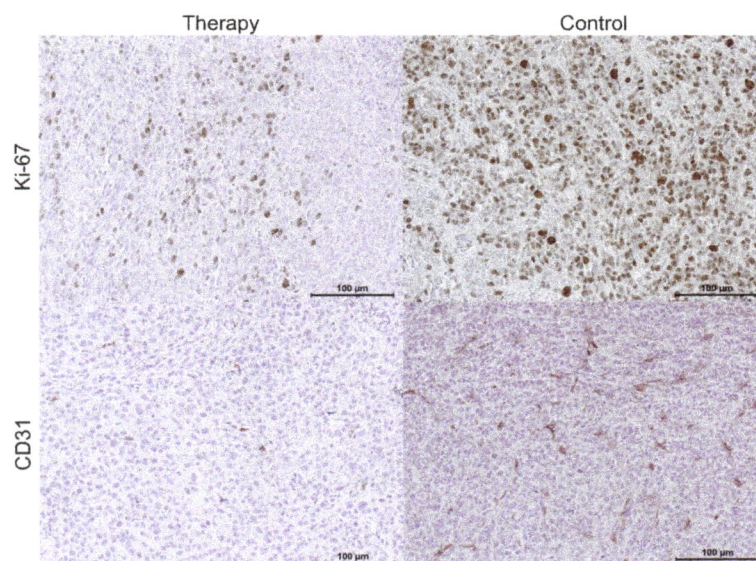

Fig. 6 Tumor cell proliferation and microvascular density in representative tumor sections. Left column: therapy. Right column: control. Top row: proliferation (Ki-67). Bottom row: microvascular density (CD31). Note the significantly lower tumor proliferation (Ki-67) and tumor microvascular density (CD31) in the therapy compared to the control group

Conclusion

In conclusion, we demonstrated that a novel BRAF and CDK 4/6 inhibitor combination therapy exhibits significant anti-angiogenic and anti-proliferative effects in experimental human melanomas in mice and that the according alterations in tumor pathophysiology can be monitored non-invasively and *in vivo* by ^{18}F–FDG-PET/CT and DW-MRI. Co-targeting the MAPK pathway using a BRAF and CDK 4/6 inhibitor combination therapy is a novel approach to potentially overcome intrinsic or de novo BRAF inhibitor resistance in BRAF-mutant melanoma and may be investigated in future clinical trials.

Abbreviations
^{18}F–FDG-PET: ^{18}F–Fluorodeoxyglucose positron emission tomography; ADC: Apparent diffusion coefficient; BRAF: B-rapidly accelerated fibrosarcoma; CDK: Cyclin-dependent kinase; CT: Computed tomography; DW-MRI: Diffusion-weighted magnetic resonance imaging; MAPK: Mitogen-activated protein kinase; MEK: Mitogen-activated extracellular signal-regulated kinase; MTV: Metabolic tumor volume; PMI: Platform for research in medical imaging; RECIST: Response evaluation criteria in solid tumors; SUV: Standardized uptake value; TTL: Tumor-to-Liver-Ratio; VOI: Volume of interest

Acknowledgements
We want to acknowledge the contribution of Rosel Oos from the Department of Nuclear Medicine (University Hospital, Ludwig-Maximilians-University Munich) for her extensive technical support.

Funding
This study was supported by a research grant from Novartis AG (Basel, Switzerland). The therapeutics (dabrafenib and ribociclib; Novartis AG, Basel, Switzerland) were supplied by the manufacturer free of charge.

Authors' contributions
RSE, PMK, AT, CCC, PB, MFR and JR were major contributors in the conception and writing of the manuscript. RSE, PMK, MMH, GK, MJS, WGK and OS performed the MRI measurements. RSE, PMK, AT, MMH, WGK, OS and JO performed the PET/CT measurements. RSE, PMK, CCC, AT, MMH, MJS, PB, MFR and JR analyzed and interpreted the imaging data, performed the postprocessing and the statistical analysis. HH-E, MMH, WGK, GK, JO and OS performed the immunohistological examinations of the tumors and the analysis of the stainings. HH-E, RSE, PMK, MMH, OS and GK administered the daily medication. All authors did substantial contributions to the conception of the work, or the acquisition, analysis, or interpretation of the data. All authors agreed to be accountable for all aspects of the work, read and revised the draft critically and approved the final manuscript.

Ethics approval
All experiments were performed in strict accordance with the Guidelines for the Care and Use of Laboratory Animals of the National Institutes of Health and with approval by the Government of Upper Bavaria Committee for Animal Research (Gz. 55.2-1-54-2532-36-2016).

Competing interests
CCC: Speakers' bureau, Siemens Healthineers. All other authors declare that they have no competing interests.

Author details
[1]Department of Radiology, Laboratory for Experimental Radiology, University Hospital, Ludwig-Maximilians-University Munich, Marchioninistr. 15, 81377 München, Germany. [2]Department of Nuclear Medicine, University Hospital, Ludwig-Maximilians-University Munich, Marchioninistr. 15, 81377 München, Germany. [3]Comprehensive Pneumology Center, German Center for Lung Research, Munich, Germany.

References
1. Amaral T, Sinnberg T, Meier F, Krepler C, Levesque M, Niessner H, et al. The mitogen-activated protein kinase pathway in melanoma part I - activation and primary resistance mechanisms to BRAF inhibition. Eur J Cancer. 2017;73:85–92.
2. Yadav V, Chen SH, Yue YG, Buchanan S, Beckmann RP, Peng SB. Co-targeting BRAF and cyclin dependent kinases 4/6 for BRAF mutant cancers. Pharmacol Ther 2015;149:139-149.
3. Hertzman Johansson C, Egyhazi BS. BRAF inhibitors in cancer therapy. Pharmacol Ther. 2014;142:176–82.
4. Chmielowski B. Is there a role for single-agent BRAF inhibition in melanoma? Clin Adv Hematol Oncol. 2017;15:108–10.
5. Manzano JL, Layos L, Buges C, de Los Llanos Gil M, Vila L, Martinez-Balibrea E, et al. Resistant mechanisms to BRAF inhibitors in melanoma. Ann Transl Med. 2016;4:237.
6. Sun C, Wang L, Huang S, Heynen GJ, Prahallad A, Robert C, et al. Reversible and adaptive resistance to BRAF(V600E) inhibition in melanoma. Nature. 2014;508:118–22.
7. Villanueva J, Vultur A, Herlyn M. Resistance to BRAF inhibitors: unraveling mechanisms and future treatment options. Cancer Res. 2011;71:7137–40.
8. Robert C, Karaszewska B, Schachter J, Rutkowski P, Mackiewicz A, Stroiakovski D, et al. Improved overall survival in melanoma with combined dabrafenib and trametinib. N Engl J Med. 2015;372:30–9.
9. da Silveira Nogueira Lima JP, Georgieva M, Haaland B, de Lima Lopes G. A systematic review and network meta-analysis of immunotherapy and targeted therapy for advanced melanoma. Cancer Med. 2017;6(6):1143–53.
10. Yadav V, Burke TF, Huber L, Van Horn RD, Zhang Y, Buchanan SG, et al. The CDK4/6 inhibitor LY2835219 overcomes vemurafenib resistance resulting from MAPK reactivation and cyclin D1 upregulation. Mol Cancer Ther. 2014; 13:2253–63.
11. Hortobagyi GN, Stemmer SM, Burris HA, Yap YS, Sonke GS, Paluch-Shimon S, et al. Ribociclib as first-line therapy for HR-positive, advanced breast cancer. N Engl J Med. 2016;375:1738–48.
12. Eisenhauer EA, Therasse P, Bogaerts J, Schwartz LH, Sargent D, Ford R, et al. New response evaluation criteria in solid tumours: revised RECIST guideline (version 1.1). Eur J Cancer. 2009;45:228–47.
13. Desar IM, van Herpen CM, van Laarhoven HW, Barentsz JO, Oyen WJ, van der Graaf WT. Beyond RECIST: molecular and functional imaging techniques for evaluation of response to targeted therapy. Cancer Treat Rev. 2009;35:309–21.
14. Teng FF, Meng X, Sun XD, Yu JM. New strategy for monitoring targeted therapy: molecular imaging. Int J Nanomedicine. 2013;8:3703–13.
15. McArthur GA, Puzanov I, Amaravadi R, Ribas A, Chapman P, Kim KB, et al. Marked, homogeneous, and early [18F]fluorodeoxyglucose-positron emission tomography responses to vemurafenib in BRAF-mutant advanced melanoma. J Clin Oncol. 2012;30:1628–34.
16. Geven EJ, Evers S, Nayak TK, Bergstrom M, Su F, Gerrits D, et al. Therapy response monitoring of the early effects of a new BRAF inhibitor on melanoma xenograft in mice: evaluation of (18) F-FDG-PET and (18) F-FLT-PET. Contrast Media Mol Imaging. 2015;10:203–10.
17. Beloueche-Babari M, Jamin Y, Arunan V, Walker-Samuel S, Revill M, Smith PD, et al. Acute tumour response to the MEK1/2 inhibitor selumetinib (AZD6244, ARRY-142886) evaluated by non-invasive diffusion-weighted MRI. Br J Cancer. 2013;109:1562–9.
18. Gaustad JV, Pozdniakova V, Hompland T, Simonsen TG, Rofstad EK. Magnetic resonance imaging identifies early effects of sunitinib treatment in human melanoma xenografts. J Exp Clin Cancer Res. 2013;32:93.
19. Kazmierczak PM, Todica A, Gildehaus FJ, Hirner-Eppeneder H, Brendel M, Eschbach RS, et al. 68Ga-TRAP-(RGD)3 hybrid imaging for the in vivo monitoring of alphavss3-Integrin expression as biomarker of anti-Angiogenic therapy effects in experimental breast cancer. PLoS One. 2016; 11:e0168248.

20. Sourbron S, Ingrisch M, Siefert A, Reiser M, Herrmann K. Quantification of cerebral blood flow, cerebral blood volume, and blood-brain-barrier leakage with DCE-MRI. Magn Reson Med. 2009;62:205–17.

21. Baudy AR, Dogan T, Flores-Mercado JE, Hoeflich KP, Su F, van Bruggen N, et al. FDG-PET is a good biomarker of both early response and acquired resistance in BRAFV600 mutant melanomas treated with vemurafenib and the MEK inhibitor GDC-0973. EJNMMI Res. 2012;2:22.

22. Schmitt RJ, Kreidler SM, Glueck DH, Amaria RN, Gonzalez R, Lewis K, et al. Correlation between early 18F-FDG PET/CT response to BRAF and MEK inhibition and survival in patients with BRAF-mutant metastatic melanoma. Nucl Med Commun. 2016;37:122–8.

23. Surov A, Meyer HJ, Wienke A. Correlation between minimum apparent diffusion coefficient (ADCmin) and tumor Cellularity: a meta-analysis. Anticancer Res. 2017;37:3807–10.

24. Flaherty KT, Infante JR, Daud A, Gonzalez R, Kefford RF, Sosman J, et al. Combined BRAF and MEK inhibition in melanoma with BRAF V600 mutations. N Engl J Med. 2012;367:1694–703.

25. Wagle N, Van Allen EM, Treacy DJ, Frederick DT, Cooper ZA, Taylor-Weiner A, et al. MAP kinase pathway alterations in BRAF-mutant melanoma patients with acquired resistance to combined RAF/MEK inhibition. Cancer Discov. 2014;4:61–8.

26. Finn RS, Crown JP, Lang I, Boer K, Bondarenko IM, Kulyk SO, et al. The cyclin-dependent kinase 4/6 inhibitor palbociclib in combination with letrozole versus letrozole alone as first-line treatment of oestrogen receptor-positive, HER2-negative, advanced breast cancer (PALOMA-1/TRIO-18): a randomised phase 2 study. Lancet Oncol. 2015;16:25–35.

27. Dummer R, Hauschild A, Lindenblatt N, Pentheroudakis G, Keilholz U, Committee EG. Cutaneous melanoma: ESMO clinical practice guidelines for diagnosis, treatment and follow-up. Ann Oncol. 2015;26(Suppl 5):v126–32.

28. Perng P, Marcus C, Subramaniam RM. (18)F-FDG PET/CT and melanoma: staging, immune modulation and mutation-targeted therapy assessment, and prognosis. AJR Am J Roentgenol. 2015;205:259–70.

8

Comparison of efficacy and complications of endoscopic and percutaneous biliary drainage in malignant obstructive jaundice

Feng Duan[*†], Li Cui[†], Yanhua Bai[†], Xiaohui Li, Jieyu Yan and Xuan Liu

Abstract

Background: Malignant obstructive jaundice is a common problem in the clinic. Currently, the generally applied treatment methods are percutaneous transhepatic biliary drainage (PTBD) and endoscopic biliary drainage (EBD). Nevertheless, there has not been a uniform conclusion published on either efficacy of the two types of drainage or the incidence rate of complications. Therefore, we conducted a systematic review and meta-analysis of studies comparing endoscopic versus percutaneous biliary drainage in malignant obstructive jaundice, to determine whether there is any difference between percutaneous and endoscopic biliary drainage, with respect to efficacy and incidence rate of overall complications.

Methods: The enrolled studies contain a total of three randomized controlled trials and eleven retrospective studies, which together encompass 2246 patients with PTBD and 8100 patients with EBD.

Results: Our analysis indicates that there is no difference between PTBD and EBD with regard to therapeutic success rate (%), overall complication (%), intraperitoneal bile leak, 30-day mortality, sepsis, or duodenal perforation (%). Cholangitis and pancreatitis after PTBD were lower than after EBD, with odds ratios (OR) of 0.48 (95% confidence interval (CI), 0.31 to 0.74) and 0.16 (95% CI, 0.05 to 0.52), respectively. Incidences of bleeding and tube dislocation for PTBD were higher than EBD, OR of 1.81 (95% CI, 1.35 to 2.44) and 3.41 (95% CI, 1.10 to 10.60).

Conclusions: This meta-analysis indicates certain advantages for both PTBD and EBD. In the clinical practice, it is advised to choose specifically either PTBD or EBD, based on location of obstruction, purpose of drainage (as a preoperative procedure or a palliative treatment) and level of experience in biliary drainage at individual treatment centers.

Keywords: Endoscopic biliary drainage, Percutaneous biliary drainage, Malignant obstructive jaundice

Background

Malignant obstructive jaundice can occur following pancreatic cancer, Ampulla of Vater, or hilar cholangiocarcinoma, etc. [1]. If it is not handled in a timely manner, it may cause lots of adverse events such as cholangitis, delay tumor treatment, reduce quality of life and increase death rate, etc. Successful biliary drainage can significantly improve prognosis in patients with malignant obstructive jaundice [2]. To date, the generally applied clinical biliary drainage methods are percutaneous transhepatic biliary drainage (PTBD) and endoscopic biliary drainage (EBD). Regarding efficacy of the two types of drainage and incidence rate of complications, interventional radiologists and gastroenterologists hold different opinions, resulting in diverging opinions on treatment approach [3, 4]. Therefore, we conducted a meta-analysis, to determine whether there is a difference with respect to efficacy and incidence rate of overall complications between PTBD and EBD.

* Correspondence: duanfeng@vip.sina.com
†Equal contributors
Department of Interventional Radiology, the General Hospital of Chinese People's Liberation Army, Beijing 100853, China

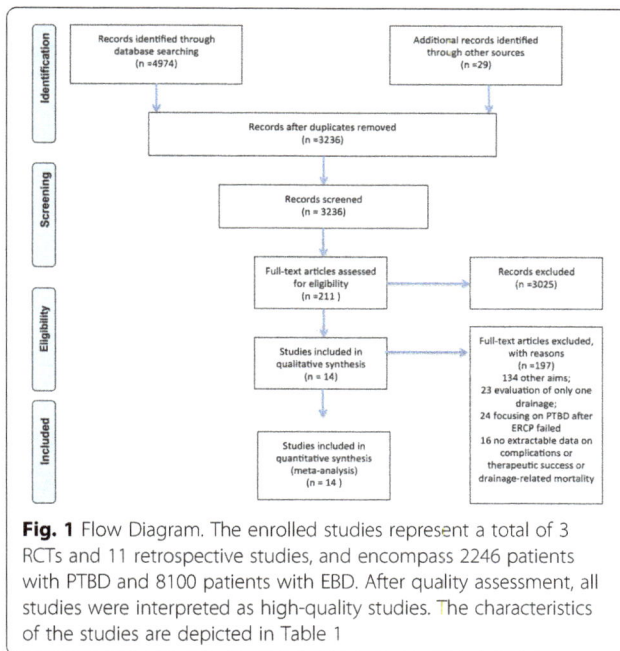

Fig. 1 Flow Diagram. The enrolled studies represent a total of 3 RCTs and 11 retrospective studies, and encompass 2246 patients with PTBD and 8100 patients with EBD. After quality assessment, all studies were interpreted as high-quality studies. The characteristics of the studies are depicted in Table 1

Methods

Search strategy

A comprehensive search of literature was conducted on Pubmed, EMBASE database and Cochrane Central Register of Controlled Trials to identify articles published until February 28th of 2017, on comparing PTBD and EBD in the management of malignant biliary tract obstruction. The search index terms were (a) 'pancreatic neoplasms' (medical subject heading, MeSH) OR 'cholangiocarcinoma', (MeSH) OR malignant biliary obstruction (title/abstract, TIAB), and with (b) 'drainage' (MeSH) OR 'percutaneous transhepatic biliary drainage' (TIAB) OR PTBD (TIAB) OR 'endoscopic retrograde biliary drainage' (TIAB) OR 'ERCP (endoscopic retrograde cholangiopancreatography)' (TIAB), and with (c) 'complications' (Subheading) OR 'adverse event' (Subheading) OR 'mortality' (MeSH) OR 'therapeutics' (MeSH). We identified additional publications by cross-checking references of the retrieved full-text articles.

Study selection

Study selection criteria were (a) written in English, (b) carried out in patients with malignant biliary obstruction, and (c) comparing PTBD and EBD for palliation of biliary obstruction. Studies were excluded when, (a) evaluations were based on only one arm of PTBD or EBD, (b) focused on PTBD after ERCP failure instead of primary PTBD, or (c) lacking data on complications, therapeutic success or drainage-related mortality. For articles reporting duplicate data, the one with the most detailed data set was selected.

Two readers independently reviewed all retrieved titles and abstracts to identify potentially eligible studies according to the selection criteria listed above, and any divergence was resolved after discussion and consensus was reached.

Data extraction

Two readers independently extracted data from the enrolled studies into a unified data extraction form, including information on author name, study year, study area, sample size, cancer type, drainage method, overall complication rate and incidence of each complication, therapeutic success rate, drainage-related mortality rate, drainage patency, length of stay and survival outcomes. Data for endoscopic drainage methods (endoscopic nasobiliary drainage and endoscopic biliary sphincterotomy) were combined prior to comparison with data for PTBD. Patients requiring conversion from one form of drainage to another were subsequently analyzed using intention-to-treat analysis. All available and relevant qualitative study measures were combined by tabulation of each drainage group. Upon any contradictory data extraction, the two readers discussed the data to reach a consensus.

Quality assessment

The quality of enrolled cohort studies was assessed by using the 9-star Newcastle-Ottawa Quality Assessment Scale, including 8 items on patient selection, comparability and outcome. Studies with 5 or more stars were interpreted as high-quality studies. The quality of enrolled randomized controlled trials (RCTs) were assessed using the 7-point Modified Jadad Score, including 7 items on randomization, allocation concealment, blinding and withdrawals, and dropouts. Studies with 4 or more points were interpreted as high-quality studies. Two readers independently conducted quality assessments, and divergence was resolved after discussion to reach consensus.

Statistical methods

Odds ratios (ORs) were calculated for each outcome and depicted as categorical variables for every comparison. The Mantel-Haenszel method for fixed effects models was applied to all comparisons exhibiting no statistical heterogeneity to determine corresponding overall effect sizes and their confidence intervals (CIs). If statistical heterogeneity was noted, the DerSimonian and Laird method for random effects was used. Forrest plots were drawn to show the point estimates in each study in relation to the pooled summary estimate. The estimated width of the point in the Forrest plots indicates the assigned weight to that study. A two-sided $P < 0.05$ was considered to indicate statistical significance for pooled

Table 1 Main characteristics of the included studies

Author	year	country	study design	No.Patients in study	No. PTBD	No. EBD	age(years, median or range)	Male (%)	Maligancy type	Quality assessment*
Speer AG	1987	Enghland	RCT	75	36	39	50–87	/	primary carcinoma of the pancreas, gallbladder, or bileducts	4
Piñol V	2002	Spain	RCT	54	28	26	73	74	primary carcinoma of the pancreas, gallbladder, or bileducts,or regional lymph node metastasis	5
Lee SH	2007	South Korea	retrospective	134(34 IPTBD)	66	34	67	69	Klatskin's tumor	8
Saluja SS	2008	India	RCT	54	27	27	51	33	Gallbladder Cancer	5
Paik WH	2009	South Korea	retrospective	85	41	44	66	68	Hilar cholangiocarcinoma	8
Kloek JJ	2010	Netherlands	retrospective	101	11	90	61	69	Hilar cholangiocarcinoma	7
Choi J	2012	South Korea	retrospective	60	31	29	59	77	hepatocellular carcinoma	7
Walter T	2013	Canada	retrospective	129	42	87	66	60	Klatskintumors	8
Huang X	2015	China	retrospective	270(170 no PBD)	45	55(ENBD 18,ERBS 37)	58	71	extrahepatic bile duct cancer	7
Kim KM	2015	South Korea	retrospective	106	62	44	42–89	64	Perihilar cholangiocarcinomas	8
Inamdar S	2016	USA	retrospective	9135	1690	7445	70	50	pancreatic cancer or cholangiocarcinoma	6
Kishi Y	2016	Japan	retrospective	171	98	72	31–86	78	biliary tract cancer	7
Jo JH	2017	South Korea	retrospective	98	43	55(13 ENBD, 42 EBS)	63.5 (29–82)	61	Klatskin tumor	8
Miura F	2017	Japan	retrospective	88	25	63	70(42–85)	70	extrahepatic bile duct cancer	7

*retrospective cohort studies was evaluated using 9-star Newcastle-Ottawa Quality Assessment Scale; RCT studies was evaluated using 7-point Modified Jadad Score

OR. The heterogeneity among studies was analyzed using a χ^2-based test of homogeneity and the inconsistency index (I^2) statistic was calculated. If the I^2 statistic indicated that heterogeneity existed between studies (>10%), a random effects model was then used. Otherwise, fixed-effects models were used. A 0.10 significance level was used to identify heterogeneity across studies. Stratified analysis was further conducted according to study design (RCT or retrospective studies). Publication bias on the summary estimates was tested by both Begg adjusted rank-correlation test and the Egger regression asymmetry test. Funnel plots were also constructed to evaluate potential publication bias. A 0.05 significance level was used to identify publication bias. All statistical analyses were done using Review Manager 5.3 and STATA 10.0.

Results

Literature search and study selection
The initial search identified 3236 titles and abstracts, of which 3025 publications were thereafter excluded, because they were not relevant with respect to drainage-related complications, therapeutic success or mortality. Therefore, a total of 211 publications were considered relevant and further evaluated. Finally, 14 publications were included in the meta-analysis (Fig. 1).

The enrolled studies represent a total of 3 RCTs and 11 retrospective studies, and encompass 2246 patients with PTBD and 8100 patients with EBD. After quality assessment, all studies were interpreted as high-quality studies. The characteristics of the studies are depicted in Table 1.

Comparison between PTBD and EBD
Ten studies report therapeutic success rate, 13 studies report overall complications, and 9 studies report 30-day mortality. All studies provide incidence data of at least one kind of complication.

PTBD was superior to EBD with respect to therapeutic success rate, incidence of overall complications, intraperitoneal bile leak, 30-day mortality, sepsis and duodenal perforation. PTBD demonstrated significant lower incidence of cholangitis and pancreatitis than EBD, with OR of 0.48 (95% CI, 0.31 to 0.74) and 0.16

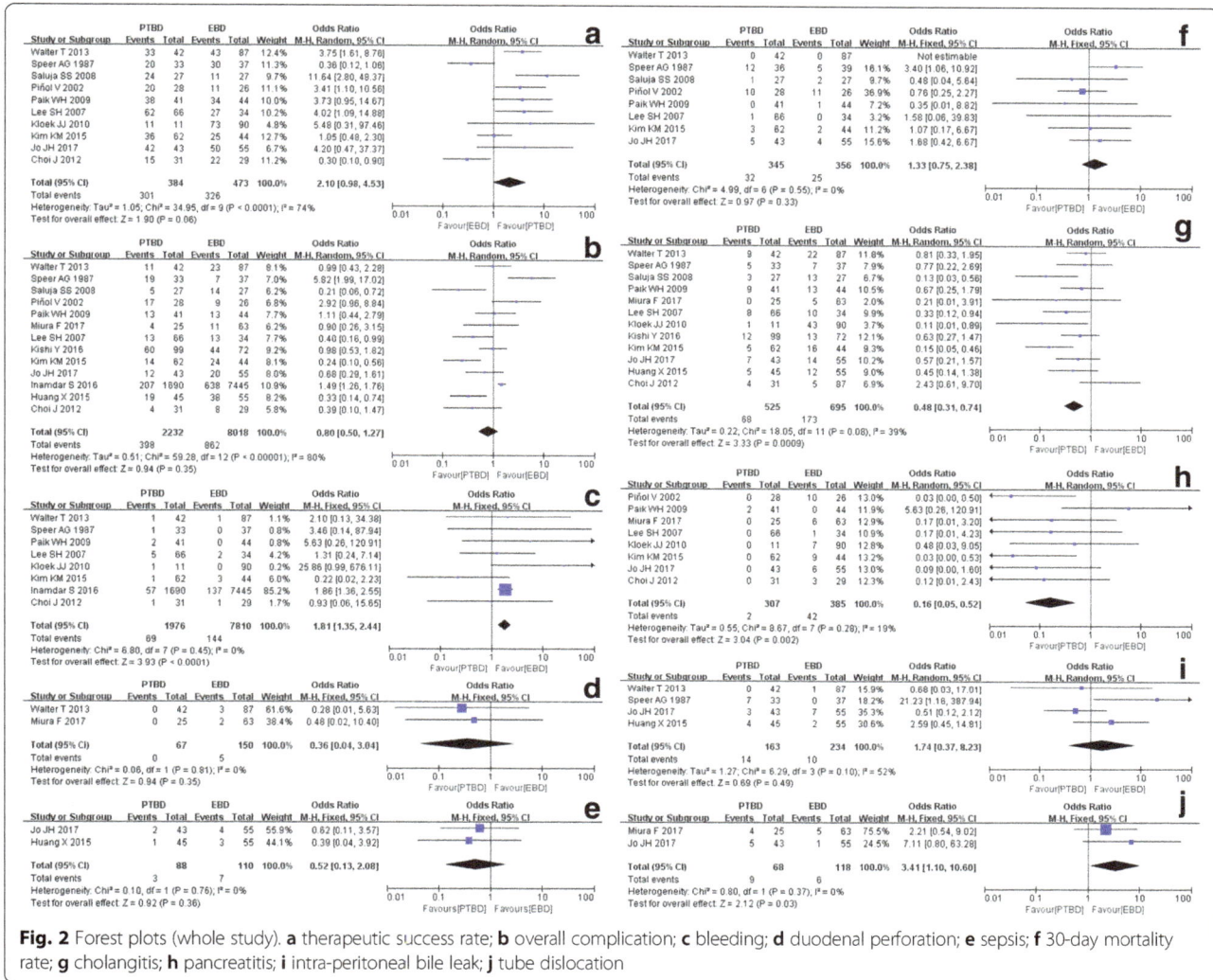

Fig. 2 Forest plots (whole study). **a** therapeutic success rate; **b** overall complication; **c** bleeding; **d** duodenal perforation; **e** sepsis; **f** 30-day mortality rate; **g** cholangitis; **h** pancreatitis; **i** intra-peritoneal bile leak; **j** tube dislocation

(95% CI, 0.05 to 0.52) for cholangitis and pancreatitis, respectively. However, incidence of bleeding and tube dislocation for PTBD was significantly higher than EBD, with OR of 1.81 (95% CI, 1.35 to 2.44) and 3.41 (95% CI, 1.10 to 10.60) for bleeding and tube dislocation, respectively (Fig. 2).

According to the stratified analysis of results from the RCT and retrospective studies (Fig. 3), there is no difference in cholangitis incidence rate between PTBD and EBD based on the RCT studies only, with an OR of 0.45 (95% CI, 0.16 to 1.21). However, based on the retrospective studies, PTBD group has a significantly lower incidence rate of cholangitis than EBD group, with an OR of 0.50 (95% CI, 0.32 to 0.80). Based on stratified analysis results of the RCT and retrospective studies, there is no difference between PTBD and EBD with respect to therapeutic success rate, overall complications or 30-day mortality rate.

Publication bias

Analysis based on the Begg adjusted rank-correlation and the Egger regression asymmetry tests presents significant publication bias for therapeutic success rate and overall complications, which indicates that studies with smaller sample size are inclined to provide results favorable to PTBD. No publication bias was detected with respect to 30-day mortality or other complications (Fig. 4).

Discussion

Although EBD has been performed much more frequently than PTBC in clinical practice on malignant obstructive jaundice, according to the results of our meta-analysis EBD did not show significant advantages over PTBD. PTBD resulted in better therapeutic success rate, and lower incidence of overall complications, intra-peritoneal bile leak, 30-day mortality, sepsis and duodenal perforation, compared to EBD. With respect to

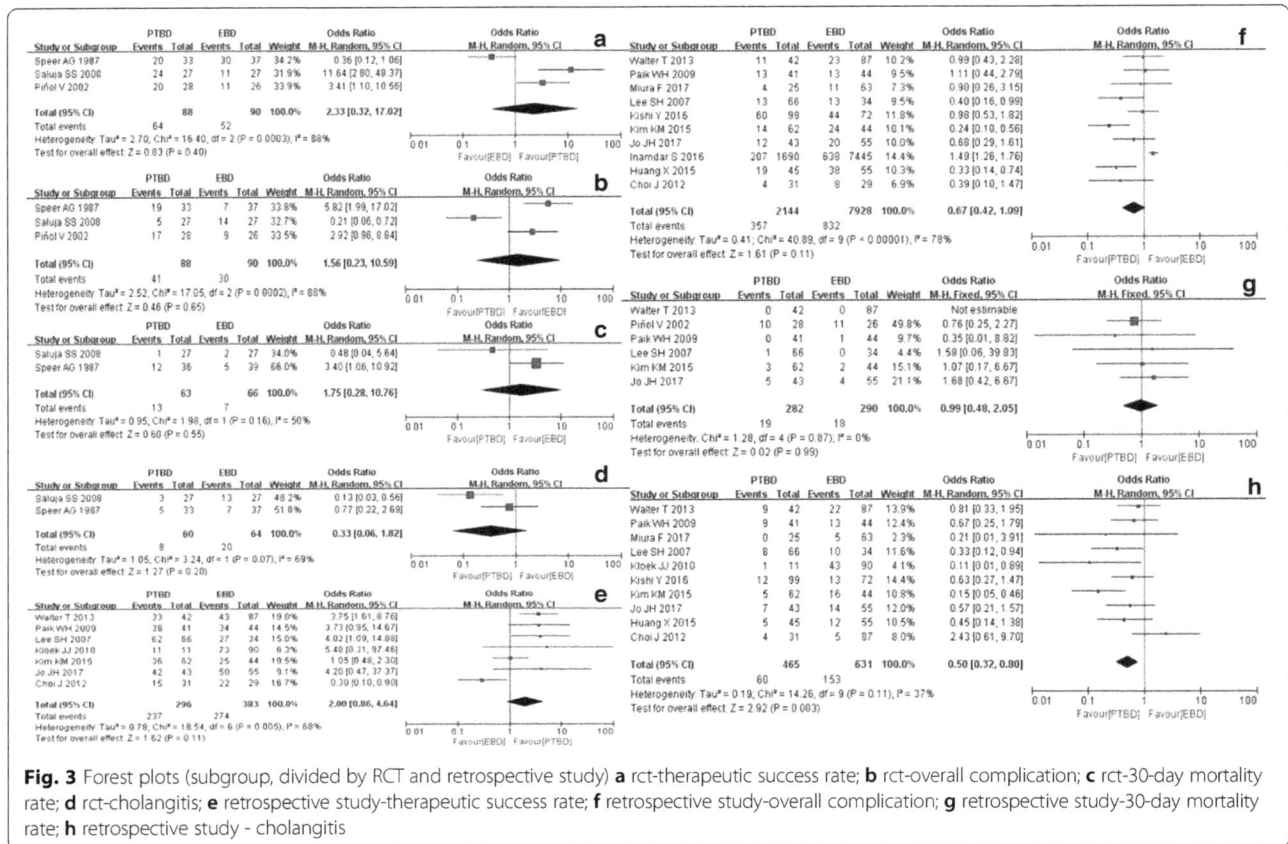

Fig. 3 Forest plots (subgroup, divided by RCT and retrospective study) **a** rct-therapeutic success rate; **b** rct-overall complication; **c** rct-30-day mortality rate; **d** rct-cholangitis; **e** retrospective study-therapeutic success rate; **f** retrospective study-overall complication; **g** retrospective study-30-day mortality rate; **h** retrospective study - cholangitis

cholangitis and pancreatitis, PTBD also showed to be a superior method.

Infection is one of the most common complication after biliary drainage. In combination with malignant biliary obstruction, patients are often in poor condition with complications such as low immunity and concurrent infection, which can have serious consequences [5–7]. Our study shows that incidence rate of cholangitis and pancreatitis was higher after EBD than after PTBD. There may be two reasons, which cause the high infection rate after EBD. Firstly, biliary drainage could be incomplete. Especially in patients with severe obstruction it is very difficult to ensure complete drainage of each biliary duct. Bacterial growth in the bile stasis after incomplete drainage causes secondary infection [8]. Secondly, incision of the duodenal papilla sometimes occurs during EBD, which damages the regular structure of duodenal papilla. As this structure prevents retrograde entering of biliary ducts or pancreatic duct by intestinal bacteria, which is the most important route of infection caused by biliary drainage. Damage to the duodenal papilla increases the chance of infection [9]. Application of antibiotics is another infection-related factor. Routine preventive administration of antibiotics is recommended prior to both PTBD and EBD [10]. Whether or not treatment with antibiotics should be continued

after biliary drainage depends on completeness of drainage. And secondly, whether there is a concomitant infection pre-operation [11]. In stratified analysis, the disparity in results between the RCT and retrospective studies was observed for cholangitis incidence rate. Retrospective studies showed PTBD yields a significantly lower incidence rate of cholangitis than EBD, while RCTs showed similar rate of cholangitis between PTBD and EBD. RCT is usually recognized to provide higher level of evidence compared with retrospective study; however, there were only two RCTs (Speer 1987 and Saluja 2008) with small sample size (60 patients) providing data of incidence rate of cholangitis. On the contrary, there were ten more recent (published from 2007 to 2017) retrospective studies with a much larger sample size (465 patients) and assessed as high quality. Considering that there were improving and more efficacious percutaneous or endoscopic techniques in recent studies, we interpret the result from retrospective studies is more reliable and can reflect the real situation.

Taken together, our study shows that incidence of tube dislocation and bleeding after PTBD was higher compared to EBD [12, 13]. PTBD is also accompanied by a higher incidence rate of metastasis, which is an important complication. It has been reported that PTBD increases the

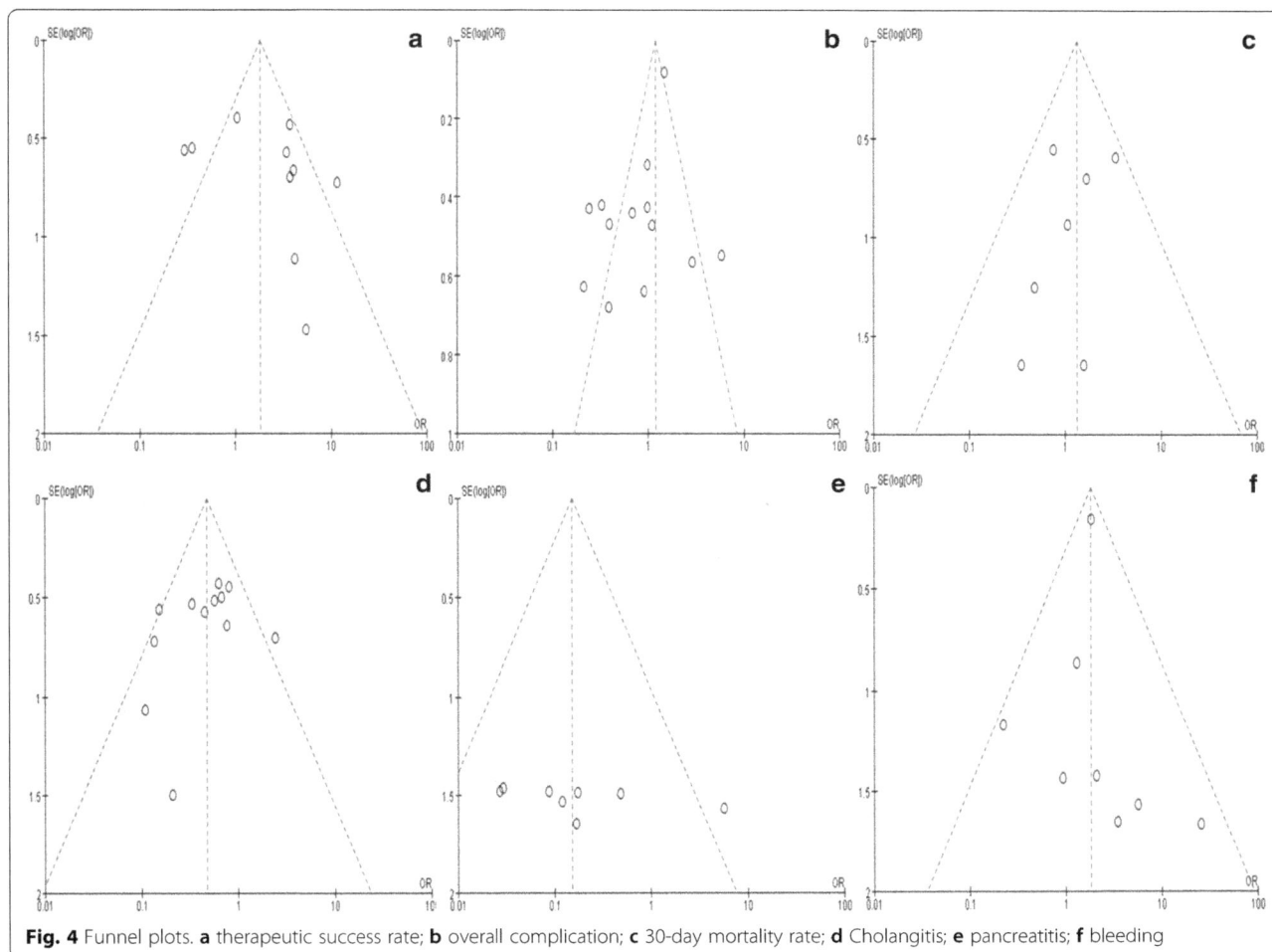

Fig. 4 Funnel plots. **a** therapeutic success rate; **b** overall complication; **c** 30-day mortality rate; **d** Cholangitis; **e** pancreatitis; **f** bleeding

incidence of metastasis after resection of distal cholangiocarcinoma and may shorten postoperative survival [14–16]. However, there are no comparison data available among the selected articles, which are suitable for meta-analysis.

Regarding the choice of biliary drainage methods, there are other factors which need to be considered, which however are not included in this study. First, regarding biliary drainage prior to surgery, PTBD (simple external drainage) is mainly performed, which is still under debate. There is a prospective randomized controlled trial currently ongoing [17], which hopefully provides convincing evidence on selection of biliary drainage methods prior to surgery. Second, quality of life after biliary drainage is also an important factor to consider. Theoretically, carrying an external drainage tube affects quality of life more than implantation of an internal stent. Nevertheless, based on a controlled study by Saluja et al., quality of life after PTBD was rated higher compared to the endoscopic biliary stent implantation group, according to World Health Organization Quality of Life physical and psychological scores at 1 and 3 months [18]. Although this study did not reach

statistical significance, there was a trend towards a better quality of life after PTBD, which may be caused by the relatively high incidence rate of fever in the biliary stent implantation group. Regarding quality of life, large scale controlled studies are needed to conclude which drainage method is better. Third, accumulation of experience on PTBD is also important. It has been reported that, for biliary obstruction caused by cholangiocarcinoma, EBD is superior in medical centers that perform limited numbers of PTBD procedures [3].

This study has several limitations. Firstly, both RCT and retrospective studies were included in the analysis. Meta-analysis of RCT studies produced high-level evidence, but there were only three RCT studies, with small sample sizes, which compared PTBD and EBD. Because of that, we also included retrospective studies, which were all evaluated as high-quality, and proceeded to conduct stratified analysis according to the study design. Secondly, there is also a significant lack of homogeneity between the different studies with respect to therapeutic success rate and occurrence of most of the complications. Thirdly, publication bias may be a factor, resulting from inclusion of studies only written in English, and inclusion of studies concerning small sample size, which likely provide results that favor PTBD.

Conclusion

This meta-analysis indicates certain advantages for both PTBD and EBD. In the clinical practice, it is advised to choose specifically either PTBD or EBD, based on location of obstruction, purpose of drainage (as a preoperative procedure or a palliative treatment) and level of experience in biliary drainage at individual treatment centers.

Abbreviations

CI: Confidence interval; EBD: Endoscopic biliary drainage; MeSH: Medical subject heading; ORs: Odds ratios; PTBD: Percutaneous trans-hepatic biliary drainage; RCTs: Randomized controlled trials; RFA: Radiofrequency ablation; TIAB: Title/abstract

Acknowledgements

We would like to extend our sincere gratitude to our departmental chair for all these support. We are deeply grateful of the help from our physicians, engineers, nurses as well as other staff of the department.

Funding

No funding exits in the submission of this manuscript.

Authors' contributions

DF, BYH and CL conceived and designed the study. DF, BYH and CL searched literatures and had study selection. YJY and LX had the data extraction part. BYH was in charge of quality assessment part. DF, CL and YJY did data analyses. DF, BYH, CL, YJY, LXH and LX wrote the paper. DF, CL and YJY reviewed and edited the manuscript. All authors read and approved the manuscript.

Competing interests

The authors declare that they have no competing interests.

References

1. Tsuyuguchi T, Takada T, Miyazaki M, et al. Stenting and interventional radiology for obstructive jaundice in patients with unresectable biliary tract carcinomas. J Hepato-Biliary-Pancreat Surg. 2008;15(1):69–73.
2. Kurniawan J, Hasan I, Gani RA, et al. Mortality-related factors in patients with malignant obstructive jaundice. Acta Med Indones. 2016;48(4):282–8.
3. Inamdar S, Slattery E, Bhalla R, et al. Comparison of adverse events for endoscopic vs Percutaneous Biliary drainage in the treatment of malignant Biliary tract obstruction in an inpatient National Cohort. JAMA Oncol. 2016;2(1):112–7.
4. Zhao XQ, Dong JH, Jiang K. Comparison of percutaneous transhepatic biliary drainage and endoscopic biliary drainage in the management of malignant biliary tract obstruction: a meta-analysis. Dig Endosc. 2015; 27(1):137–45.
5. Boursier J, Cesbron E, Tropet AL, et al. Comparison and improvement of MELD and child-Pugh score accuracies for the predietion of 6-month mortality in cirrhotic patients. J Clin Gastroenterol. 2009;43(6):580–5.
6. Dambraukas Z, Paskauskas S, Lizdenis P, et al. Percutaneous transhepatic biliary stenting: the first experience and results of the Hospital of Kaunas University of medicine. Medicina (Kaunas). 2008;44(12):969–76.
7. Namias N, Demoya M, Sleeman D, et al. Risk of postoperative infection in patients with bactibilia undergoing surgery for obstructive jaundice. Surg Infect. 2005;6(3):323–8.
8. Herzog T, Belyaev O, Hessam S, et al. (2012). Bacteribilia with resistant microorganisms after preoperative biliary drainage the influence of bacteria on postoperative outcome. Scand J Gastroenterol. 2012;47(7):827–35.
9. Dumonceau J-M, Macias-Gomez C. Endoscopic management of complications of chronic pancreatitis. World J Gastroenterol. 2013;19(42): 7308–15.
10. Banerjee S, Shen B, Baron TH, et al. Antibiotic prophylaxis for GI endoscopy. Gastrointest Endosc. 2008;67:791–8.
11. Jacobson BC, Baron TH, Adler DG, et al. ASGE guideline: the role of endoscopy in the diagnosis and the management of cystic lesions and inflammatory fluid collections of the pancreas. Gastrointest Endosc. 2005;61:363–70.
12. Van Delden OM, Lameris JS. Percutaneous drainage and stenting for palliation of malignant bile duct obstruction. Eur Radiol. 2008;18:448–56.
13. Nimura Y, Kamiya J, Kondo S, et al. Aggressive preoperative management and extended surgery for hilar cholangiocarcinoma: Nagoya experience. J Hepato-Biliary-Pancreat Surg. 2000;7:155–62.
14. Komaya K, Ebata T, Fukami Y, et al. Percutaneous biliary drainage is oncologically inferior to endoscopic drainage: a propensity score matching analysis in resectable distal cholangiocarcinoma. J Gastroenterol. 2016;51(6):608–19.
15. Takahashi Y, Nagino M, Nishio H, et al. Percutaneous transhepatic biliary drainage catheter tract recurrence in cholangiocarcinoma. Br J Surg. 2010;97:1860–6.
16. Sakata J, Shirai Y, Wakai T, et al. Catheter tract implantation metastases associated with percutaneous biliary drainage for extrahepatic cholangiocarcinoma. World J Gastroenterol. 2005;11:7024–7.
17. Wiggers JK, Coelen RJ, Rauws EA, et al. Preoperative endoscopic versus percutaneous transhepatic biliary drainage in potentially resectable perihilar cholangiocarcinoma (DRAINAGE trial): design and rationale of a randomized controlled trial. BMC Gastroenterol. 2015;15:20.
18. Saluja SS, Gulati M, Garg PK, et al. Endoscopic or percutaneous biliary drainage for gallbladder cancer: a randomized trial and quality of life assessment. Clin Gastroenterol Hepatol. 2008;6(8):944–950.e3.

9

Changes in biodistribution on ^{68}Ga-DOTA-Octreotate PET/CT after long acting somatostatin analogue therapy in neuroendocrine tumour patients may result in pseudoprogression

Martin H. Cherk[1,3,4], Grace Kong[1], Rodney J. Hicks[1,2] and Michael S. Hofman[1,2*]

Abstract

Background: To evaluate the effects of long-acting somatostatin analogue (SSA) therapy on ^{68}Ga-DOTA-octreotate (GaTate) uptake at physiological and metastatic sites in neuroendocrine tumour (NET) patients.

Methods: Twenty-one patients who underwent GaTate PET/CT before and after commencement of SSA therapy were reviewed. Maximum standardized uptake values (SUVmax) were measured in normal organs. Changes in uptake of 49 metastatic lesions in 12 patients with stable disease were also compared. Serum chromogranin-A (CgA) levels were available for correlation between scans in 17/21 patients.

Results: Mean thyroid, spleen and liver SUVmax decreased significantly following SSA therapy from a baseline of 5.9 to 3.5, 30.3 to 23.1 and 10.3 to 8.0, respectively ($p = < 0.0001$ for all). Pituitary SUVmax increased from 10.2 to 11.0 ($p = 0.004$) whereas adrenal and salivary gland SUVmax did not change. Tumour SUVmax increased in 7 of 12 patients with stable disease; CgA was stable or decreasing in 5 of these patients. 30/49 (61%) metastatic lesions had an increase in SUVmax and lesion-to-liver uptake ratio increased in 40/49 (82%) following SSA therapy.

Conclusion: Long-acting SSA therapy decreases GaTate uptake in the thyroid, spleen and liver but in most cases increases intensity of uptake within metastases. This has significant implications for interpretation of GaTate PET/CT following commencement of therapy as increased intensity alone may not represent true progression. Our findings also suggest pre-dosing with SSA prior to PRRT may enable higher doses to be delivered to tumour whilst decreasing dose to normal tissues.

Keywords: Somatostatin, Octreotate, Ga-68, Neuroendocrine tumour, Positron emission tomography, DOTATATE, PET/CT, Octreotide

Background

Neuroendocrine tumours (NETs) are a heterogeneous group of tumours, which arise most commonly in the gastreoenteropancreatic tract but can arise from any organ where neuroendocrine cells reside [1, 2]. These tumours have several biological properties in common including the presence of somatostatin receptor (SSTR) expression in the majority of tumours [3]. Five SSTRs have been characterized to date with SSTR-2 and SSTR-5 expression exhibited in 70–90% of all NETs [4].

The high prevalence of SSTR overexpression in NETs has enabled the use of synthetic somatostatin analogues (SSA) to control symptoms related to over production of biologically active amines and peptide hormones frequently associated with NETs and to possibly delay disease progression [5–8]. These are generally administered as slow-release formulations to increase patient convenience.

* Correspondence: michael.hofman@petermac.org
[1]Centre for Cancer Imaging, Peter MacCallum Cancer Centre, 305 Grattan Street, Melbourne, VIC 3000, Australia
[2]Department of Medicine / Sir Peter MacCallum Department of Oncology, University of Melbourne, Melbourne, Australia
Full list of author information is available at the end of the article

Available long-acting SSA (LA-SSA) currently include octreotide (Sandostatin-LAR, Novartis, Switzerland) and lanreotide (Somatuline, Ipsen, France).

^{68}Ga-DOTA-Octreotate (GaTate) PET, which binds to SSTR-2, is becoming increasingly available as a superior diagnostic technique to stage and restage patients with NET. It is also used to determine suitability for peptide receptor radionuclide therapy (PRRT) based on the degree of radiotracer uptake in the tumour [9]. PRRT using ^{177}Lu-DOTA-octreotate or ^{90}Y–DOTA-octreotate have significant efficacy in controlling NETs that have progressed despite SSA therapy and is considered when GaTate PET uptake at tumour sites is greater than background liver uptake, indicating a sufficient target [10–14].

Administration of SSA therapy prior to GaTate PET/CT has the potential to alter radiotracer biodistribution. The EANM procedure guidelines recommend a time interval of 3–4 weeks after administration of long-acting analogues before performing GaTate PET/CT [15]. The guidelines, however, acknowledge that the effects of SSA therapy have not been well characterised. The aim of this study was to perform intra-individual comparison of radiotracer uptake on GaTate PET/CT in both physiologic and sites of metastatic disease at baseline and following LA-SSA therapy.

Methods
Study population
We retrospectively identified 21 (13 M; 8 F, Age 30–89) patients with histologically-proven metastatic NET who had a GaTate PET/CT at baseline whilst treatment naïve (scan 1) and a restaging scan after commencing LA-SSA (scan 2) without any other intervening therapies such as chemotherapy or PRRT. All studies were performed at the Peter MacCallum Centre between June 2010 and February 2014. Scan 2 was performed after a variable amount of time of SSA therapy (mean and median 6 months, range 2–12 months) at the discretion of the referring physician. We recommend different intervals before restaging depending on the grade of the tumour. For European Neuroendocrine Tumour Society (ENETS) Grade 2 tumours which may progress more rapidly there is a greater imperative to restage earlier (eg. 3–6 months) so that other therapies such as peptide receptor radionuclide therapy (PRRT) can be used in the event of rapid progression. For ENETS Grade 1 tumours, the likelihood of progression within such a short period is remote, and we therefore recommend anatomic restaging in 6 months and GaTate PET/CT restaging in 12 months intervals, unless clinical or biochemical assessment raises suspicion of earlier disease progression. Serum chromogranin-A levels at the time of PET scans were available for comparison in 17 of 21 patients. Chromogranin-A levels were performed within 1, 2 and 3 months of the follow-up PET

scan in 82%, 15% and 3%, respectively. Patient characteristics are presented in Table 1. The study constituted a clinical audit and quality assurance activity and institutional ethics approval was therefore not required. The study was undertaken in accordance with the Helsinki Declaration of 1975, as revised in 2008.

^{68}Ga-DOTA-Octreotate (GaTate) PET/CT
^{68}Ga-DOTA-Octreotate was synthesized as previously described [16, 17]. For each production, 42µg of peptide was used but the product was divided and administered to several patientsdepending on patient weight, generator yield and number of patients scheduled. The administered peptide mass therefore ranged from 10-40µg. Beginning 35–88 min after intravenous injection of 85–307 MBq ^{68}Ga-DOTA-Octreotate (GaTate), patients were imaged from vertex to proximal thighs on a PET/CT scanner (Discovery 690 GE Healthcare, USA or Siemens Biograph Siemens Healthcare, Germany). A low-dose CT acquisition was obtained first followed by the PET acquisition. No fasting was required. Patients were encouraged to void during the uptake phase. For patients on LA-SSA therapy, we perform GaTate PET/CT in the week prior to next LA-SSA administration, i.e. 3–4 weeks after LA-SSA administration. A longer period after LA-SSA injection before repeating GaTate PET/CT is not feasible, particularly in patients with symptoms from hormone secretion deriving symptomatic benefit. A shorter period is more likely to result in competitive effects between LA-SSA and radiotracer. Therefore, the time period just before the next administration is most pragmatic. Importantly, the uptake time of second scan in relation to LA-SSA injection was consistent throughout the cohort. 14/21 scan pairs were performed on the same PET/CT machine with both PET/CT machines calibrated and standardized for SUV measurements.

Image analysis
A 3-D fusion workstation (MIMvista 5.0, MIMvista Corp. Cleveland, OH, USA) was used for image analysis. For quantitation at sites of physiological GaTate uptake and metastatic disease, a 3-D volume of interest (VOI) tool was used to draw VOIs around the pituitary gland, thyroid gland, parotid and sub-mandibular glands, adrenal glands, liver, spleen and metastatic deposits to measure maximum standardized uptake value (SUVmax). Splenic activity was not analysed in one patient owing to prior splenectomy. Four small VOIs were drawn over the proximal limbs and combined together to calculate the average body background. Using an automated SUV threshold of 10 to encompass all tumour with adjustment to exclude any sites of physiologic uptake such as spleen and kidney, total body tumour volume (mL) was also measured.

Table 1 Patient Characteristics

Pt	Age	NET Type	Sites of SSTR-Positive Disease	Rx	Dose	Vol 1	Vol 2	CG1	CG2
1	40	SB Carcinoid	Nodes	12	30 S	3.22	5.1	< 1.6	< 1.6
2	61	Pancreatic	Pancreas, Lungs	8	30 S	4.3	11	51	16
3	55	SB Carcinoid	Small Bowel, Nodes, Peritoneal	6	30 S	6.1	5.1	62	32
4	53	SB Carcinoid	Liver, Peritoneum, Nodes	12	30 S	7.9	10.6	345	175
5	62	SB Carcinoid	Nodes	3	120 L	9.5	9.8	40	23
6	41	Bronchial	Lungs, Bones, Salivary Glands	6	30 S	12.5	12.8	9.3	< 6
7	52	SB Carcinoid	Breasts, Nodes, Liver, Peritoneal	4	30 S	13.6	14.6	NA	NA
8	39	SB Carcinoid	Bone, Liver	6	30 S	14.8	15.2	NA	NA
9	56	SB Carcinoid	Liver, Peritoneal, Ovary	5	30 S	19.2	19.8	35	14
10	89	SB Carcinoid	Small bowel, Nodes, Peritoneal	4	90 L	29.4	27.6	265	48
11	55	SB Carcinoid	Peritoneal, Nodes, Liver	5	30 S	51.8	46.7	99	101
12	66	SB Carcinoid	Small Bowel, Peritoneal	4	30 S	67.2	62.4	454	111
13	80	Pancreatic	Pancreas, Liver	6	30 S	1.4	100	77	243
14	49	SB Carcinoid	Liver, Bones, Peritoneum	6	40 S	3	46.4	82	212
15	30	Pancreatic	Liver	13	30 S	7.8	45	79	640
16	66	Paraganglioma	Pelvic / Peri-hepatic masses, Bone	3	20 S	38.6	75.1	14	26
17	73	SB Carcinoid	Ileum, Nodes, Liver	5	30 S	44.1	201.2	267	NA
18	65	Bronchial	Bone, Liver	10	30 S	45.2	120.5	< 121	130
19	68	SB Carcinoid	Liver, Nodes	6	30 S	86.7	472.3	144	750
20	67	SB Carcinoid	Liver, Bones	2	30 S	205.3	297.6	NA	NA
21	65	Pancreatic	Pancreas, Liver	6	20 S	338	783	129	133

Pt = Patient Number, NET = Neuroendocrine Tumour, SSTR = Somatostatin Receptor, Rx = Months SSA therapy, Dose = Monthly SSA (mg), S = Sandostatin LAR, L = Lanreotide, Vol 1 = Total body tumour volume scan 1 (mL), Vol 2 = Total body tumour volume scan 2 (mL), CG1 = Chromogranin level (μg/L) scan 1 CG2 = Chromogranin level (μg/L) scan 2. The first 12 numbered patients are those without tumour progression between the two scans and are further detailed in Table 2

Subanalysis to account for potential confounders

Distribution of GaTate is potentially confounded by a 'tumour sink effect' [16] whereby higher tumour volumes act as a 'sink' for the injected radiotracer resulting in decreased bioavailability and lower SUV measurements at other physiologic body sites. Therefore, if significant disease progression or regression occurred between scans, this could potentially result in changes of uptake at physiologic sites. To minimize this bias, a subgroup analysis was performed in patients with stable disease between the two studies as defined by < 10% change in total body tumour volume or low (< 20 ml) total body tumour volume on both scans (Patients 1–12 Table 1). An additional sub-analysis on the cohort was performed in patients with longer or shorter uptake times following radiotracer administration.

Statistical analysis

Statistical analysis was performed using Analyse-it (Analyse-it Software Ltd., Leeds, UK). Comparisons were made using paired student's t tests for normally distributed variables with a two-sided p-value of 0.05 considered statistically significant. Bland Altman analysis was performed to evaluate variability in GaTate uptake time between scans.

Results

Changes in physiologic distribution

Splenic, thyroid and hepatic SUVmax decreased significantly for all patients ($n = 21$) between baseline GaTate PET/CT and following SSA therapy (Fig. 1). For the overall cohort, splenic SUVmax decreased by 24% from 30.3 to 23.1 ($p = < 0.0001$) (Fig. 2), thyroid by 41% from 5.9 to 3.5 ($p < 0.0001$) (Fig. 3) and liver by 22% from 10.3 to 8.0 ($p = < 0.0001$) (Fig. 4). Adrenal ($n = 42$) and salivary gland ($n = 84$, 2 glands with possible metastatic deposits excluded) SUVmax did not change significantly following SSA therapy, from 16.6 to 17.7 ($p = 0.24$) and 3.9 to 4.0 ($p = 0.11$), respectively. Pituitary gland SUVmax increased slightly following SSA therapy from a baseline of 10.2 to 11.9 ($p = 0.004$).

In the subgroup analysis of patients with stable disease ($n = 12$), findings were similar with mean splenic activity decreasing from 31.2 to 24.9 ($p = 0.0006$), thyroid from 5.8 to 3.4 ($p = 0.0006$) and liver from 10.4 to 8.3 ($p = < 0.0001$). No change was seen in adrenal or salivary gland SUVmax and pituitary gland SUVmax increased from 10.0 to 12.2 ($p = 0.02$).

Variability of intra-individual GaTate uptake time between scans did not appear to influence findings with

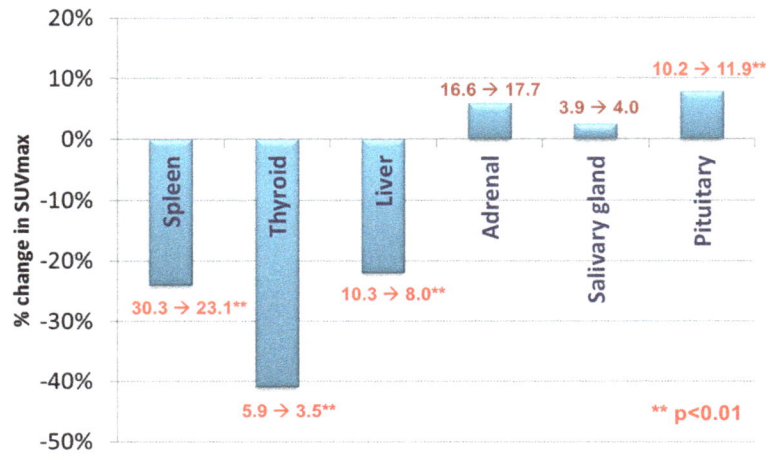

Fig. 1 Change in mean SUVmax from baseline to repeat GaTate PET/CT after SSA therapy

significant reduction in mean splenic, thyroid and hepatic SUVmax demonstrated in patients with either longer (n = 12) or shorter (n = 9) uptake times on their second GaTate scan (Additional file 1: Figure S1, Additional file 2: Figure S2 and Additional file 3: Figure S3).

Changes in metastatic lesion uptake

SUVmax of 49 metastatic lesions in patients with stable disease (n = 12) were measured at baseline and following long acting somatostatin analogue therapy (1–5 lesions measured per patient) (Table 2). 30/49 (61%) of metastatic lesions had an increase in SUVmax following SSA therapy. On a per patient analysis, metastatic lesion SUVmax increased in 7/12 (58%) patients. In 5/7 of these patients chromogranin-A levels were available for correlation and all 5 demonstrated stable or decreasing serum levels at the time of scan 2. Average metastatic lesion SUVmax decreased in 5/12 (42%) of patients with all 5 of these patients also demonstrating stable/ decreasing serum chromogranin-A levels at the time of

scan 2. For bone, nodal and liver disease the SUVmax increased by 5.0 ± 11.6, 3.0 ± 10.9 and 6.2 ± 5.9, respectively.

An analysis of metastatic lesion SUV relative to hepatic activity was also performed. In patients with stable disease, 40/49 (82%) had a SUVmax higher than liver at baseline compared to 44/49 (90%) following SSA therapy, resulting in a change in Krenning Score. Metastatic lesion:liver SUVmax ratio increased in 40/49 (82%) of lesions following SSA therapy (Table 3).

Discussion

Our findings demonstrate that long-acting SSA therapy has variable effects on physiological ^{68}Ga-DOTA-Octreotate uptake in different organs with reduction of uptake in the thyroid gland, spleen and liver, slight increase in uptake in the pituitary gland and no effect on salivary and adrenal gland uptake. By performing a subanalysis in patients with relatively stable disease between scans, we were able to confidently exclude 'tumour sink

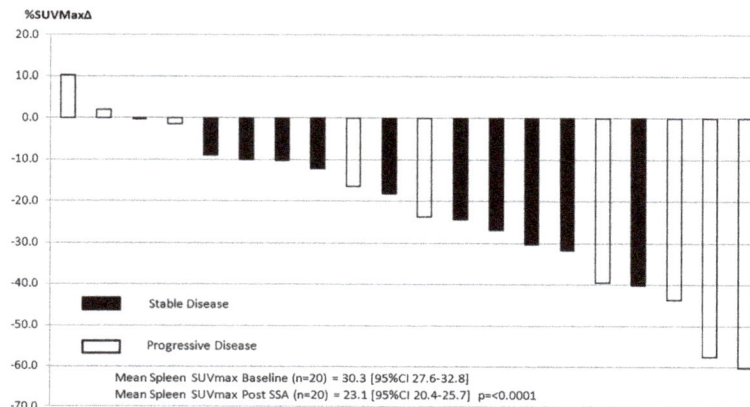

Fig. 2 Spleen SUVMax % Δ Post SSA (n = 20, 1 patient prior splenectomy)

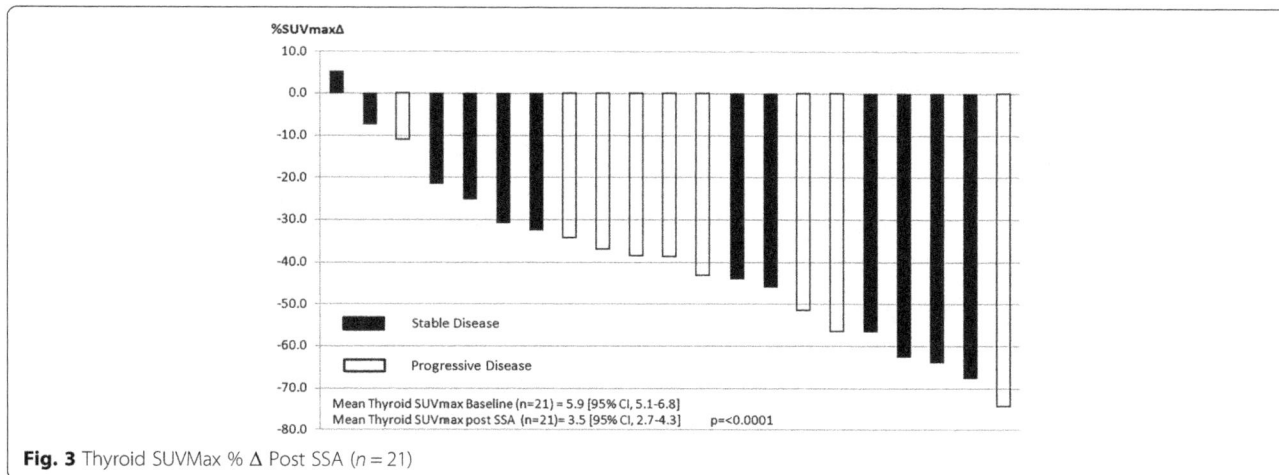

Fig. 3 Thyroid SUVMax % Δ Post SSA (*n* = 21)

effect' as a contributing cause for these changes. The changes were also not explained by differences in uptake period.

The approximate 25% and 20% reduction in physiologic splenic and hepatic GaTate SUVmax demonstrated following SSA therapy has implications for both interpretation of imaging and management of patients for PRRT. Our study demonstrated SSA therapy increased metastatic lesion:liver uptake ratio in 82% of lesions, thereby potentially increasing the Krenning score, a visual scoring system which uses tumour intensity relative to liver and spleen to grade uptake [18]. Although originally developed for interpretation for planar Indium-111 octreotide scanning, we and other groups apply the same scoring for GaTate PET/CT. The increase in metastatic lesion:liver uptake ratio was primarily due to a decrease in liver SUVmax.

These results have significant implications for interpretation of GaTate PET/CT for response assessment following commencement of SSA therapy. Increased tumour to hepatic and splenic ratio may thereby result in increase in Krenning Score which may be misinterpreted as disease progression. Moreover, SUVmax of metastatic lesions increased in 58% patients with stable disease. Correlation with stable or decreasing Chromogranin-A in these patient support the rationale that the change in uptake intensity merely reflected altered biodistribution. In patients without interval disease progression in whom tumour SUVmax increased, the change did not meet the EORTC criteria of 25% increase [19] in intensity to define progressive disease. Furthermore, the increased sensitivity could result in visualization of small volume disease not seen at baseline. In our experience, this is most likely to occur with sub-cm lesions subject to partial volume effects. Our findings also suggest that SSA therapy increases the likelihood of a patient being considered suitable for PRRT, as most groups use a Krenning Score of 3 or greater

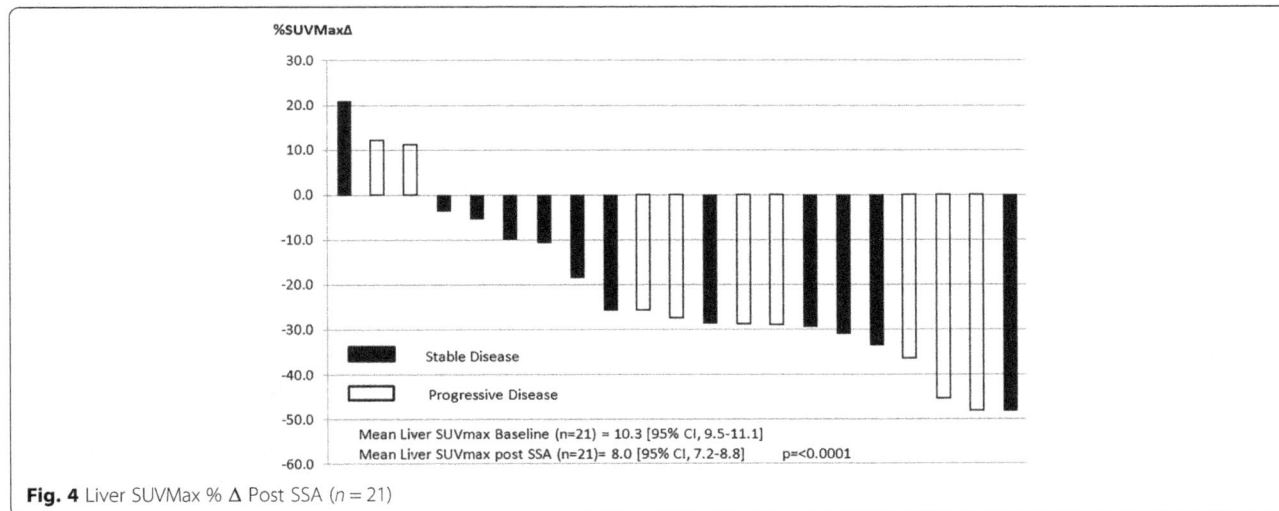

Fig. 4 Liver SUVMax % Δ Post SSA (*n* = 21)

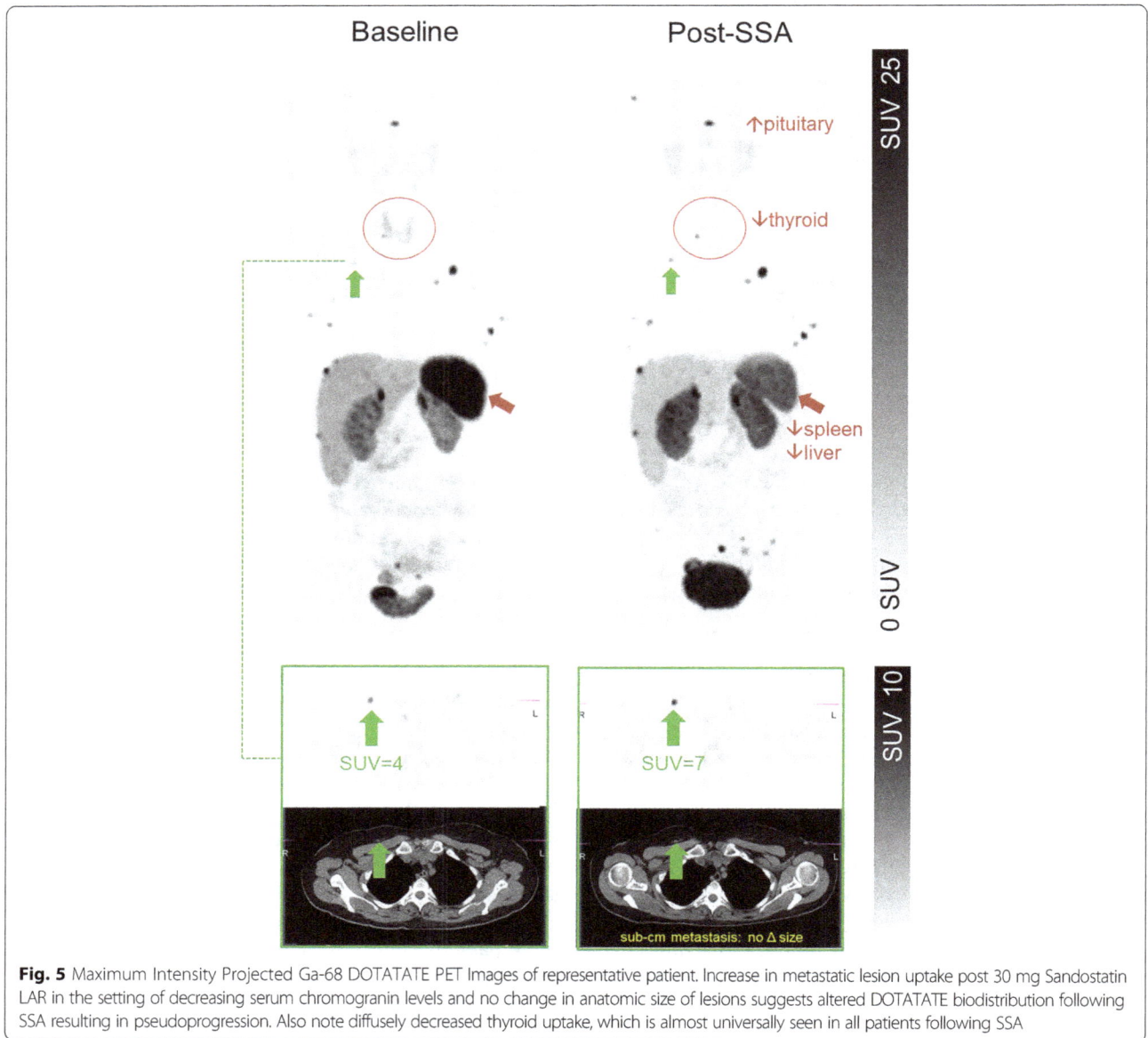

Fig. 5 Maximum Intensity Projected Ga-68 DOTATATE PET Images of representative patient. Increase in metastatic lesion uptake post 30 mg Sandostatin LAR in the setting of decreasing serum chromogranin levels and no change in anatomic size of lesions suggests altered DOTATATE biodistribution following SSA resulting in pseudoprogression. Also note diffusely decreased thyroid uptake, which is almost universally seen in all patients following SSA

(uptake greater than background liver activity) to determine suitability [10].

Our results also have significant implications for delivery of PRRT, with agents such as ^{177}Lu or ^{90}Y DOTA-octreotate. Of most relevance is the decrease in splenic uptake following SSA therapy, as myelosuppression secondary to bystander splenic irradiation may be a potential dose limiting factor of PRRT [20, 21]. Our findings suggest pretreatment with SSA therapy reduces physiologic splenic uptake, and therefore may reduce total splenic radiation exposure from PRRT and related myelosuppression. The higher tumour uptake potentially increasesthe therapeutic index of PRRT. These findings raise the possibility that is somewhat analogous to the administration of 'cold' Rituximab to saturate physiological

binding sites prior to treatment with radiolabelled Rituximab in patients with B cell lymphoma to increase binding at sites of disease [22]. The administration of LA-SSA therapy prior to PRRT may improve efficacy of PRRT in a proportion of patients by altering biodistribution and increasing binding in metastatic lesions (Fig. 5). On the contrary, however, it does appear to decrease metastatic lesion uptake in a proportion of patients potentially rendering PRRT less effective in some patients.

The increase in pituitary gland uptake, decrease in thyroid uptake and lack of change in the salivary and adrenal glands following SSA therapy indicate that SSTR-uptake kinetics vary in different organs. The clinical relevance of these changes are uncertain but the authors note that absent or faint thyroid uptake on GaTate

Table 2 SUVmax change in 49 Metastatic Lesions in 12 patients without Progression between baseline and restaging scan

Patient	Mets	Met 1	SUVmax Δ	Met 2	SUVmax Δ	Met 3	SUVmax Δ	Met 4	SUVmax Δ	Met 5	SUVmax Δ	Av SUVmax Δ
1	1	Node	11.6	NA	NA	NA	NA	NA	NA	NA	NA	11.6
2	3	Lung	−13.9	Node	3.4	Node	−2	NA	NA	NA	NA	−4.2
3	2	Node	−13	Bone	−9	NA	NA	NA	NA	NA	NA	−11.0
4	5	Liver	8.7	Liver	2.9	Bowel	3.1	Peritoneal	9.1	Bowel	0	4.8
5	4	Bowel	−1.3	Bowel	−1.7	Node	−0.7	Bone	−1.2	NA	NA	−1.2
6	5	Bone	2.5	Bone	−4.6	Saliv Gland	−2.5	Bone	−0.9	Bone		−8.7 -2.8
7	5	Bone	1.9	Bone	2.2	Bowel	14.1	Bone	15.2	Liver	−2.1	6.3
8	5	Liver	9.8	Liver	18.4	Liver	3.6	Liver	6.8	Bone	2.9	8.3
9	4	Bowel	5	Liver	1.6	Bone	6.5	Bone	4.5	NA	NA	4.4
10	5	Node	19.7	Bone	˙8	Bone	9.4	Node	16.8	Bone	37	20.2
11	5	Bowel	−7.4	Bowel	−4.7	Node	−6.2	Bowel	−10.1	Node	−2.3	−6.1
12	5	Liver	6.5	Bowel	1.4	Bowel	−1	Bowel	−1.2	Bowel	−3.2	0.5

Mets = Total number of metastases assessed per patient, Met 1–5 = Location of metastasis, Av SUVmax Δ = Average SUV Max Δ for all measured lesions in each patient

PET/CT is a feature that the patient is likely receiving SSA therapy. The significant change in splenic and liver intensity also cautions against using these in isolation as reference organs for windowing nuclear medicine images; scaling images according to a fixed SUV threshold may be preferred.

Our results are supported by Velikyan et al. [23] in which different doses of short-acting SSA administered immediately prior to injection of ^{68}Ga-DOTATOC for PET scanning influenced the degree of NET uptake, with a dose of 50 μg Octreotide associated with increased NET uptake and higher doses of 250 μg and 500 μg associated with a decrease in NET uptake in the same patient. The majority of patients (16/21) in our study were receiving 30 mg Sandostatin LAR monthly, with the remainder (5/21) on 20 or 40 mg Sandostatin LAR or 90-120 mg of Lanreotide monthly that was ceased at least 4 weeks prior to the second PET scan. It is uncertain

how much biologically active SSA was present in each patient at the time of the second PET scan and whether changes demonstrated were due to residual biologically active SSA or whether they were longer term effects of prior SSA exposure that was no longer active at the time of scanning.

We acknowledge there are several significant limitations of this retrospective study including variability of GaTate uptake times between scans performed in each patient and 7/21 scan pairs being performed on different PET scanners. All PET/CT cameras at our institution are calibrated and standardized for SUVmax measurements so any differences between machines would be expected to be minimal. Differences in intra-individual GaTate uptake times between scans appeared to have minimal influence on findings with significant reduction in mean splenic, thyroid and hepatic SUVmax demonstrated in patients with either

Table 3 Metastasis:Liver SUVmax ratio 12 Stable patients

Patient	Met 1	R1	R2	Met 2	R1	R2	Met 3	R1	R2	Met 4	R1	R2	Met 5	R1	R2
1	Node	2.72	3.51	NA	NA	NA	NA	NA	NA	NA	NA	NA	NA	NA	NA
2	Lung	3.29	1.93	Node	0.93	1.36	Node	1.44	1.30	NA	NA	NA	NA	NA	NA
3	Node	1.67	0.84	Bone	1.42	0.96	NA	NA	NA	NA	NA	NA	NA	NA	NA
4	Liver	2.62	4.04	Liver	1.57	2.12	Bowel	1.53	2.11	Peritoneal	1.43	2.77	Bowel	1.06	1.18
5	Bowel	2.39	2.76	Bowel	1.22	1.29	Node	0.90	1.01	Bone	0.76	0.78	NA	NA	NA
6	Bone	0.76	1.08	Bone	1.05	0.54	Saliv Gland	2.28	2.06	Bone	0.92	0.85	Bone	4.60	3.73
7	Bone	2.26	3.48	Bone	2.62	4.04	Bowel	1.58	4.36	Bone	1.47	4.37	Liver	2.47	3.18
8	Liver	1.73	3.83	Liver	1.61	4.89	Liver	1.38	2.44	Liver	1.18	2.63	Bone	0.72	1.43
9	Bowel	0.72	1.29	Liver	2.16	2.57	Bone	1.58	2.40	Bone	3.44	4.28	NA	NA	NA
10	Node	2.20	5.70	Bone	1.76	4.83	Bone	0.83	2.39	Node	1.51	4.32	Bone	2.20	7.80
11	Bowel	1.71	1.52	Bowel	2.64	3.05	Node	3.22	3.69	Bowel	2.78	2.68	Node	3.10	3.93
12	Liver	1.43	3.71	Bowel	0.96	2.06	Bowel	1.30	2.35	Bowel	1.05	1.84	Bowel	2.91	5.13

Met 1–5 = Location of metastasis, R1 = Baseline Metastasis:Liver SUVmax ratio R2 = Post SSA Metastasis:Liver Uptake ratio

longer or shorter uptake times on their second GaTate scan. A further limitation was the large variation in time (2–13 months) that had elapsed between baseline and post SSA PET scans with any tumour progression or regression occurring during this interval likely to directly affect metastatic lesion uptake. We accounted for this as best possible by only measuring changes in metastatic lesion uptake in patients with relatively stable disease between scans.

Despite the above limitations, we believe our findings are important and contribute to the paucity of literature evaluating the effects SSA therapy has on GaTate uptake at physiological and metastatic sites in NET patients and potential implications this has for PRRT. Based on these results, it is quite possible that the EANM procedure guideline recommendations of waiting 3–4 weeks after administration of long-acting somatostatin analogues before performing GaTate PET/CT may not be justified as an earlier timepoint could provide greater sensitivity in some patients [15]. It does, however, appear appropriate to perform GaTate PET/CT at a consistent timing relative to administration of long-acting somatostatin analogues. Nevertheless, given the changes that in biodistribution it appears that a consistent time point follow LA-SSA should be used for consistency. Further prospective, more controlled research of cohorts at multiple time points following differing doses and preparation of long-acting SSA would provide further insights.

Conclusion

Long-acting SSA therapy decreases GaTate uptake in the thyroid gland, spleen and liver but in most cases increases metastatic lesion:liver uptake ratio. This has significant implications for interpretation of GaTate PET/CT as SSA therapy may thereby increase Krenning Score or other quantitative parameters resulting in apparent progression. In patients on therapy, consistent timing of GaTate PET/CT in relation to LA-SSA administration is pragmatic to minimise any bias attributable to competitive or other effects of LA-SSA at time of imaging. Caution should be made not to interpret changes in intensity of uptake alone as progression when comparing a post-therapy to baseline LA-SSA naïve patient or when the dose of LA-SSA is changed. The changes observed after LA-SSA therapy,may increase the likelihood of a patient being deemed suitable for PRRT. Our findings also suggest predosing with SSA prior to PRRT may enable higher doses to be delivered to tumour whilst decreasing dose to normal tissues in a proportion of patients, potentially reducing myelosuppression as a consequence of lower splenic irradiation.

Abbreviations

CgA: Chromogranin-A; ENETS: European Neuroendocrine Tumour Society; GaTate: 68Ga-DOTATATE; LA-SSA: Long-acting somatostatatin analogue; NET: Neuroendocrine tumour; PRRT: Peptide receptor radionuclide therapy; SSA: Somatostatatin analogue; SSTR: Somtatostatin receptor; SUV: Standarised uptake value

Acknowledgements

We wish to thank our radiochemistry team, including Dr. Peter Roselt, for 68Ga-DOTATATE production.

Funding

Not applicable

Authors' contributions

All authors reviewed the final manuscript prior to submission. All authors contributed to trial design, analysis and manuscript review. MC performed quantitative analysis and review of PET scans, and authored the first draft of the manuscript. All authors read and approved the final manuscript.

Competing interests

The authors declare that they have no competing interests

Author details

1Centre for Cancer Imaging, Peter MacCallum Cancer Centre, 305 Grattan Street, Melbourne, VIC 3000, Australia. 2Department of Medicine / Sir Peter MacCallum Department of Oncology, University of Melbourne, Melbourne, Australia. 3Department of Medicine, Monash University, Melbourne, Australia. 4Department of Nuclear Medicine, The Alfred, 55 Commercial Rd, Prahan, VIC 3181, Australia.

References

1. Yao JC, Hassan M, Phan A, Dagohoy C, Leary C, Mares JE, Abdalla EK, Fleming JB, Vauthey JN, Rashid A, Evans DB. One hundred years after "carcinoid": epidemiology of and prognostic factors for neuroendocrine tumors in 35,825 cases in the United States. J Clin Oncol. 2008;26:3063–72.
2. Caplin ME, Buscombe JR, Hilson AJ, Jones AL, Watkinson AF, Burroughs AK. Carcinoid tumour. Lancet. 1998;352:799–805.
3. Reubi JC, Schar JC, Waser B, Wenger S, Heppeler A, Schmitt JS, Macke HR. Affinity profiles for human somatostatin receptor subtypes SST1-SST5 of somatostatin radiotracers selected for scintigraphic and radiotherapeutic use. Eur J Nucl Med. 2000;27:273–82.
4. Papotti M, Bongiovanni M, Volante M, Allia E, Landolfi S, Helboe L, Schindler M, Cole SL, Bussolati G. Expression of somatostatin receptor types 1-5 in 81 cases of gastrointestinal and pancreatic endocrine tumors. A correlative immunohistochemical and reverse-transcriptase polymerase chain reaction analysis. Virchows Arch. 2002;440:461–75.
5. Wild D, Macke HR, Waser B, Reubi JC, Ginj M, Rasch H, Muller-Brand J, Hofmann M. 68Ga-DOTANOC: a first compound for PET imaging with high affinity for somatostatin receptor subtypes 2 and 5. Eur J Nucl Med Mol Imaging. 2005;32:724.
6. Waser B, Tamma ML, Cescato R, Maecke HR, Reubi JC. Highly efficient in vivo agonist-induced internalization of sst2 receptors in somatostatin target tissues. J Nucl Med. 2009;50:936–41.
7. Caplin ME, Pavel M, Cwikla JB, Phan AT, Raderer M, Sedlackova E, Cadiot G, Wolin EM, Capdevila J, Wall L, et al: Lanreotide in metastatic enteropancreatic neuroendocrine tumors. N Engl J Med 2014, 371:224–233.
8. Rinke A, Muller HH, Schade-Brittinger C, Klose KJ, Barth P, Wied M, Mayer C, Aminossadati B, Pape UF, Blaker M, et al. Placebo-controlled, double-blind, prospective, randomized study on the effect of octreotide LAR in the control of tumor growth in patients with metastatic neuroendocrine midgut tumors: a report from the PROMID study group. J Clin Oncol. 2009;27:4656–63.

9. Kayani I, Bomanji JB, Groves A, Conway G, Gacinovic S, Win T, Dickson J, Caplin M, Ell PJ. Functional imaging of neuroendocrine tumors with combined PET/CT using 68Ga-DOTATATE (DOTA-DPhe1,Tyr3-octreotate) and 18F-FDG. Cancer. 2008;112:2447–55.

10. Kwekkeboom DJ, de Herder WW, Kam BL, van Eijck CH, van Essen M, Kooij PP, Feelders RA, van Aken MO, Krenning EP. Treatment with the radiolabeled somatostatin analog [177 Lu-DOTA 0,Tyr3]octreotate: toxicity, efficacy, and survival. J Clin Oncol. 2008;26:2124–30.

11. Bodei L, Cremonesi M, Kidd M, Grana CM, Severi S, Modlin IM, Paganelli G. Peptide receptor radionuclide therapy for advanced neuroendocrine tumors. Thorac Surg Clin. 2014;24:333–49.

12. Seregni E, Maccauro M, Chiesa C, Mariani L, Pascali C, Mazzaferro V, De Braud F, Buzzoni R, Milione M, Lorenzoni A, et al. Treatment with tandem [90Y]DOTA-TATE and [177Lu]DOTA-TATE of neuroendocrine tumours refractory to conventional therapy. Eur J Nucl Med Mol Imaging. 2014;41: 223–30.

13. Strosberg J, El-Haddad G, Wolin E, Hendifar A, Yao J, Chasen B, Mittra E, Kunz PL, Kulke MH, Jacene H, et al. Phase 3 trial of 177Lu-Dotatate for midgut neuroendocrine tumors. N Engl J Med. 2017;376:125–35.

14. Hicks RJ, Kwekkeboom DJ, Krenning E, Bodei L, Grozinsky-Glasberg S, Arnold R, Borbath I, Cwikla J, Toumpanakis C, Kaltsas G, et al. ENETS consensus guidelines for the standards of Care in Neuroendocrine Neoplasia: peptide receptor radionuclide therapy with radiolabeled somatostatin analogues. Neuroendocrinology. 2017;105(3):295–309.

15. Virgolini I, Ambrosini V, Bomanji JB, Baum RP, Fanti S, Gabriel M, Papathanasiou ND, Pepe G, Oyen W, De Cristoforo C, Chiti A. Procedure guidelines for PET/CT tumour imaging with 68Ga-DOTA-conjugated peptides: 68Ga-DOTA-TOC, 68Ga-DOTA-NOC, 68Ga-DOTA-TATE. Eur J Nucl Med Mol Imaging. 2010;37:2004–10.

16. Beauregard JM, Hofman MS, Kong G, Hicks RJ. The tumour sink effect on the biodistribution of 68Ga-DOTA-octreotate: implications for peptide receptor radionuclide therapy. Eur J Nucl Med Mol imaging. 2012;39:50–6.

17. Zhernosekov KP, Filosofov DV, Baum RP, Aschoff P, Binl H, Razbash AA, Jahn M, Jennewein M, Rosch F. Processing of generator-produced 68Ga for medical application. J Nucl Med. 2007;48:1741–8.

18. Kwekkeboom DJ, Teunissen JJ, Bakker WH, Kooij PP, de Herder WW, Feelders RA, van Eijck CH, Esser JP, Kam BL, Krenning EP. Radiolabeled somatostatin analog [177Lu-DOTA0,Tyr3]octreotide in patients with endocrine gastroenteropancreatic tumors. J Clin Oncol. 2005;23:2754–62.

19. Young H, Baum R, Cremerius U, Herholz K, Hoekstra O, Lammertsma AA, Pruim J, Price P. Measurement of clinical and subclinical tumour response using [18F]-fluorodeoxyglucose and positron emission tomography: review and 1999 EORTC recommendations. European Organization for Research and Treatment of Cancer (EORTC) PET Study Group. Eur J Cancer. 1999;35: 1773–82.

20. Sabet A, Ezziddin K, Pape UF, Ahmadzadehfar H, Mayer K, Poppel T, Guhlke S, Biersack HJ, Ezziddin S. Long-term hematotoxicity after peptide receptor radionuclide therapy with 177Lu-octreotate. J Nucl Med. 2013;54:1857–61.

21. Kesavan M, Claringbold PG, Turner JH. Hematological toxicity of combined 177Lu-octreotate radiopeptide chemotherapy of gastroenteropancreatic neuroendocrine tumors in long-term follow-up. Neuroendocrinology. 2014; 99:108–17.

22. Kaminski MS, Tuck M, Estes J, Kolstad A, Ross CW, Zasadny K, Regan D, Kison P, Fisher S, Kroll S, Wahl RL. 131I-tositumomab therapy as initial treatment for follicular lymphoma. N Engl J Med. 2005;352:441–9.

23. Velikyan I, Sundin A, Eriksson B, Lundqvist H, Sorensen J, Bergstrom M, Langstrom B. In vivo binding of [68Ga]-DOTATOC to somatostatin receptors in neuroendocrine tumours–impact of peptide mass. Nucl Med Biol. 2010;37:265–75.

10

Additional value of ^{18}F-FDG PET/CT evaluation in axillary nodes during neoadjuvant therapy for triple-negative and HER2-positive breast cancer

Mette S. van Ramshorst[1], Suzana C. Teixeira[2], Bas B. Koolen[2,3], Kenneth E. Pengel[4], Kenneth G. Gilhuijs[5], Jelle Wesseling[6], Sjoerd Rodenhuis[1], Renato A. Valdés Olmos[2], Emiel J. Rutgers[3], Wouter V. Vogel[2], Gabe S. Sonke[1] and Marie-Jeanne T. Vrancken Peeters[3*]

Abstract

Background: ^{18}F-FDG PET/CT can monitor metabolic activity in early breast cancer during neoadjuvant systemic therapy (NST), but it is unknown if the metabolic breast and axillary response differ. We evaluated the correlation between metabolic breast and axillary response at various time points during NST. Furthermore, we analysed if the combined metabolic response improves pathologic complete response (pCR) prediction compared to using the metabolic breast response alone.

Methods: ^{18}F-FDG PET/CT was performed at baseline (PET1), 2–3 weeks (PET2), and 6–8 weeks (PET3) of NST in patients with triple-negative (TN) and HER2-positive node-positive breast cancer. SUVmax and ΔSUVmax were determined separately for breast and axilla. Spearman's correlation coefficients (r) between both localisations were calculated. The accuracy of pCR total (ypT0/is,ypN0) prediction using the metabolic response in breast, axilla or both was examined using logistic regression analysis.

Results: Hundred-five patients were included: 45 TN and 60 HER2-positive tumours. The metabolic response in breast and axilla correlated moderately in TN tumours ($r = 0.57$) using ΔSUVmax between PET1-PET3 and poorly in HER2-positive tumours ($r = 0.49$) using SUVmax at PET2. In TN tumours, metabolic breast response predicted pCR well without improvement after adding axillary response (c-index 0.82 versus 0.85, $p = 0.63$). In HER2-positive tumours, metabolic breast response predicted pCR poorly with improvement after adding axillary response (c-index 0.64 versus 0.72, $p = 0.06$).

Conclusions: ^{18}F-FDG PET/CT response during NST differs between breast and axilla. In TN tumours, pCR total prediction can be made independent of metabolic axillary response. In HER2-positive tumours, axillary response may improve pCR total prediction. These findings may help guide PET/CT-response-based changes during NST.

Keywords: Breast cancer, ^{18}F-FDG PET/CT, Neoadjuvant treatment, Early response monitoring

* Correspondence: m.vrancken@nki.nl
[3]Department of Surgical Oncology, Netherlands Cancer Institute, Plesmanlaan 121, 1066 CX Amsterdam, The Netherlands
Full list of author information is available at the end of the article

Background

Neoadjuvant systemic treatment (NST) is increasingly used in early breast cancer to allow down-staging of the primary tumour to facilitate breast-conserving surgery [1]. Initially tumour-positive lymph nodes may convert into tumour-negative lymph nodes during NST which permits less aggressive treatment of the axilla as well [2]. In vivo response monitoring and adapting ineffective therapy regimens may become important additional assets of a neoadjuvant approach [3, 4].

Magnetic resonance imaging (MRI) is increasingly used as standard of care for response evaluation in the breast during NST in the Netherlands. Functional imaging with radiolabelled fluor-18-deoxyglucose (^{18}F-FDG) positron emission tomography combined with computed tomography (PET/CT) can visualise the glucose metabolism in the primary tumour and affected lymph nodes. Furthermore, detection of changes in tumour glucose metabolism in response to treatment enables early response monitoring [5]. Optimal long-term outcome is seen after pathologic complete response in breast and axilla (pCR total) [6] but the sensitivity to NST may differ between both sites [7, 8]. Nevertheless, most previous neoadjuvant PET/CT studies focussed on the metabolic response of the breast alone [9–15]. Substantially fewer studies evaluated the early metabolic response of the axilla [8, 16–18], the combined response in breast and axilla [7, 9, 19, 20] or the agreement between both [21].

Therefore, the aim of our study, performed in HER2-positive and triple-negative (TN) breast cancer patients, was twofold. First, we assessed the correlation between the metabolic response in breast and axilla. Second, we evaluated the additional value of incorporating the metabolic axillary response over the breast response alone in predicting pCR total.

Methods

We performed a prospective single-centre study with sequential PET/CT scanning before and during NST in women with primary stage II-III HER2-positive or TN breast cancer. Patients were included from September 2008 until June 2014. The institutional review board approved the study protocol and all included patients provided written informed consent. Only patients with a visible primary tumour and affected lymph nodes at baseline PET/CT were included in this analysis. Forty-five of these patients were included in a previous report [19].

Pathological evaluation

At baseline, core biopsies were obtained from the primary tumour for pathologic diagnosis and oestrogen receptor, progesterone receptor, and HER2-status, according to Dutch national guidelines (http://www.oncoline.nl/). A marker was placed at the primary tumour site to guide surgery and pathologic evaluation. Breast conserving surgery or a mastectomy was performed based on tumour characteristics, and patient's preference. Baseline nodal status was assessed by physical, ultrasound, and PET/CT examination with cytological evaluation by fine needle aspiration of suspicious lymph nodes. Biopsies of the primary tumour and fine needle aspiration of the lymph nodes were aimed to be obtained prior to baseline PET/CT. Patients with clinical node-negative disease underwent a sentinel node procedure (SNP) either before or after NST. In case of node-positive disease at baseline a level I-II axillary lymph node dissection was performed or the initially positive marked lymph node(s) was removed guided by marking the dominant axillary node(s) with radioactive iodine seeds (MARI-procedure) [2]. PCR was assessed by experienced breast pathologists, and was defined as no residual invasive tumour cells irrespective of in-situ lesions [6]. PCR breast, pCR axilla, and their combination (pCR total) were determined.

Treatment

Patients with TN tumours received three cycles dose-dense doxorubicin/cyclophosphamide (AC) followed by MRI-evaluation. Patients with an unfavourable MRI response, defined as <25% reduction of the largest diameter of late enhancement, switched to three cycles capecitabine/docetaxel [CD] or three cycles carboplatin/paclitaxel [CP] [22]. Patients with a favourable response were randomized between three additional cycles of AC or CD/CP. Patients with homologous recombination deficient (HRD) tumours were randomized between three cycles CD/CP or an additional AC-cycle followed by intensified alkylating chemotherapy consisting of cyclophosphamide/thiotepa/carboplatin (CTC). Patients with HER2-positive tumours received 24 cycles weekly paclitaxel/trastuzumab/carboplatin (PTC) with trastuzumab only in weeks 7, 8, 15, 16, 23, and 24 [23]. In case of an unfavourable MRI response after 8 weeks of NST patients switched to four cycles 5-fluorouracil/epirubicin/cyclophosphamide/trastuzumab (FEC-T).

PET/CT procedures

A PET/CT was performed at baseline (PET1), after 2 to 3 weeks of treatment (PET2), and after 6 to 8 weeks (PET3). Patients were instructed to fast for 6 hours prior to the scan and blood glucose levels were required to be <10mmol/L. Based on the patient's body mass index 180-240MBq ^{18}F-FDG was administered intravenously and 10mg diazepam was given orally to reduce ^{18}F-FDG-uptake by brown fat. Following a resting period of 60 ± 10 min, in accordance with EANM procedure guidelines, a PET-scan (3.00 min per bed position and image reconstruction to 2x2x2mm voxels) of the thorax was performed according to the hanging breast protocol, using a whole-body scanner (Gemini TF; Philips, Cleveland, OH) [24]. A low-dose CT-scan (2mm slices) without intravenous contrast preceded the PET acquisition for anatomical localisation. In order to be able to make a valid comparison between scans within an individual and between individuals the same imaging system and protocol including the target time interval between ^{18}F-FDG injection and PET acquisition were used throughout the study. At baseline a standard supine whole-body PET/CT was performed as well as part of disease staging.

Image reading

The acquired PET/CT images were evaluated by a panel of experienced reviewers (BK, MvR, ST), supervised by two nuclear medicine specialists (RVO, WV). All baseline scans were qualitatively assessed for sufficient ^{18}F-FDG-uptake of the primary tumour and lymph node metastases, defined as the ability to visually distinguish known tumour locations from adjacent non-malignant tissue (i.e. pathological versus physiological uptake, respectively) with an estimated ratio of >2.0, to allow subsequent quantitative response evaluation. Quantitative ^{18}F-FDG-uptake of the primary tumour and the most active level I-II axillary lymph node was measured as the maximum standardised uptake value (SUVmax) within a 3D region of interest (ROI). Level III lymph nodes were not included, as these are not routinely resected during axillary clearance. If the automated ROI generation was unreliable due to a low tumour-to-background ratio, the ROI was manually drawn. In case of a complete metabolic response on the subsequent scans the baseline ROI localisation was used for calculation of the SUVmax.

Statistical analyses

All analyses were performed separately for TN and HER2-positive tumours. Descriptive statistics were used to outline patient, tumour, and treatment characteristics. For response analyses the most active axillary lymph node was included. The absolute SUVmax values at the different time points and the relative percentage changes in SUVmax (hereafter referred to as SUVmax and ΔSUVmax respectively) were determined in breast and axilla, and their association was calculated using Spearman's correlation coefficient (r). The association of the various PET/CT parameters at different time points with pCR was tested using logistic regression analyses and presented as the c-index (equivalent of the area under the curve [AUC] in ROC analyses). Correlation and c-index results were interpreted according to previously described classifications [25, 26]. The change in c-index when adding axillary response to a model including breast response alone was tested for significance based on the algorithm proposed by DeLong et al [27].

Data were analysed using SPSS version 22.0 (SPSS Inc. Chicago, USA) and STATA (version 13; StataCorp, College Station, TX, USA). P-value of <0.05 was considered statistically significant. No adjustment for multiple testing was made.

Results
Baseline and treatment characteristics
In total 169 patients were included. Sixteen were ineligible because of stage I disease (n = 5), stage IV disease (n = 3), missing baseline PET/CT (n = 4), or no trastuzumab use in case of HER2-positive disease (n = 4). Of the remaining 153 patients, 105 had a primary tumour and positive axillary lymph nodes, both pathologically proven and visible on PET/CT. Forty-five patients had TN and 60 HER2-positive disease (Additional file 1: Figure S1). Positive nodal status was pathologically proven in all but one patient by fine needle aspiration (Table 1). In this one patient lymph node metastases were detected by a pre-treatment SNP, however one positive axillary lymph node remained in-situ and showed ^{18}F-FDG-uptake on PET/CT. Nineteen patients changed treatment after 6 to 8 weeks of therapy (i.e. after PET3). In the TN subgroup, six patients changed because of insufficient MRI response and none of them achieved a pCR breast or pCR axilla. Eleven patients switched therapy according to study protocol (ten with an HRD tumour, and one without), and one patient switched because of patient's preference. Of these 12 patients eight achieved pCR breast and six pCR axilla and pCR total. In the HER2-positive subgroup one patient changed treatment based on an insufficient MRI response. Neither pCR breast nor pCR axilla was achieved.

Surgery and pathologic response
With the exception of one patient with progressive disease during chemotherapy who refused further treatment, all patients underwent surgery. This patient was classified as having no pCR. Thus, 104 patients underwent breast surgery: 66 breast conserving surgery and 38 a mastectomy. Pathologic axillary lymph node response was assessed by axillary lymph node dissection in 89, MARI-procedure in 13, and post-treatment SNP in two patients.

In TN tumours pCR breast was achieved in 53% (24/45), pCR axilla in 47% (21/45), and pCR total in 40% (18/45). In the HER2-positive subgroup the rate of pCR breast was 65% (39/60), pCR axilla 75% (45/60), and pCR total 57% (34/60). In total 25 patients had a discrepant pathologic response of the breast and axilla: 11 pCR breast/no pCR axilla, and 14 pCR axilla/no pCR breast.

Triple-negative disease
Baseline PET/CT was performed in all 45 patients with TN disease, PET2 in 35, and PET3 in 38. Thirty-two

Table 1 Baseline and treatment characteristics according to subtype

	TN (n = 45)		HER2+ (n = 60)		All (n = 105)	
	n	(%)	n	(%)	n	(%)
Age (years)						
Median (IQR)	50	(36–55)	45	(37–52)	47	(37–54)
Tumour size on MRI (mm)						
Median (IQR)	31	(22–45)	38	(22–60)	33	(22–50)
Disease stage						
II	19	(42%)	26	(43%)	45	(43%)
III	26	(58%)	34	(57%)	60	(57%)
Baseline axillary staging method						
Positive, pre-SNP[a]	1	(2%)	0	(0%)	1	(1%)
Positive, FNA	44	(98%)	60	(100%)	104	(99%)
Grade						
1–2	13	(29%)	25	(42%)	38	(36%)
3	16	(36%)	14	(23%)	30	(29%)
Unknown	16	(36%)	21	(35%)	37	(35%)
Histology						
Ductal	43	(96%)	55	(92%)	98	(93%)
Lobular	0	(0%)	4	(7%)	4	(4%)
Other	2	(4%)	1	(2%)	3	(3%)
HR-status						
ER- and PR-	45	(100%)	29	(48%)	74	(71%)
ER+ and/or PR+	0	(0%)	31	(52%)	31	(30%)
Treatment						
AC[b]	45	(100%)	0	(0%)	45	(43%)
PTC[c]	0	(0%)	60	(100%)	60	(57%)
PET assessment						
PET1 performed	45	(100%)	60	(100%)	105	(100%)
PET2 performed	35	(78%)	45	(75%)	80	(76%)
PET3 performed	38	(84%)	47	(78%)	84	(80%)

TN triple-negative, HER2+ HER2-positive, n number of patients, PA pathology, SNP sentinel node procedure, FNA fine needle aspiration, ER oestrogen receptor, PR progesterone receptor, AC doxorubicin/cyclophosphamide, PTC paclitaxel/trastuzumab/carboplatin
[a]SNP performed before PET1, but remaining positive axillary lymph node in situ outside surgical region
[b]Nineteen patients switched treatment after PET3: six to capecitabine/docetaxel, ten to high-dose carboplatin/thiotepa/cyclophosphamide, three to paclitaxel (+/- carboplatin)
[c]Two patients received paclitaxel/trastuzumab/carboplatin plus pertuzumab, and one patients switched to 5-fluorouracil/epirubicin/cyclophosphamide plus trastuzumab after PET3

Table 2 Correlation coefficients between the metabolic response in breast and axilla with different SUVmax variables according to subtype

	TN (n = 45)			HER2+ (n = 60)		
	median	(IQR)	r	median	(IQR)	r
SUVmax PET1						
Breast	10.7	(6.5 – 16.5)	0.42	6.8	(4.7 – 9.3)	0.38
Axilla	8.0	(4.9 – 13.8)		5.3	(3.3 – 7.6)	
SUVmax PET2						
Breast	7.9	(5.1 – 10.0)	0.36	2.8	(2.2 – 3.6)	0.49
Axilla	4.2	(3.1 – 7.2)		2.1	(1.7 – 2.5)	
SUVmax PET3						
Breast	3.5	(2.5 – 5.0)	0.33	2.0	(1.5 – 2.4)	0.14
Axilla	2.1	(1.3 – 3.6)		1.7	(1.3 – 2.4)	
ΔSUVmax (%) PET1-PET2						
Breast	-32%	(-49 – -16)	0.49	-56%	(-68 – -47)	0.30
Axilla	-33%	(-58 – -13)		-56%	(-70 – -38)	
ΔSUVmax (%) PET1-PET3						
Breast	-67%	(-77 – -49)	0.57	-69%	(-78 – -52)	0.27
Axilla	-70%	(-84 – -48)		-66%	(-79 – -50)	

TN triple-negative, HER2+ HER2-positive, n number of patients, IQR interquartile range, r Spearman's correlation coefficient

and axilla was found with ΔSUVmax between PET1-PET3, and although all patients showed a decrease in ΔSUVmax in both locations at PET3 the correlation was moderate ($r = 0.57$) (Additional file 2: Figure S2a).

PCR breast prediction was most accurate using ΔSUVmax breast between PET1-PET3 (c-index 0.85) (Additional file 3: Table S1). Likewise, ΔSUVmax axilla between PET1--PET3 was best for pCR axilla prediction (c-index 0.82). The metabolic breast response, using ΔSUVmax between PET1-PET3, was well predictive for pCR total and the addition of metabolic response in the axilla using ΔSUVmax between PET1-PET3 did not further improve pCR total prediction (c-index 0.82 versus 0.85, $p = 0.63$) (Table 3).

HER2-positive disease

Baseline PET/CT was performed in all 60 patients with HER2-positive disease, PET2 in 45, and PET3 in 47. Forty patients underwent three PET/CT-scans. The median time between last chemotherapy and PET2 was 6 days (IQR 5-7), and between last chemotherapy and PET3 12 days (IQR 8-14). The best correlation between metabolic response in breast and axilla was found with SUVmax at PET2, although poor ($r = 0.49$) (Additional file 2: Figure S2b). In addition, an inverse response in terms of an increase in SUVmax in one location and a decrease or no difference in the other was observed in four patients at time of PET2.

patients underwent three PET/CT-scans. The median time between last chemotherapy and PET2 was 13 days (interquartile range [IQR] 13-14), and between last chemotherapy and PET3 7 days (IQR 7-8). The median SUVmax and ΔSUVmax at the different time points are summarized in Table 2, including correlation coefficients between metabolic response in breast and axilla. The best correlation between metabolic response in breast

Table 3 C-indices (95% confidence interval) for the prediction of pathologic complete response by metabolic response in TN and HER2-positive breast cancer

	Pathologic complete response		
	Breast	Axilla	Total
TN: ΔSUVmax PET1-PET3			
Breast	0.85 (0.72 – 0.98)	0.83 (0.69 – 0.98)	0.82 (0.66 – 0.98)
Axilla	0.82 (0.68 – 0.95)	0.82 (0.68 – 0.97)	0.83 (0.67 – 0.98)
Breast + axilla	0.86 (0.74 – 0.98)	0.86 (0.72 – 0.99)	0.85 (0.69 – 1.00)
p-value*	0.78	0.60	0.63
HER2-positive: SUVmax PET2			
Breast	0.62 (0.44 – 0.81)	0.65 (0.47 – 0.84)	0.64 (0.47 – 0.81)
Axilla	0.68 (0.52 – 0.84)	0.77 (0.62 – 0.92)	0.67 (0.51 - 0.83)
Breast + axilla	0.72 (0.56 – 0.89)	0.78 (0.63 – 0.92)	0.72 (0.57 – 0.88)
p-value*	0.11	0.06	0.06

*p-value for the improvement in c-index by the addition of metabolic response in the axilla

The metabolic response in the breast poorly discriminates patients who will achieve a pCR breast from patients who will not. The difference in SUVmax (ΔSUVmax) in the breast between PET1-PET2 had the best discriminating performance of all PET-parameters assessed (c-index 0.64), although absolute SUVmax in the breast at PET2 showed an almost similar performance (c-index 0.62) (Additional file 4: Table S2). In the axilla, SUVmax at PET2 had the best discriminating performance to predict pCR axilla (c-index 0.77). Prediction of total pCR by SUVmax in the breast at PET2 was poor but improved to fair, although not statistically significant, when both the metabolic breast and axillary response using SUVmax at PET2 were included (c-index 0.64 versus 0.72, p = 0.06) (Table 3).

Discussion

This study shows that the correlation between ^{18}F-FDG PET/CT responses during NST in breast and axillary lymph nodes is moderate in triple-negative and poor in HER2-positive breast cancer. In TN disease, PET/CT response can be used to predict pCR and the breast response alone suffices to predict pCR total. Conversely, in HER2-positive disease, the accuracy of PET/CT to predict pCR is limited, while incorporating the metabolic response of both the breast and axilla may improve pCR total prediction.

Lymph node involvement at baseline and after NST is an important prognostic factor in non-metastatic breast cancer [28, 29]. Furthermore, pCR defined as no invasive tumour cells in breast and axilla is best related to long-term outcome [6]. Despite this knowledge, many previous PET/CT studies evaluated the metabolic response of the breast alone to predict pCR total, without examining if the metabolic response of the primary tumour and lymph nodes is the same [4, 11–15]. Adding information about the metabolic response of axilla may aid to predict pCR total. Studies, that did evaluate the metabolic response in breast and axilla, used different strategies to combine response information of both locations to predict pCR total. Some evaluated the response of the baseline lesion with highest FDG-uptake alone [9, 30, 31] and others used ΔSUVmax between the lesion with the highest FDG-uptake at baseline and at the subsequent scan [32, 33]. However, information may be missed if the response differs between both sites or may result in comparing a breast lesion with an axillary lymph node or vice versa if the lesion with the highest FDG-uptake changes during treatment. Dalus et al. found different SUVmax measurements for breast and lymph nodes, possibly reflecting a different biological behaviour in these two sites which may relate to selection of a sub-clone of tumour cells that spreads to the lymph nodes. Therefore, they proposed to evaluate the response of the primary tumour and axilla separately [21]. We agree with this proposal until a valid combined variable has been established. Only a few studies have described the metabolic response in breast and axilla separately and its respective association with pCR breast and pCR axilla within the same cohort [7, 34]. These studies did not evaluate the correlation between the metabolic response in both locations. Therefore our study is unique and provides important new insights for PET/CT interpretation.

We found a moderate correlation between the metabolic breast and axillary response in TN breast cancer (r = 0.57) without significant improvement in pCR total prediction with adding the metabolic axillary response to the breast response alone. This suggests that chemotherapy sensitivity in breast and axilla corresponds well. Therefore, the metabolic breast response alone suffices to guide NST decisions. In accordance with this, Groheux et al. did not find a better prediction of pCR total in TN disease if the axillary response was incorporated in addition to the breast response [9, 31]. Koolen et al. previously described a part of our study population and found the strongest association between the combined metabolic breast and axillary response and pCR total with an AUC of 0.93 versus 0.87 for breast response alone [19]. The statistical significance of this improvement was not tested. With the inclusion of additional patients in the current analysis, the association between the combined metabolic response and pCR total was somewhat weaker, although still good with a non-significant improvement using the combination over the breast alone (c-index 0.85 versus 0.82, p = 0.63) [19].

In HER2-positive breast cancer the metabolic responses in breast and axilla correlate poorly (r = 0.49). The ability to predict pCR breast, and pCR total by the metabolic breast response was poor (c-index 0.62, and 0.64, respectively). The addition of metabolic response in the axilla improved the pCR total prediction compared to the use of breast response alone, which was statistically near-significant (c-index 0.64 versus 0.72, p = 0.06). Lack of statistical significance despite a relatively large increase in c-index, might be attributable to the small sample size, and larger studies are needed to determine the added value of including the metabolic response in both locations for pCR total prediction in this subtype. In line with our results, Groheux and colleagues found an improvement in pCR total prediction in node-positive patients if the axillary response was included [30]. These and our findings suggest that if PET/CT is used for response monitoring in HER2-positive breast cancer, it should evaluate both breast and axilla, and we recommend separate evaluation of both sites rather than an unconfirmed combined parameter as described above. The use of targeted therapy in HER2-positive tumours may explain why the different response according to tumour location was more pronounced in this subtype, as it may differentially affect sub-clones with varying HER2-expression. Also, we cannot exclude that in selected cases non-specific ^{18}F-FDG uptake related to regional inflammatory processes or tissue sampling may have contaminated the pathological uptake. Although we recognize this as a limitation of our study the impact on our results will be limited, especially after FNA. Furthermore, non-specific ^{18}F-FDG uptake is likely to have affected both subtypes equally. Lastly, with the relatively small sample size we cannot exclude that the poor and moderate correlation of metabolic responses between locations is due to chance rather than a biological finding. However, despite only four inverse responses in the HER2-positive subtype, in relative terms, this constitutes 9% of HER2-positive cases with a PET2. Additionally, the poor correlation between metabolic and axillary response despite a decrease in both locations seems relevant as it may have implications for defining metabolic responders with different thresholds for different localizations.

In accordance with the literature we found that the best prognostic PET/CT response parameter for both pCR breast and pCR axilla is ΔSUVmax between baseline PET/CT and PET/CT after 6 weeks in TN tumours and the absolute SUVmax value at PET/CT after 3 weeks of therapy in HER2-positive tumours [9, 12, 30, 31, 35].

Our data reinforce that it is important to describe results according to breast cancer subtype due to different tumour behaviour. Subgroup analysis based on hormone receptor status within the HER2-positive cohort would have been valuable, but was not feasible due to the limited number of patients.

The inclusion of patients with sufficiently high baseline FDG-uptake for response evaluation, may have led to selection of relatively aggressive tumour types and an associated higher response rate reflecting the high pCR rate in our study. Nevertheless, sufficient baseline activity is required for PET/CT-evaluation and thus this selection reflects daily practice. Furthermore, a substantial number of patients with TN tumours switched therapy, and PET/CT-scans were only performed during the initially applied regimen. However, switches based on insufficient MRI response are assumed to have had little impact on our results as all these patients remained a pathological non-responder despite the change in treatment and it is unlikely that they would have achieved total pCR if they had continued their initially applied regimen.

Clear definitions of responders and non-responders will aid the clinical use of PET/CT during neoadjuvant breast cancer treatment. The optimal cut-off value depends on several factors as described by others including treatment regimen, timing of evaluation, breast cancer subtype, and mainly depends on the purpose of the response evaluation: identifying non-responders to change ineffective treatment or identifying responders to reduce overtreatment [35].

Several PET-parameters exist but no superiority of one over the other has been established so far. This study started in 2008 and we used the region with the highest metabolic activity (i.e. SUVmax) instead of the entire metabolically active tumour volume which has been introduced more recently. However, SUVmax has important benefits as it is convenient to use and has good reproducibility [9, 32].

PET/CT for response evaluation during NST in breast cancer is not the current standard of care and probably awaits a direct comparison with other imaging modalities. In the current study we focused on the use of PET/CT only and how to optimally use this to predict pCR total. Therefore, we cannot make a statement about the relative value of PET/CT compared to other imaging modalities, but this has been described by others [36, 37]. Nowadays, trastuzumab-labelled PET/CT scans are available with visualisation of HER2-positive lesions. This modality may improve selection of patients for anti-HER2 treatment, but its role in monitoring response is undetermined [38]. Furthermore, trials to confirm the benefit of PET/CT-response-based treatment adaptations in terms of outcome are needed [3, 4].

Conclusion

Our study demonstrates that the correlation between metabolic response in the breast and axilla is moderate in TN and poor in HER2-positive breast cancer. Furthermore, ^{18}F-FDG PET/CT can be used to evaluate the response to neoadjuvant chemotherapy in TN disease. The metabolic breast response alone, using ΔSUVmax between PET/CT at baseline and after 6 weeks treatment, predicts pCR total well and adding metabolic axillary response has no additional value. In HER2-

positive tumours, pCR total prediction by the metabolic breast response alone, using SUVmax at PET/CT after 3 weeks treatment, is poor. This may be improved by evaluating both the primary tumour and axillary lymph node metabolic response in this subtype, and separate evaluation is recommended.

Abbreviations
^{18}F-FDG: Fluor-18-deoxyglucose; AC: Doxorubicine/cyclophosphamide; AUC: Area under the curve; CD: Capecitabine/docetaxel; CP: Carboplatin/paclitaxel; CTC: Cyclophosphamide/thiotepa/carboplatin; FEC-T: Fluorouracil/epirubicin/cyclophosphamide/trastuzumab; HER2: Human epidermal growth factor receptor-2; HRD: Homologous recombination deficient; MARI: Marking the axilla with radioactive iodine seeds; MRI: Magnetic resonance imaging; NST: Neoadjuvant systemic treatment; pCR: Pathologic complete response; PET/CT: Positron emission tomography combined with computed tomography; PTC: Paclitaxel/trastuzumab/carboplatin; ROI: Region of interest; SNP: Sentinel node procedure; SUVmax: Maximum standardised uptake value; TN: Triple-negative

Acknowledgements
The authors thank the patients and their families for participating in this study, and the medical doctors and clinical research nurses for their effort and committment.
No additional data are available upon request as all data are represented in the manuscript.

Funding
This study was funded by CTMM, Centre for Translational Molecular Medicine (http://www.ctmm.nl/), project Breast CARE (grant 030-104). The funding source did not have a role in the design of the study, collection, analysis, and interpretation of data and in writing the manuscript.

Authors' contributions
Study concepts: ER, KG, MVP, RVO. Study design: ER, KG, MVP, RVO. Data acquisition: BK, ER, GS, KP, MvR, RVO, SR, ST, WV. PET/CT evaluation: BK, MvR, RVO, SR, ST, WV. Quality control of data and algorithms: BK, KP, MvR, ST, WV. Data analysis and interpretation: GS, MVP, MvR, WV. Statistical analyses: MvR. Manuscript preparation: BK, GS, MvR, ST, WV. Manuscript editing: BK, ER, JW, KG, KP, GS, MVP, MvR, RVO, SR, ST, WV. Manuscript review: BK, ER, JW, KG, KP, GS, MVP, MvR, RVO, SR, ST, WV. All authors read and approved the final manuscript

Competing interests
The authors declare that they have no conflicting interests.

Author details
[1]Department of Medical Oncology, Netherlands Cancer Institute, Plesmanlaan 121, 1066 CX Amsterdam, The Netherlands. [2]Department of Nuclear Medicine, Netherlands Cancer Institute, Plesmanlaan 121, 1066 CX Amsterdam, The Netherlands. [3]Department of Surgical Oncology, Netherlands Cancer Institute, Plesmanlaan 121, 1066 CX Amsterdam, The Netherlands. [4]Department of Radiology, Netherlands Cancer Institute, Plesmanlaan 121, 1066 CX Amsterdam, The Netherlands. [5]Department of Department of Radiology/Image Sciences Institute, University Medical Centre Utrecht, Heidelberglaan 100, 3584 CX Utrecht, The Netherlands. [6]Department of Pathology and Division of Molecular Pathology, Netherlands Cancer Institute, Plesmanlaan 121, 1066 CX Amsterdam, The Netherlands.

References
1. Mieog JS, van der Hage JA, van de Velde CJ. Preoperative chemotherapy for women with operable breast cancer. Cochrane Database Syst Rev. 2007;(2): CD005002.
2. Donker M, Straver ME, Wesseling J, Loo CE, Schot M, Drukker CA, et al. Marking axillary lymph nodes with radioactive iodine seeds for axillary staging after neoadjuvant systemic treatment in breast cancer patients: the MARI procedure. Ann Surg. 2015;261:378–82.
3. von Minckwitz G, Blohmer JU, Costa SD, Denkert C, Eidtmann H, Eiermann W, et al. Response-guided neoadjuvant chemotherapy for breast cancer. J Clin Oncol. 2013;31:3623–30.
4. Coudert B, Pierga JY, Mouret-Reynier MA, Kerrou K, Ferrero JM, Petit T, et al. Use of [(18)F]-FDG PET to predict response to neoadjuvant trastuzumab and docetaxel in patients with HER2-positive breast cancer, and addition of bevacizumab to neoadjuvant trastuzumab and docetaxel in [(18)F]-FDG PET-predicted non-responders (AVATAXHER): an open-label, randomised phase 2 trial. Lancet Oncol. 2014;15:1493–502.
5. Avril S, Muzic Jr RF, Plecha D, Traughber BJ, Vinayak S, Avril N. 18F-FDG PET/CT for Monitoring of Treatment Response in Breast Cance. J Nucl Med. 2016;57 suppl 1:34s–9s.
6. Cortazar P, Zhang L, Untch M, Mehta K, Costantino JP, Wolmark N, et al. Pathological complete response and long-term clinical benefit in breast cancer: the CTNeoBC pooled analysis. Lancet. 2014;384:164–72.
7. Garcia Vicente AM, Amo-Salas M, Relea Calatayud F, Munoz Sanchez MD, Pena Pardo FJ, Jimenez Londono GA, et al. Prognostic Role of Early and End-of-Neoadjuvant Treatment 18F-FDG PET/CT in Patients With Breast Cancer. Clin Nucl Med. 2016;41:e313–22.
8. Rousseau C, Devillers A, Campone M, Campion L, Ferrer L, Sagan C, et al. FDG PET evaluation of early axillary lymph node response to neoadjuvant chemotherapy in stage II and III breast cancer patients. Eur J Nucl Med Mol Imaging. 2011;38:1029–36.
9. Groheux D, Majdoub M, Sanna A, de Cremoux P, Hindie E, Giacchetti S, et al. Early Metabolic Response to Neoadjuvant Treatment: FDG PET/CT Criteria according to Breast Cancer Subtype. Radiology. 2015;277:358–71.
10. Groheux D, Hindie E, Giacchetti S, Delord M, Hamy AS, de Roquancourt A, et al. Triple-negative breast cancer: early assessment with 18F-FDG PET/CT during neoadjuvant chemotherapy identifies patients who are unlikely to achieve a pathologic complete response and are at a high risk of early relapse. J Nucl Med. 2012;53:249–54.
11. Humbert O, Berriolo-Riedinger A, Riedinger JM, Coudert B, Arnould L, Cochet A, et al. Changes in 18F-FDG tumor metabolism after a first course of neoadjuvant chemotherapy in breast cancer: influence of tumor subtypes. Ann Oncol. 2012;23:2572–7.
12. Humbert O, Cochet A, Riedinger JM, Berriolo-Riedinger A, Arnould L, Coudert B, et al. HER2-positive breast cancer: (1)(8)F-FDG PET for early prediction of response to trastuzumab plus taxane-based neoadjuvant chemotherapy. Eur J Nucl Med Mol Imaging. 2014;41:1525–33.
13. Humbert O, Riedinger JM, Charon-Barra C, Berriolo-Riedinger A, Desmoulins I, Lorgis V, et al. Identification of biomarkers including 18FDG-PET/CT for early prediction of response to neoadjuvant chemotherapy in Triple Negative Breast Cancer. Clin Cancer Res. 2015;21:5460–8.
14. Pahk K, Kim S, Choe JG. Early prediction of pathological complete response in luminal B type neoadjuvant chemotherapy-treated breast cancer patients: comparison between interim 18F-FDG PET/CT and MRI. Nucl Med Commun. 2015;36:887–91.
15. Lee HW, Lee HM, Choi S-E, Yoo H, Ahn SG, Lee M-K, et al. The Prognostic Impact of Early Change in Standardized Uptake Value of 18F-fluorodeoxy-glucose Positron Emission Tomography after Neoadjuvant Chemotherapy in Locally Advanced Breast Cancer Patients. J Nucl Med. 2016;57:1183–8. doi: 10.2967/jnumed.115.166322.
16. Straver ME, Aukema TS, Olmos RA, Rutgers EJ, Gilhuijs KG, Schot ME, et al. Feasibility of FDG PET/CT to monitor the response of axillary lymph node metastases to neoadjuvant chemotherapy in breast cancer patients. Eur J Nucl Med Mol Imaging. 2010;37:1069–76.
17. Koolen BB, Valdes Olmos RA, Wesseling J, Vogel WV, Vincent AD, Gilhuijs KG, et al. Early assessment of axillary response with (1)(8)F-FDG PET/CT during neoadjuvant chemotherapy in stage II-III breast cancer: implications for surgical management of the axilla. Ann Surg Oncol. 2013;20:2227–35.
18. Garcia Vicente AM, Soriano Castrejon A, Leon Martin A, Relea Calatayud F, Munoz Sanchez Mdel M, Cruz Mora MA, et al. Early and delayed prediction of axillary lymph node neoadjuvant response by (18)F-FDG PET/CT in patients with locally advanced breast cancer. Eur J Nucl Med Mol Imaging. 2014;41:1309–18.

Additional value of 18F-FDG PET/CT evaluation in axillary nodes during neoadjuvant therapy...

89

19. Koolen BB, Pengel KE, Wesseling J, Vogel WV, Vrancken Peeters MJ, Vincent AD, et al. Sequential (18)F-FDG PET/CT for early prediction of complete pathological response in breast and axilla during neoadjuvant chemotherapy. Eur J Nucl Med Mol Imaging. 2014;41:32–40.

20. Garcia Garcia-Esquinas MA, Arrazola Garcia J, Garcia-Saenz JA, Furio-Bacete V, Fuentes Ferrer ME, Ortega Candil A, et al. Predictive value of PET-CT for pathological response in stages II and III breast cancer patients following neoadjuvant chemotherapy with docetaxel. Rev Esp Med Nucl Imagen Mol. 2014;33:14–21.

21. Dalus K, Rendl G, Rettenbacher L, Pirich C. FDG PET/CT for monitoring response to neoadjuvant chemotherapy in breast cancer patients. Eur J Nucl Med Mol Imaging. 2010;37:1992–3.

22. Loo CE, Teertstra HJ, Rodenhuis S, van de Vijver MJ, Hannemann J, Muller SH, et al. Dynamic contrast-enhanced MRI for prediction of breast cancer response to neoadjuvant chemotherapy: initial results. AJR Am J Roentgenol. 2008;191:1331–8.

23. Sonke GS, Mandjes IA, Holtkamp MJ, Schot M, van Werkhoven E, Wesseling J, et al. Paclitaxel, carboplatin, and trastuzumab in a neo-adjuvant regimen for HER2-positive breast cancer. Breast J. 2013;19:419–26.

24. Boellaard R, O'Doherty MJ, Weber WA, Mottaghy FM, Lonsdale MN, Stroobants SG, et al. FDG PET and PET/CT: EANM procedure guidelines for tumour PET imaging: version 1.0. Eur J Nucl Med Mol Imaging. 2010;37:181–200.

25. El Khouli RH, Macura KJ, Barker PB, Habba MR, Jacobs MA, Bluemke DA. Relationship of temporal resolution to diagnostic performance for dynamic contrast enhanced MRI of the breast. J Magn Reson Imaging. 2009;30:999–1004.

26. Hinkle DE, Wiersma W, Jurs SG. Applied Statistics for the Behavioral Sciences. 5th ed. Boston: Houghton Mifflin; 2003.

27. DeLong ER, DeLong DM, Clarke-Pearson DL. Comparing the areas under two or more correlated receiver operating characteristic curves: a nonparametric approach. Biometrics. 1988;44:837–45.

28. Donegan WL. Tumor-related prognostic factors for breast cancer. CA Cancer J Clin. 1997;47:28–51.

29. Mougalian SS, Hernandez M, Lei X, Lynch S, Kuerer HM, Symmans WF, et al. Ten-Year Outcomes of Patients With Breast Cancer With Cytologically Confirmed Axillary Lymph Node Metastases and Pathologic Complete Response After Primary Systemic Chemotherapy. JAMA Oncol. 2016;2:508–16.

30. Groheux D, Giacchetti S, Hatt M, Marty M, Vercellino L, de Roquancourt A, et al. HER2-overexpressing breast cancer: FDG uptake after two cycles of chemotherapy predicts the outcome of neoadjuvant treatment. Br J Cancer. 2013;109:1157–64.

31. Groheux D, Hindie E, Giacchetti S, Hamy AS, Berger F, Merlet P, et al. Early assessment with 18F-fluorodeoxyglucose positron emission tomography/computed tomography can help predict the outcome of neoadjuvant chemotherapy in triple negative breast cancer. Eur J Cancer. 2014;50:1864–71.

32. Wahl RL, Jacene H, Kasamon Y, Lodge MA. From RECIST to PERCIST: Evolving Considerations for PET response criteria in solid tumors. J Nucl Med. 2009;50(suppl 1):122S–50S.

33. JH O, Lodge MA, Wahl RL. Practical PERCIST: A Simplified Guide to PET Response Criteria in Solid Tumors 1.0. Radiology. 2016;280:576–84.

34. Jung SY, Kim SK, Nam BH, Min SY, Lee SJ, Park C, et al. Prognostic Impact of [18F] FDG-PET in operable breast cancer treated with neoadjuvant chemotherapy. Ann Surg Oncol. 2010;17:247–53.

35. Groheux D, Mankoff D, Espie M, Hindie E. F-FDG PET/CT in the early prediction of pathological response in aggressive subtypes of breast cancer: review of the literature and recommendations for use in clinical trials. Eur J Nucl Med Mol Imaging. 2016;43:983–93.

36. Liu Q, Wang C, Li P, Liu J, Huang G, Song S. The Role of (18)F-FDG PET/CT and MRI in Assessing Pathological Complete Response to Neoadjuvant Chemotherapy in Patients with Breast Cancer: A Systematic Review and Meta-Analysis. Biomed Res Int. 2016;2016:3746232.

37. Hieken TJ, Boughey JC, Jones KN, Shah SS, Glazebrook KN. Imaging response and residual metastatic axillary lymph node disease after neoadjuvant chemotherapy for primary breast cancer. Ann Surg Oncol. 2013;20:3199–204.

38. Gebhart G, Lamberts LE, Wimana Z, Garcia C, Emonts P, Ameye L, et al. Molecular imaging as a tool to investigate heterogeneity of advanced HER2-positive breast cancer and to predict patient outcome under trastuzumab emtansine (T-DM1): the ZEPHIR trial. Ann Oncol. 2016;27:619–24.

11

Can morphological MRI differentiate between primary central nervous system lymphoma and glioblastoma?

H. Malikova[1,2]*, E. Koubska[1], J. Weichet[1,2], J. Klener[3], A. Rulseh[1,4], R. Liscak[5] and Z. Vojtech[6,7]

Abstract

Background: Primary central nervous system lymphoma (PCNSL) is a rare, aggressive brain neoplasm that accounts for roughly 2-6% of primary brain tumors. In contrast, glioblastoma (GBM) is the most frequent and severe glioma subtype, accounting for approximately 50% of diffuse gliomas. The aim of the present study was to evaluate morphological MRI characteristics in histologically-proven PCNSL and GBM at the time of their initial presentation.

Methods: We retrospectively evaluated standard diagnostic MRI examinations in 54 immunocompetent patients (26 female, 28 male; age 62.6 ± 11.5 years) with histologically-proven PCNSL and 54 GBM subjects (21 female, 33 male; age 59 ± 14 years).

Results: Several significant differences between both infiltrative brain tumors were found. PCNSL lesions enhanced homogenously in 64.8% of cases, while nonhomogeneous enhancement was observed in 98.1% of GBM cases. Necrosis was present in 88.9% of GBM lesions and only 5.6% of PCNSL lesions. PCNSL presented as multiple lesions in 51.9% cases and in 35.2% of GBM cases; however, diffuse infiltrative type of brain involvement was observed only in PCNSL (24.1%). Optic pathways were infiltrated more commonly in PCNSL than in GBM (42.6% vs. 5.6%, respectively, $p < 0.001$). Other cranial nerves were affected in 5.6% of PCNSL, and in none of GBM. Signs of bleeding were rare in PCNSL (5.6%) and common in GBM (44.4%); $p < 0.001$. Both supratentorial and infratentorial localization was present only in PCNSL (27.7%). Involvement of the basal ganglia was more common in PCNSL (55.6%) than in GBM (18.5%); ($p < 0.001$). Cerebral cortex was affected significantly more often in GBM (83.3%) than in PCNSL (51.9%); mostly by both enhancing and non-enhancing infiltration.

Conclusion: Routine morphological MRI is capable of differentiating between GBM and PCNSL lesions in many cases at time of initial presentation. A solitary infiltrative supratentorial lesion with nonhomogeneous enhancement and necrosis was typical for GBM. PCNSL presented with multiple lesions that enhanced homogenously or as diffuse infiltrative type of brain involvement, often with basal ganglia and optic pathways affection.

Keywords: Conventional MRI, Enhancement, Initial evaluation

* Correspondence: hanamalikova123@gmail.com
[1]Department of Radiology, Na Homolce Hospital, Roentgenova 2, Prague 15000, Czech Republic
[2]Department of Radiology, Third Faculty of Medicine, Charles University in Prague and Faculty Hospital Kralovske Vinohrady, Ruska 87, Prague 10000, Czech Republic
Full list of author information is available at the end of the article

Background

Although glioblastoma (GBM) and primary central nervous lymphoma (PCNSL) differ in many respects, it is often reported that morphological differentiation between them by MRI is difficult [1]. PCNSL is a rare, aggressive brain neoplasm that may involve the brain, leptomeninges, spinal cord and eyes without systematic lymphomatous involvement, and accounts for approximately 2-6% of primary brain tumors [2]. PCNSL is typically diffuse large B-cell lymphoma (DLBCL), and rarely other types such as Burkitt lymphoma, T cell lymphoma or Hodgkin lymphoma [3, 4]. In immunocompetent patients, PCNSL usually affects older individuals with a slight male predilection and its incidence has been increasing in recent years [5–8]. Immunocompromised patients especially with AIDS have an increased risk of PCNSL, which develops at younger age [5]. The treatment of choice for PCNSL is radiation therapy and/or chemotherapy [9]. In contrast, gliomas are the most common primary brain tumors, accounting for roughly 70% of all primary brain tumors in adults. GBM is the most frequent and severe glioma subtype and accounts for about approximately 50% of diffuse gliomas. It is characterized by infiltration beyond the enhancing margin and with rapid growth [10, 11]. The primary treatment for GBM is surgical resection followed by radiation therapy and chemotherapy [12].

It has been suggested that MRI has limited potential in differentiating between PCNSL and GBM [1], and several studies have employed advanced MRI techniques such as diffusion-weighed imaging (DWI), MR spectroscopy or dynamic contrast enhancement [13–16]. Systematic evaluation of conventional morphological MRI manifestations of both tumors is, however, lacking. Therefore, we endeavored to compare morphological signs on MRI in sufficiently large groups of GBM and PCNSL patients at their initial presentation, thus on the first diagnostic MRI. Only immunocompetent PCNSL subjects were included due to potential confounding effects of pharmacotherapy in immunocompromised patients, such as corticosteroid therapy.

Methods

Patient selection

We retrospectively evaluated all available MRI examinations and medical records in patients with histologically proven PCNSL and GBM. All patients provided written, informed consent to treatment and agreed with publishing medical data in scientific literature in anonymous form. This retrospective study was approved by the Ethics committee of Na Homolce Hospital, Prague, Czech Republic.

Group A (PCNSL) Patients with histologically-proven CNS lymphoma acquired at our institution from 2007–2015 were included. DLBCL was histologically proven in all patients, and systemic lymphoma was excluded by bone marrow biopsy, whole-body computed tomography (CT) or whole-body positron emission tomography/CT. From 64 subjects with PCNSL, 54 were immunocompetent while 10 were excluded due to known immunodeficiency. Thus, 54 immunocompetent PCNSL patients were included. Histological specimens were obtained by stereotactic biopsy ($N = 43$), open surgical biopsy ($N = 6$) or by open surgical resection ($N = 5$).

Group B (GBM) Fifty-four consecutive patients with histologically proven GBM (WHO grade IV) acquired at our institution from 2012-2013 were additionally included. Subjects with secondary upgrade of previously known low grade glioma were excluded. The diagnosis was confirmed by histological examination of specimens obtained by open surgery with one exception, in which the specimen was obtained by stereotactic biopsy.

MRI examination

All MRI examinations were performed at different whole-body 1.5 T scanners and included the following sequences: fast spin echo (FSE) T2-weighted images (T2 WI), T2-weighted fluid-attenuated inversion recovery (FLAIR), susceptibility-weighted images (SWI) or T2* gradient echo (GE). Inconstantly diffusion-weighted images (DWI; b-value 1000) and ADC maps were available (in 35 PCNSL patients and in 51 GBM patients). After intravenous gadolinium contrast administration, spin echo (SE) T1 WI or GE T1 3D were always performed. All MRI examinations were evaluated by consensual reading by 2 experienced radiologists.

The following signs were assessed on the initial MRI examination (for details, see Table 3): lesion localization; quantity (solitary, multiple and diffuse infiltrative) and quality (demarcated, infiltrative and diffuse infiltrative) of the lesions; type of enhancement and necrosis presence; diffusion restriction presence; meningeal and/or ependymal involvement; cranial nerve involvement; involvement of the corpus callosum, butterfly pattern; involvement of the basal ganglia; presence of perifocal vasogenic edema; signs of bleeding. Inclusion criteria for solitary or multiple infiltrative lesions were as follows (at least one criterion): ill-defined borders; non-enhancing portions of tumor beyond enhancing portion; infiltration of the ependyma, meninges or cranial nerves. Diffuse infiltrative lesions were defined as follows: involvement of both white and grey matter by enhancing tumorous affection (which was nonhomogenous, patchy, worm-like, stripy, etc.) and non-enhancing tumorous infiltration, which was spread along to large white matter tracts and continuously affected at least a) more than 2/3 of one cerebral hemisphere and/or b) different extend of both supratentorial and infratentorial regions. See also

Fig. 1. Inclusion criteria for meningeal and ependymal involvement were thickening and enhancing meningeal /ependymal surfaces, which can be smooth, irregular or nodular.

Statistics

Data were expressed as mean $\pm$ SD and as median. Categorical values were analyzed using the chi-squared test. Unpaired t-test was used for the comparison of the time intervals. P-values <0.05 were considered significant. Analyses were performed using STATISTICA software version 12.

Results

Patient and clinical data

Patient demographic data are summarized in Table 1. In the Table 1 you can also find detailed data about the time intervals from clinical onset to initial brain MRI and initial MRI to intervention (open surgery or stereotactic biopsy). The time interval between clinical onset and initial brain MRI did not significantly differ between PCNSL and GBM; however interval between the initial MRI and stereotactic biopsy/surgery was significantly

Table 1 Patient selection data

	PCNSL	GBM
NO of patients	54	54
Sex	26 female, 28 male	21 female, 33 male
Age	62.6 ± 11.5 years (median 65 years)	59 ± 14 years (median 62 years)
Interval from the first clinical manifestation to the first MRI	46 ± 89 days (median 30 days) min. 0 day max. 180 days	49 ± 63 days (median 25 days) min. 0 day max. 270 days
Interval from the first MRI to stereobiopsy or surgery	59 ± 118 days (median 30 days) min. 1 day max. 660 days	9 ± 7 days (median 8 days) min. 1 day max. 30 days

Max maximum, *min* minimum, *NO* number

longer in PCNSL subjects (mean 59 ± 118 days, median 30 days) in comparison to GBM patients (mean 9 ± 7 days, median 8 days), ($p = 0.002$).

The patients presented with various clinical manifestations (in some patients a combination of multiple manifestations were present; see Table 2). The most common manifestations included organic brain syndrome, signs

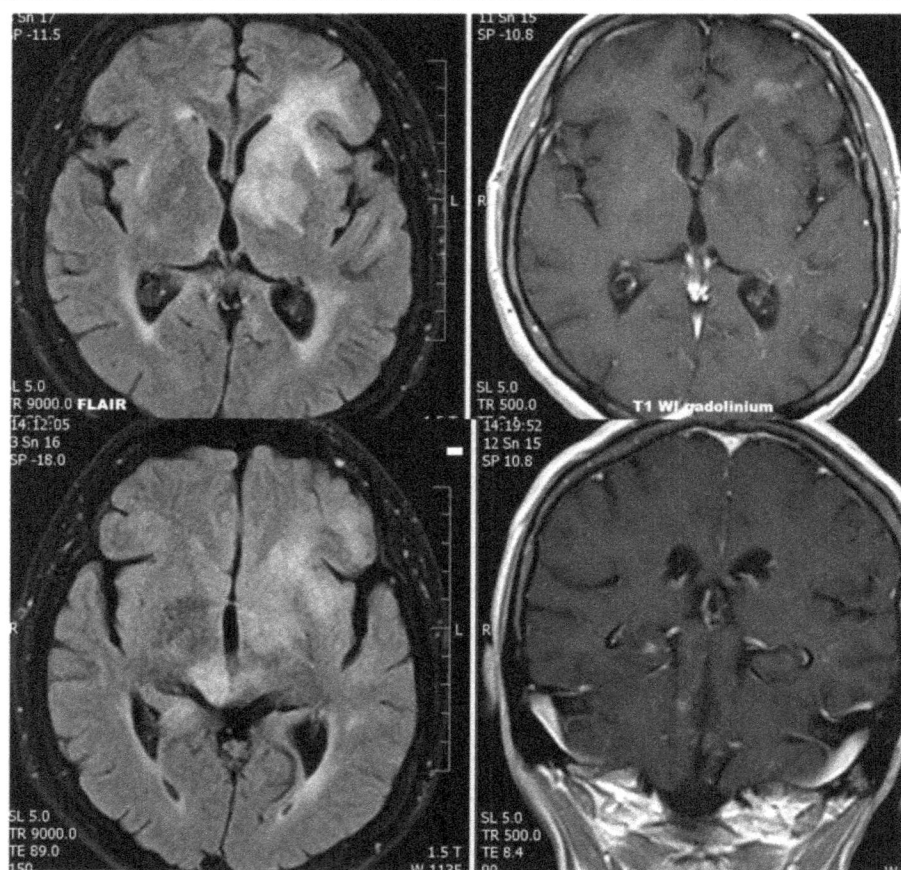

Fig. 1 PCNSL. Diffuse infiltrative brain affection

Table 2 Clinical presentation

Clinical symptoms	PCNSL (NO of patients)	GBM (NO of patients)
Organic brain syndrome	22	12
Signs of intracranial hypertension	16	23
Paresis	16	19
Vertigo	12	13
Phatic disorder	11	14
Visual disturbances	7	3
Cranial nerve dysfunction other than visual disturbance	5	0
Fatigue	4	7
Dysesthesia or hypesthesia	4	1
Seizure	1	9

NO number

of intracranial hypertension, paresis, vertigo or phatic disorder. PCNSL patients presented significantly more often with cranial nerve dysfunction and visual disturbance then GBM subjects, ($p = 0.012$) and also in organic brain syndrome, ($p = 0.038$). GBM patients presented significantly more often by seizures then PCNSL patients, ($p = 0.008$).

MRI findings

Initial diagnostic MRI results for both groups are summarized in Table 3. PCNSL lesions were generally localized supratentorially (66.7%). PCNSL affected both white and grey matter, basal ganglia involvement was present in 55.6%, and cortical grey matter was affected in 51.9%. Cortical grey matter was involved by both enhancing and non-enhancing tumorous infiltration in 37.1% of cases, only enhancing portion was present in 3.7% of cases, only non-enhancing infiltration was seen in 11.1% of cases. Solitary affection of white matter was found only in 7.4%; in 3.8% an isolated involvement of basal ganglia was present and in one case (1.9%) solitary

Table 3 MRI findings in PCNSL and GBM at the time of initial evaluation

MRI finding		PCNSL	GBM	*p*-value
Localization	only supratentorial	**66.7%**	**98.1%**	**<0.001**
	only infratentorial	5.5%	1.9%	0.308
	supra- and infratentorial	**27.7%**	**0%**	**<0.001**
Type of lesions	solitary demarcated lesion	**3.7%**	**13%**	**0.046**
	solitary infiltrative type	20.4%	51.9%	0.121
	multiple infiltrative lesions	51.9%	35.2%	0.081
	diffuse infiltrative type	**24.1%**	**0%**	**<0.001**
Type of enhancement	homogeneous	**64.8%**	**0%**	**<0.001**
	nonhomogeneous	**14.8%**	**98.1%**	**<0.001**
	diffuse infiltrative – worm-like, patchy, stripy…	**20.4%**	**0%**	**<0.001**
	presence of necrosis	**5.6%**	**88.9%**	**<0.001**
Involvement of brain surface	without reaching brain surface	12.9%	11.1%	0.567
	reaching brain surface	87%	88.9%	0.846
	meningeal infiltration	35.2%	46.3%	0.240
	ependymal infiltration	53.7%	37%	0.054
Optic nerves, chiasma or tracts involvement		**42.6%**	**5.6%**	**<0.001**
Cranial nerves involvement (optical nerves and tracts excluded)		5.6%	0%	0.079
Corpus callosum infiltration		42.6%	44.4%	0.846
Butterfly pattern		24.1%	14.8%	0.224
Basal ganglia involvement		**55.6%**	**18.5%**	**<0.001**
Cerebral cortex involvement		**83.3%**	**51.9%**	**<0.001**
[a]DWI	free diffusion	1.9%	10.4%	0.189
	restricted diffusion in some part of the solid	97%	89.6%	0.189
Signs of bleeding		**5.6%**	**44.4%**	**<0.001**
Presence of vasogenic edema		92.6%	83.3%	0.139

[a]DWI was available in 35 PCNSL patients and 51 GBM patients. Statisticaly significant results are in bold (*p* less than 0.05)

infiltration of hypothalamus or vestibular nerve was found. At time of initial MRI, PCNSL appeared as multiple infiltrative lesions in 51.9% of cases, as a solitary infiltrative lesion in 20.4% of cases and as a diffuse infiltrative affection in 24.1% (Fig. 1). Solitary demarcated lesions were rare (3.7%). PCNSL enhanced homogenously (64.8%), vasogenic perifocal edema was present in most cases (92.6%), and diffusion restriction was detected in 97% of cases (Fig. 2). Optic nerves and tracts were infiltrated in 42.6% of cases (Fig. 3). Other cranial nerves were affected in 5.6% of PCNSL cases; in one case (1.9%) the optic and trigeminal nerve was affected, and in one case (1.9%) the optic nerves and both auditory and facial nerves were involved and in one case (1.9%) solitary infiltration of the auditory nerve was present without other brain lesions (Fig. 4a, b). PCNSL typically reached the surface of the brain (87%) with meningeal infiltration present in 35.2% of cases and ependymal infiltration in 53.7% of cases. Signs of bleeding (5.6%) were rare.

Nearly all lesions in GBM subjects were localized supratentorially (98.1%); solitary infiltrative lesions were present in 51.9% of cases and multiple lesions in 35.2%.

Nonhomogeneous enhancement of GBM lesions was detected in 98.1% of cases and necrosis was present in 88.9% of cases (Fig. 5). GBM dominantly affected white matter; however, in most cases also cortical grey matter was affected (83.3%). In case of cortical involvement by GBM (83.3%), in 63% of cases cortex was affected by enhancing and also non-enhancing portion of tumorous infiltration; in 20.3% of cases cortex was affected only by non-enhancing portion of tumor. Basal ganglia were target in 18.5% and mostly in their margins. Isolated involvement of cortical grey matter was not found. GBM very often reached the surface of the brain (88.9%), and meningeal infiltration was found in 46.3% of cases and ependymal infiltration in 37% of cases (Fig. 6). Vasogenic edema was present in 83.3% of cases. Diffusion restriction was detected in solid portions of the tumor in 89.6% of cases, while no diffusion restriction was observed in the necrotic portion of the tumor. Signs of bleeding were found in 44.4% of cases. In GBM cases optic nerves, chiasma or tracts were infiltrated in 5.6%; the affection of other cranial nerves was not found. Only 2 cases were exceptional. In one case, the lesion was

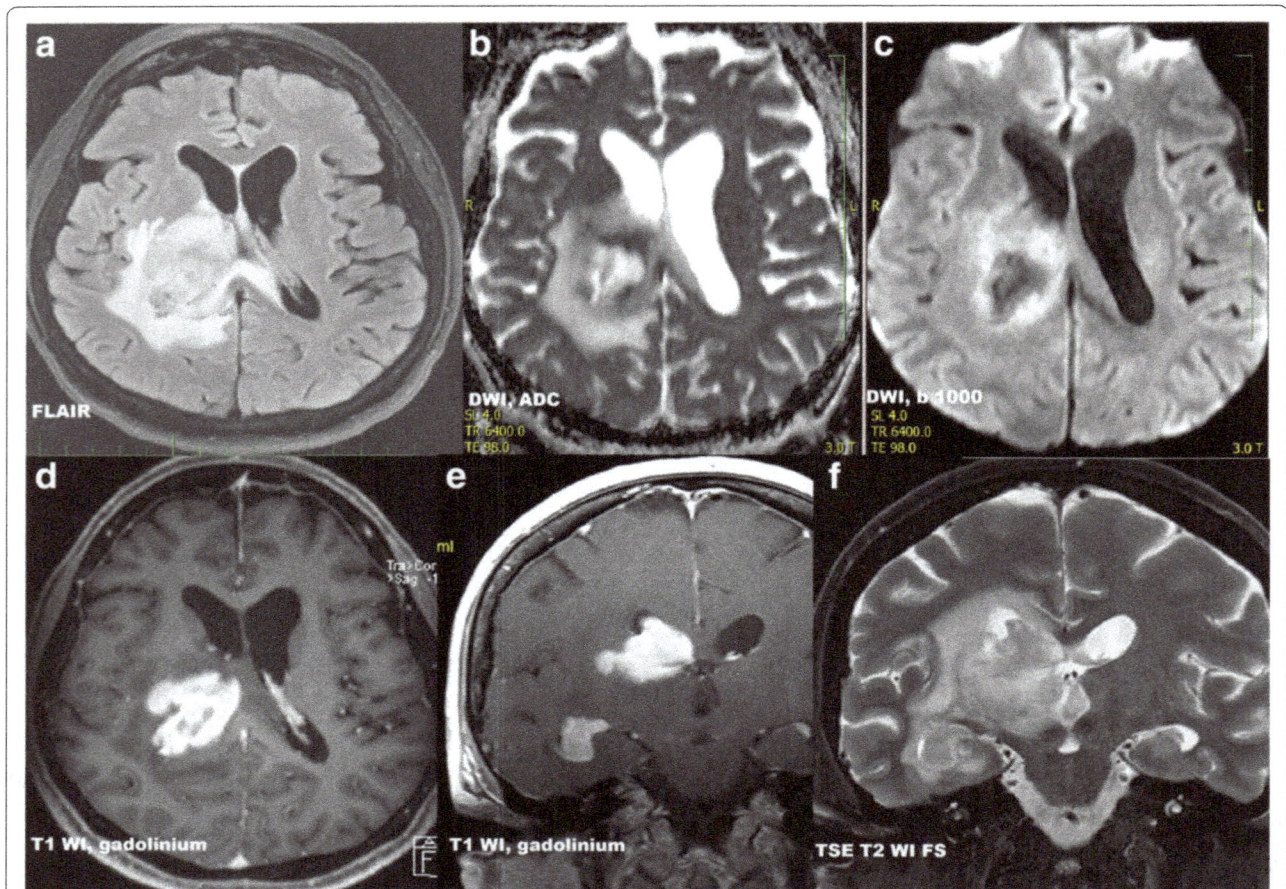

Fig. 2 a) FLAIR, axial scan **b)** DWI, ADC map, axial scan **c)** DWI, b=1000, axial scan **d)** SE T1 WI after intravenous gadolinium contrast administration, axial scan **e)** SE T1 WI after intravenous gadolinium contrast administration, coronal scan **f)** FSE T2 WI with fat saturation, coronal scan

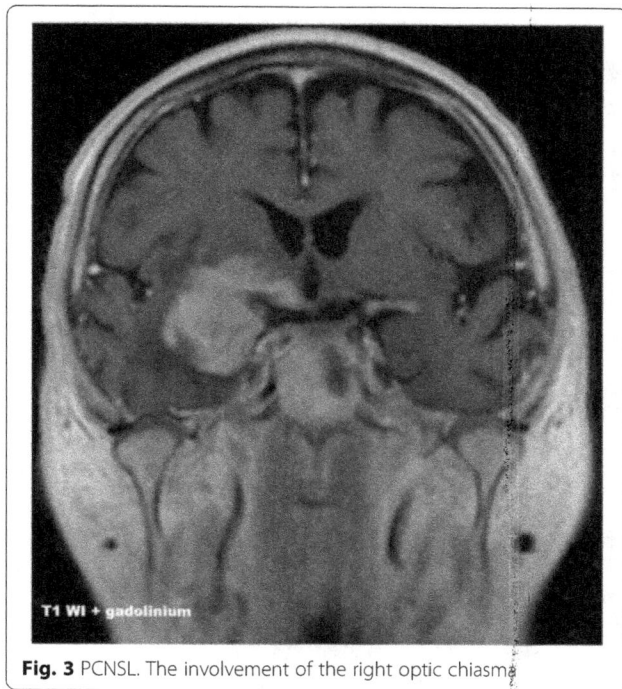

Fig. 3 PCNSL. The involvement of the right optic chiasma

localized infratentorially with nonhomogeneous enhancement (Fig. 7). In the second exceptional case, a non-enhancing supratentorial lesion was present suspected to be low-grade glioma; however, histology confirmed the diagnosis of GBM (WHO Grade IV).

Several significant differences between both brain infiltrative tumors were found (see Table 3). Notably, no homogenous enhancement was found in GBM, in contrast to homogeneous enhancement detected in 64.8% of PCNSL lesions ($p < 0.001$). Enhancement in GBM was nonhomogeneous in 98.1% of cases (no enhancement in 1 case) and necrosis was present in 88.9% of cases. Conversely, necrosis was present only in 5.6% of PCNSL cases and nonhomogeneous enhancement in 14.8% of PCNSL cases (both $p < 0.001$). Diffuse infiltrative type of brain involvement was observed only in PCNSL (24.1% of cases). Additionally, optic pathways infiltration was more frequent in PCNSL than in GBM ($p < 0.001$); present in 42.6% of PCNSL cases and only in 5.6% of GBM cases. Signs of bleeding were more common in GBM (44.4%) than PCNSL (5.6%); $p < 0.001$. Both supratentorial and infratentorial localization was present only in PCNSL (27.7%). The basal ganglia were involved more often in PCNSL (55.6%) than in GBM (18.5%); $p < 0.001$. Finally, cerebral cortex was affected significantly often in GBM (83.3%) than in PCNSL (51.9%); mostly by both enhancing and non-enhancing infiltration. In the Table 4 you can find combinations of several MRI findings and their occurrence in both groups. According those findings we constructed the diagram of the decision tree

analysis (Fig. 8). According to Tables 3 and 4, major criteria in decision making process between PCNSL and GBM are the type of enhancement and presence or absence of necrosis. As minor criteria we considered basal ganglia and optic pathways affections, signs of bleeding, both supratentorial and infratentorial localization and diffuse infiltrative type of lesion.

Discussion

In the present study, we compared morphological MRI characteristics in PCNSL and GBM at time of initial MRI. At initial evaluation, PCNSL lesions were presented as multiple infiltrative lesions, which enhanced homogenously or as diffuse infiltrative affection of the brain. GBM typically manifested as a supratentorial solitary infiltrative tumor nearly in all cases nonhomogeneous enhancement was present with evident necrosis. Both GBM and PCNSL lesions reached the surface of the brain in most cases; meningeal and ependymal infiltration was not uncommon.

We detected several significant differences between PCNSL and GBM lesions. The most striking difference was in enhancement patterns; while homogeneous enhancement was not detected in GBM, most PCNSL lesions (64.8%) enhanced homogeneously. Additionally, necrosis was observed in most GBM lesions (88.9%) but was rare in PCNSL (5.6%). Optic pathways infiltration was common in PCNSL and rare in GBM. Other cranial nerves infiltrations were not frequent and were found only in PCNSL (5.6%). Signs of bleeding were rare in PCNSL and common in GBM. The basal ganglia involvement occurred more frequently in PCNSL than in GBM. Diffuse infiltrative type of brain involvement was observed only in PCNSL (24.1%) and also only PCNSL was localized both supratentorial and infratentorial (27.7%). Finally, cerebral cortex was affected significantly often in GBM (83.3%) than in PCNSL (51.9%); mostly by both enhancing and non-enhancing tumorous infiltration. Solitary non-enhancing tumorous affection of cerebral cortex in both diagnoses was uncommon.

Our MRI findings in GBM are in agreement with those reported previously [17]. However, our findings in PCNSL are only partially consistent with those reported by Haldorsen et al. [18]. In the present study, immunocompetent PCNSL patients presented with multiple lesions in 51.9% of cases, and with involvement of the basal ganglia in 55.6% cases. In contrast, Haldorsen et al. reported multiple lesions in only 35% of PCNSL cases, with basal ganglia involvement in 32% of cases [18]. However, they also reported disseminating lesions in 7% of cases [18]. In our study we used category diffused infiltrative affection and probably this category is equal to Haldorsen's disseminating lesions. We found diffuse infiltrative brain affection by PCNSL in 24.1% of cases.

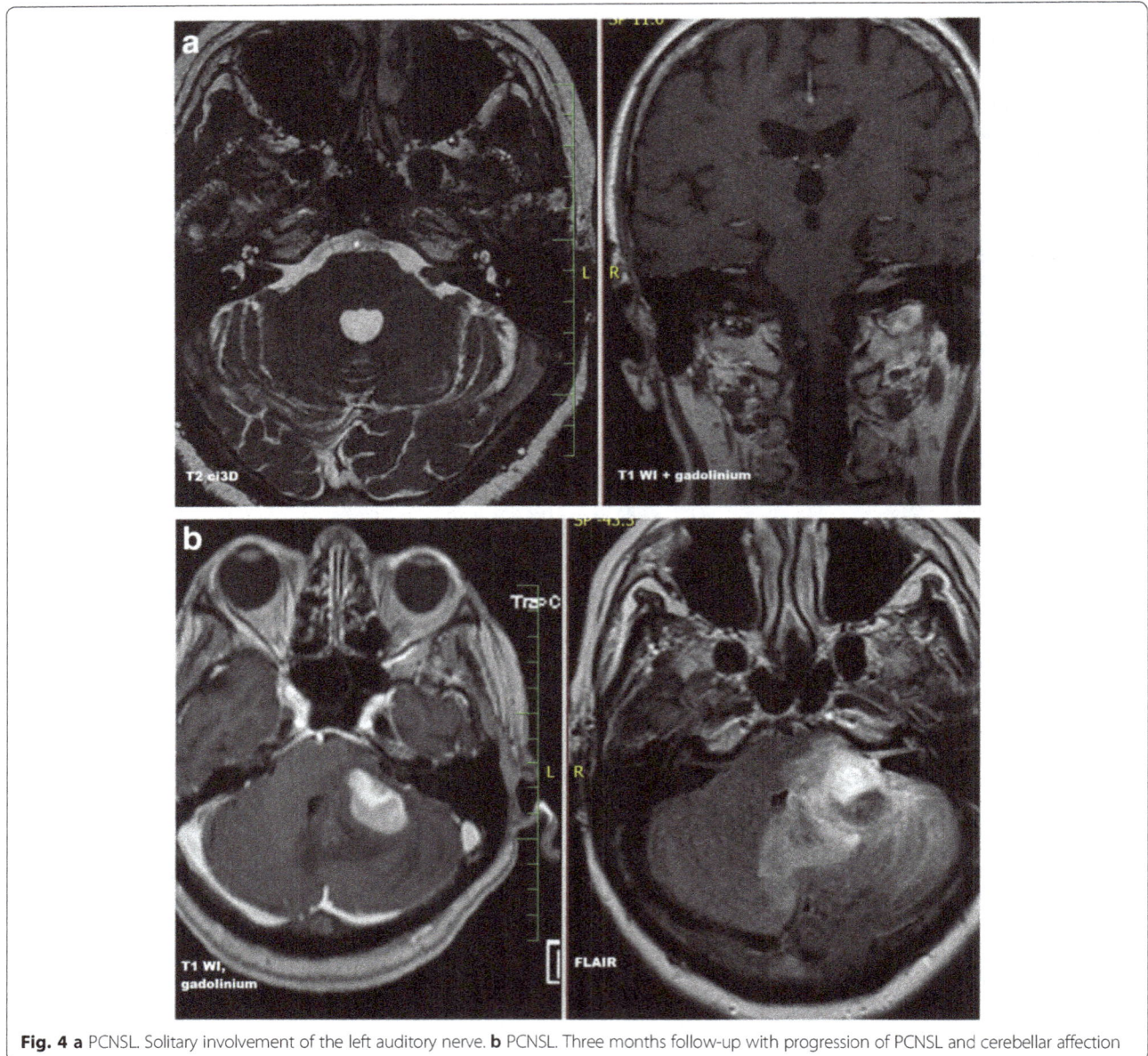

Fig. 4 a PCNSL. Solitary involvement of the left auditory nerve. **b** PCNSL. Three months follow-up with progression of PCNSL and cerebellar affection

They also did not report the presence or absence of cranial nerve infiltration [18]. In our study, optic pathways involvement was present in 42.6% of PCNLS cases, other cranial nerves were affected in 5.6%. In one case, solitary auditory nerve involvement was present without other lesions. Several case reports have been published describing solitary involvement of the auditory nerves in PCNSL manifesting by sudden hearing lost [19, 20]. Cranial nerve and leptomeningeal involvement is considered very common in secondary CNS lymphoma [21]; however, systematic lymphoma was excluded in our patients. One difficulty in comparing our results to those reported previously is that many studies are limited by small sample sizes [22, 23]. Therefore, we consider the study of

Haldorsen et al. as the most reliable for comparison with our results [18]. Their population-based study evaluated CT/MRI features in 75 AIDS-negative patients in Norway between the years 1989-2003 [18]. However, only 52 patients underwent MRI, the rest of patients were examined only by CT, and considering the fact that sensitivity of CT is significantly lower than MRI, some lesions may have been missed [18]. Haldorsen et al. also included patients with immunosuppression therapy (5%) and also 6 patients, in whom only imaging after corticosteroid therapy was available. Differences between our results are partly explainable by designs of patient selection. We could also a little bit hypothesize about changing imaging findings in the time.

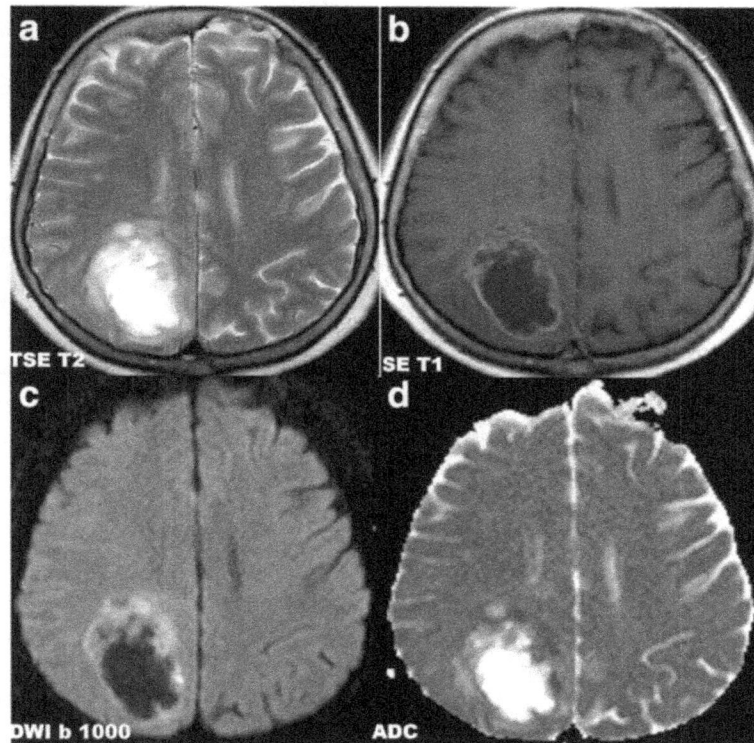

Fig. 5 a) FSE T2 WI, axial scan **b)** SE T1 WI after intravenous gadolinium contrast administration, axial scan **c)** DWI, b=1000, axial scan **d)** DWI, ADC map, axial scan

A number of studies have explored advanced MRI techniques such as DWI, perfusion imaging and MR spectroscopy [15, 24]. As PCNSL is highly cellular, diffusion is often restricted. We detected diffusion restriction in 97% of our PCNSL cases. Accordingly, Toh et al. reported significantly lower fractional anisotropy (FA) and apparent diffusion coefficient (ADC) in PCNSL compared to GBM [25]. Although diffusion restriction is also often present in the solid portion of GBM tumors (89.6% in our GBM group), it is important to note than there is generally free diffusion in the necrotic or cystic portions of GBM tumors. The importance of revascularization through angiogenesis for tumor growth has led to a growing interest in novel imaging techniques such as the assessment of tumor vascularity. MR perfusion imaging can visualize nutritive delivery of arterial blood to

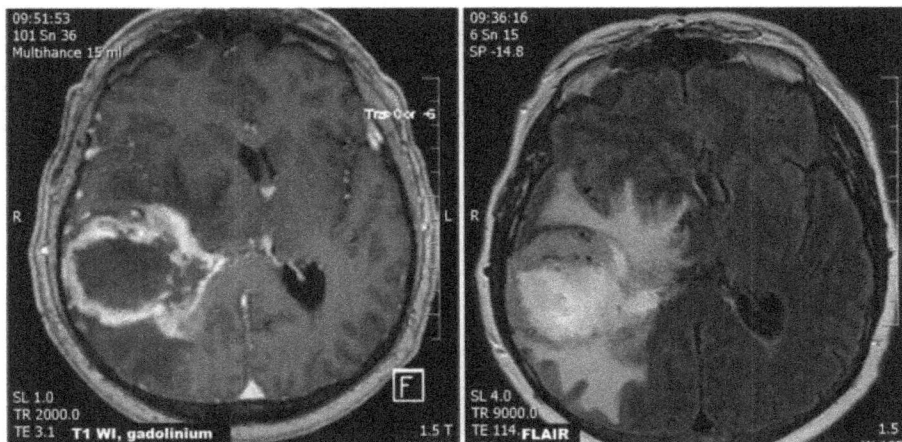

Fig. 6 GBM. GBM with ependymal involvement

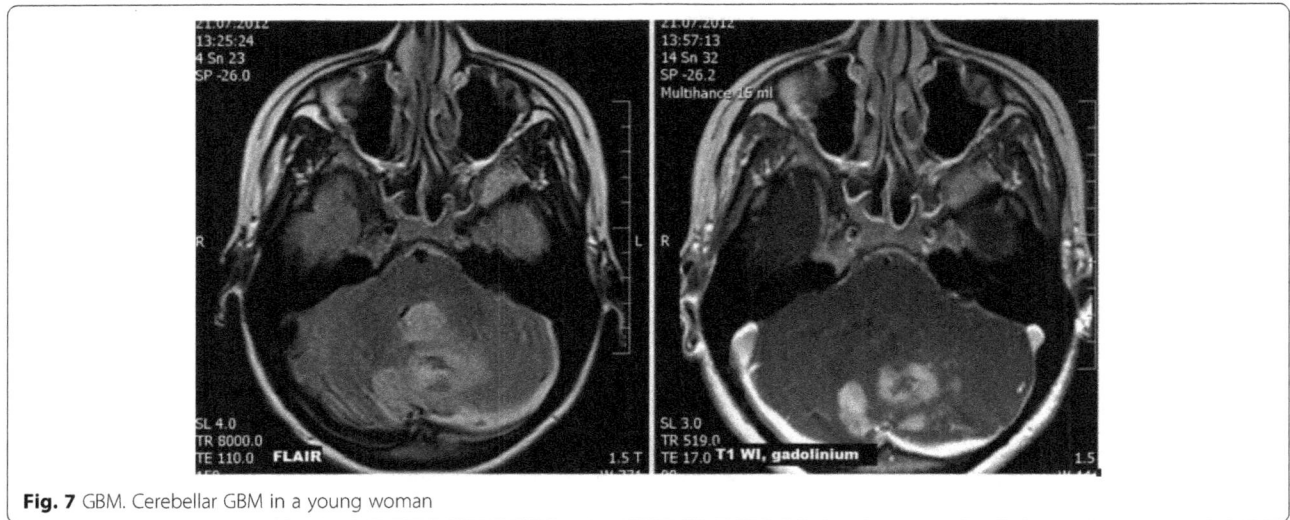

Fig. 7 GBM. Cerebellar GBM in a young woman

the capillary bed in tumors. According to published data, PCNSL demonstrates lower relative mean cerebral blood volume than GBM; likely due to massive leakage of contrast media into the interstitial space [15]. In the MR spectroscopy study by Yamasaki et al., a large lipid peak on ^{1}H-MR spectroscopy images in PCNSL and small or absent lipid peak in GBM without necrosis was found [24]. MR perfusion and spectroscopic data were available only in few cases in the present study, thus we did not have sufficient data for comparison.

PCNSL and GBM are serious malignant brain tumors with different therapeutic management. Histological verification of PCNSL before oncological treatment is mandatory. Open surgery in PCNSL is not necessary; the diagnostic method of choice is stereotactic biopsy, which is not without complication [26]. We believe that the MRI morphological differences between PCNSL and GBM reported in the present study may be useful in daily radiological practice and may help to differentiate between both malignant entities.

The present study has several limitations. Due to its retrospective nature, some MRI examinations were of lower quality and acquired on different whole-body systems. As stated above, we did not have sufficient data for reviewing advanced MRI techniques such as MR spectroscopy or perfusion, also we do not have sufficient data for FA evaluation and not all patients underwent DWI and for measurement of ADC value. In limitations of the study we must mention the fact of relative incidence of both conditions. PCNSL occur less frequently than GBM. This fact makes the diagnosis more complex as no simple morphological feature is able to discriminate between these conditions. We tried to extract combinations of relevant features and provide radiological clues for further work-up.

Conclusions

Routine morphological MRI is capable of differentiating between GBM and PCNSL lesions in many cases at time of initial presentation. PCNSL often presented as

Table 4 Combinations of several MRI findings and their occurrence in PCNSL and GBM at the time of their initial evaluation

Combinations of findings	PCNSL	GBM	p - value
• Supratentorial • Solitary infiltrative • Non-homogenous enhancement • Necrosis presence	3 (23.1%) of 13 solitary cases (5.6% of all PCNSL)	28 (77.8%) of 36 solitary cases (51.9% of all GBM)	**<0.001**
• Supratentorial • Solitary infiltrative • Non-homogenous enhancement	4 (30.8%) of 13 solitary cases (7.4% of all PCNSL)	34 (94.4%) of 36 solitary cases (63% of all GBM)	**<0.001**
• Multiple infiltrative • Homogenous enhancement	27 (96.4%) of 28 multiple cases (50% of all PCNSL)	0 (0%) of 18 multiple cases (0% of all GBM)	**<0.001**
• Diffuse infiltrative type • No necrosis	13 cases (24.1% of all PCNSL)	0 (0%) of all GBM cases	**<0.001**
• Multiple infiltrative • Non-homogenous enhancement	1(3.6%) of 28 multiple cases (1.9% of all PCNSL)	18 (100%) of 18 multiple cases (33.3% of all GBM)	**<0.001**

Statisticaly significant results are in bold (p less than 0.05)

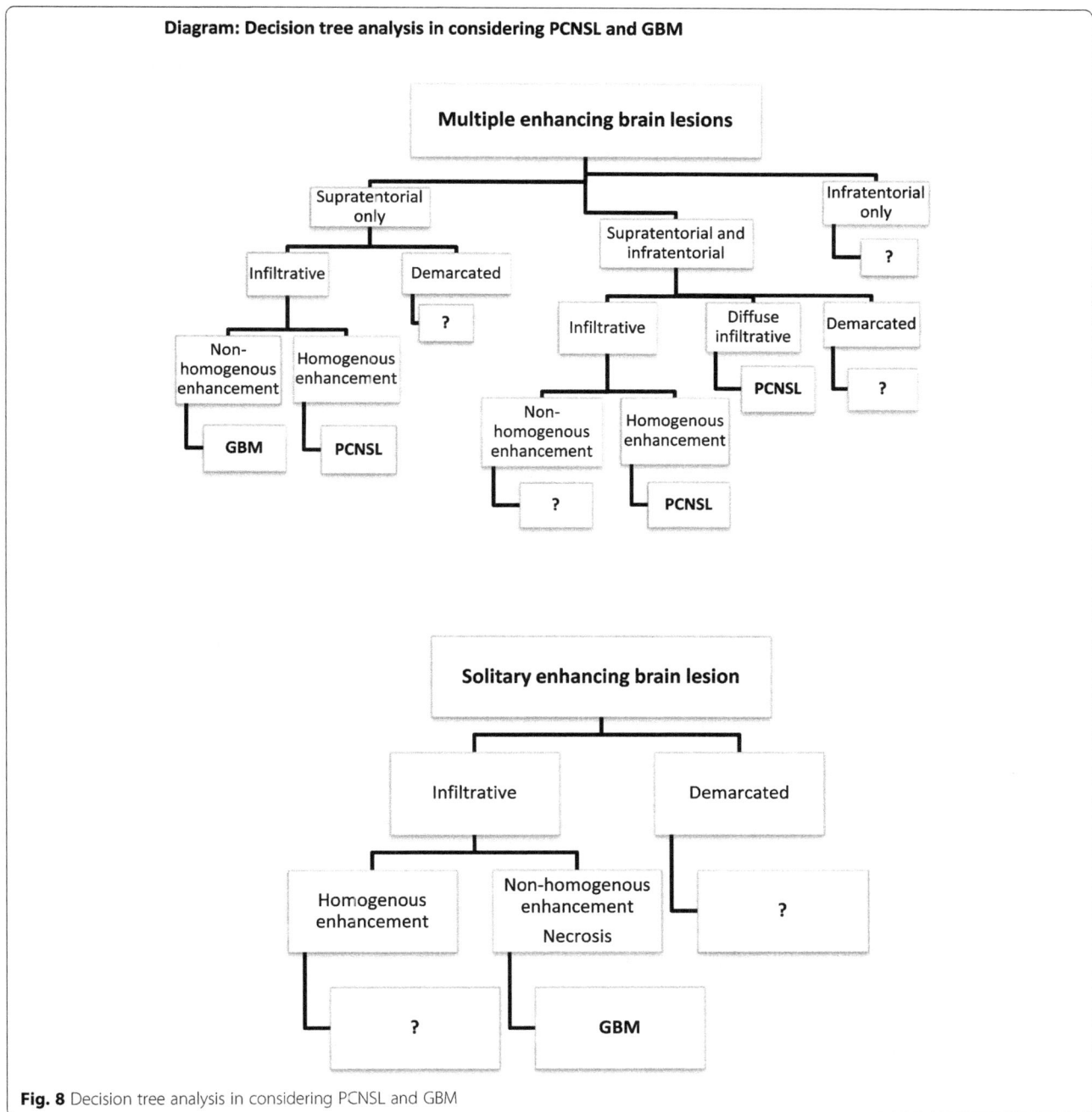

Diagram: Decision tree analysis in considering PCNSL and GBM

Fig. 8 Decision tree analysis in considering PCNSL and GBM

multiple lesions that enhanced homogenously, often with optic pathways infiltration and involvement of the basal ganglia or as diffuse infiltrative type of brain involvement. A solitary supratentorial lesion with nonhomogeneous enhancement and necrosis presence was typical for GBM.

Abbreviations
ADC: apparent diffusion coefficient; CNS: central nervous system; DLBCL: diffuse large B-cell lymphoma; DWI: diffusion-weighted images; FLAIR: T2-weighted fluid-attenuated inversion recovery; FSE: fast spin echo; GBM: glioblastoma; GE: gradient echo; MRI: magnetic resonance imaging; PCNSL: primary central nervous system lymphoma; SWI: susceptibility-weighted images; T: tesla; T1 WI: T1 weighted images; T2 WI: weighted images

Acknowledgements
None.

Funding
The research at Na Homolce Hospital is supported by Ministry of Health, Czech Republic - conceptual development of research organization (Nemocnice Na Homolce - NNH, 00023884, IG 154303), from this support the open access fee is paid.

Authors' contributions

JK and EK collected GBM patients; RL and EK collected PCNSL patients; HM and JW evaluated MRI; HM, ZV and AR prepared manuscript; HM performed statistical analysis. All authors read and approved the final manuscript.

Competing interest

The authors declare that they have no competing interests.

Author details

[1]Department of Radiology, Na Homolce Hospital, Roentgenova 2, Prague 15000, Czech Republic. [2]Department of Radiology, Third Faculty of Medicine, Charles University in Prague and Faculty Hospital Kralovske Vinohrady, Ruska 87, Prague 10000, Czech Republic. [3]Department of Neurosurgery, Na Homolce Hospital, Roentgenova 2, Prague 15000, Czech Republic. [4]Department of Radiology, 1st Faculty of Medicine and General University Hospital, Charles University, Prague, Czech Republic. [5]Department of Stereotactic and Radiation Neurosurgery, Na Homolce Hospital, Roentgenova 2, Prague 15000, Czech Republic. [6]Department of Neurology, Na Homolce Hospital, Roentgenova 2, Prague 15000, Czech Republic. [7]Department of Neurology, Third Faculty of Medicine, Charles University in Prague, Ruska 87, Prague 10000, Czech Republic.

References

1. Al-Okaili RN, Krejza J, Woo JH, Wolf RL, O'Rourke DM, Judy KD, Poptani H, Melhem ER. Intraaxial brain masses: MR imaging-based diagnostic strategy–initial experience. Radiology. 2007;243(2):539–50.
2. van der Sanden GA, Schouten LJ, van Dijck JA, van Andel JP, van der Maazen RW, Coebergh JW, Working Group of Specialists in Neuro-Oncology in the Southern and Eastern Netherlands. Primary central system lymphomas: incidence and survival in the Southern and Eastern Netherlands. Cancer. 2002;94(5):1547–56.
3. Da Silva AN, Lopez MB, Schiff D. Rare pathological variants and presentations of primary central nervous system lymphomas. Neurosurg Focus. 2006;21(5), E7.
4. Bhagavathi S, Wilson JD. Primary central nervous system lymphoma. Arch Pathol Lab Med. 2008;132(11):1830–4.
5. Schabet M. Epidemiology of primary CNS lymphoma. J Neurooncol. 1999; 43(3):199–201.
6. Olson JE, Janney CA, Rao RD, Cerhan JR, Kurtin PJ, Schiff D, Kaplan RS, O'Neill BP. The continuing increase in the incidence of primary central nervous system non-Hodgkin lymphoma: a surveillance, epidemiology, and end results analysis. Cancer. 2002;95(7):1504–10.
7. Hoffman S, Propp JM, McCarthy BJ. Temporal trends in incidence of primary brain tumors in the United States, 1985-1999. Neuro Oncol. 2006;8(1):27–37.
8. Partovi S, Karimi S, Lyo JK, Esmaeili A, Tan J, DeAngelis LM. Multimodality imaging of primary CNS lymphoma in immunocompetent patients. Br J Radiol. 2014;87(1036):20130684.
9. Batchelor T, Loeffler JS. Primary CNS lymphoma. J Clin Oncol. 2006;24(8): 1281–8.
10. Ricard D, Idbaih A, Ducray F, Lahutte M, Hoang-Xuan K, Delattre J-Y. Primary brain tumours in adults. Lancet. 2012;379(9830):1984–96.
11. Stupp R, Mason WP, van den Bent MJ, Weller M, Fisher B, Taphoorn MJ, Belanger K, Brandes AA, Marosi C, Bogdahn U, Curschmann J, Janzer RC, Ludwin SK, Gorlia T, Allgeier A, Lacombe D, Cairncross JG, Eisenhauer E, Mirimanoff RO, European Organisation for Research and Treatment of Cancer Brain Tumor and Radiotherapy Groups; National Cancer Institute of Canada Clinical Trials Group. Radiotherapy plus concomitant and adjuvant temozolomide for glioblastoma. N Engl J Med. 2005;352(10):987–96.
12. Giese A, Westphal M. Treatment of malignant glioma: a problem beyond the margins of resection. J Cancer Res Clin Oncol. 2001;127(4):217–25.
13. Stadnik TW, Chaskis C, Michotte A, Shabana WM, van Rompaey K, Luypaert R, Budinsky L, Jellus V, Osteaux M. Diffusion-weighted MR Imaging of Intracerebral Masses: Comparison with Conventional MR Imaging and Histologic Findings. AJNR. 2001;22(5):969–76.
14. Weber MA, Zoubaa S, Schlieter M, Jüttler E, Huttner HB, Geletneky K, Ittrich C, Lichy MP, Kroll A, Debus J, Giesel FL, Hartmann M, Essig M. Diagnostic

performance of spectroscopic and perfusion MRI for distinction of brain tumors. Neurology. 2006;66(12):1899–906.
15. Kickingereder P, Sahm F, Wiestler B, Roethke M, Heiland S, Schlemmer HP, Wick W, von Deimling A, Bendszus M, Radbruch A. Evaluation of microvascular permeability with dynamic contrast-enhanced MRI for the differentiation of primary CNS lymphoma and glioblastoma: radiologic-pathologic correlation. AJNR. 2014;35(8):1503–8.
16. Ahn SJ, Shin HJ, Chang J-H, Lee S-K. Differentiation between Primary Cerebral Lymphoma and Glioblastoma Using the Apparent Diffusion Coefficient: Comparison of Three Different ROI Methods. PLoS One. 2014;9(11), e112948.
17. Osborn AG, Salzman KL, Jhaveri MD, editors. Diagnostic Imaging Brain. 3rd ed. Philadelphia: Elsevier; 2016.
18. Haldorsen IS, Kråkenes J, Krossness BK, Mella O, Espeland A. CT and MR imaging features of primary central nervous system lymphoma in Norway, 1989-2003. AJNR. 2009;30(4):744–51.
19. Lenarz M, Durisin M, Becker H, Lenarz T, Nejadkazem M. Primary Central Nervous System Lymphoma Presenting as Bilateral Tumors of the Internal Auditory Canal. Skull Base. 2007;17(6):409–12.
20. Wang ZT, Su HH, Hou Y, Chu ST, Lai PH, Tseng HH, Lin SJ, Chou YW. Diffuse Large B-cell Lymphoma of the Cerebellopontine Angle in a Patient with Sudden Hearing Loss and Facial Palsy. J Chin Med Assoc. 2007;70(7):294–7.
21. Haldorsen IS, Espeland A, Larsson EM. Central nervous system lymphoma: characteristic findings on traditional and advanced imaging. AJNR. 2011; 32(6):984–92.
22. Senocak E, Oguz KK, Ozgen B, Mut M, Ayhan S, Berker M, Ozdemir P, Cila A. Parenchymal lymphoma of the brain on initial MR imaging: a comparative study between primary and secondary brain lymphoma. Eur J Radiol. 2011; 79(2):288–94.
23. Mansour A, Qandeel M, Abdel-Razeq H, Abu Ali HA. MR imaging features of intracranial primary CNS lymphoma in immune competent patients. Cancer Imaging. 2014;14(1):22.
24. Yamasaki F, Takayasu T, Nosaka R, Amatya VJ, Doskaliyev A, Akiyama Y, Tominaga A, Takeshima Y, Sugiyama K, Kurisu K. Magnetic resonance spectroscopy detection of high lipid levels in intraaxial tumors without central necrosis: a characteristic of malignant lymphoma. J Neurosurg. 2015; 122(6):1370–4.
25. Toh CH, Castillo M, Wong AM, Wei KC, Ng SH, Wan YL. Primary Cerebral Lymphoma and Glioblastoma Multiforme: Differences in Diffusion Characteristics Evaluated with Diffusion Tensor Imaging. AJNR. 2008;29:471–5.
26. Malikova H, Liscak R, Latnerova I, Guseynova K, Syrucek M, Pytlik R. Complications of MRI-guided stereotactic biopsy of brain lymphoma. Neuro Endocrinol Lett. 2014;35(7):613–8.

12

Diagnostic performance of ^{18}F-FDG PET/CT using point spread function reconstruction on initial staging of rectal cancer: a comparison study with conventional PET/CT and pelvic MRI

Masatoshi Hotta[1][*] (iD), Ryogo Minamimoto[1], Hideaki Yano[2], Yoshimasa Gohda[2] and Yasutaka Shuno[2]

Abstract

Background: Accurate staging is crucial for treatment selection and prognosis prediction in patients with rectal cancer. Point spread function (PSF) reconstruction can improve spatial resolution and signal-to-noise ratio of PET imaging. The aim of this study was to evaluate the effectiveness of ^{18}F-FDG PET/CT with PSF reconstruction for initial staging in rectal cancer compared with conventional PET/CT and pelvic MRI.

Methods: A total of 59 patients with rectal cancer underwent preoperative ^{18}F-FDG PET/CT and pelvic MRI. The maximum standardized uptake value (SUVmax) and lesion to background (L/B) ratio of possible metastatic lymph nodes, and metabolic tumor volumes (MTVs) of primary tumors were calculated. For N and T (T1-2 vs T3-4) staging, sensitivities, specificities, positive predictive values, negative predictive values, and accuracies were compared between conventional PET/CT [reconstructed with ordered subset expectation maximization (OSEM)], PSF-PET/CT (reconstructed with OSEM+PSF), and pelvic MRI. Histopathologic analysis was the reference standard.

Results: For N staging, PSF-PET/CT provided higher sensitivity (78.6%) than conventional PET/CT (64.3%), and pelvic MRI (57.1%), and all techniques showed high specificity (PSF-PET: 95.4%, conventional PET: 96.7%, pelvic MRI: 93.5%). SUVmax and L/B ratio were significantly higher in PSF-PET/CT than conventional-PET/CT ($p < 0.001$). The accuracy for T staging in PSF-PET/CT (69.4%) was not significantly different to conventional PET/CT (73.5%) and pelvic MRI (73.5%). MTVs of PSF and conventional PET showed a significant difference among T stages ($p < 0.001$), with higher values in advanced stages. In M staging, both PSF and conventional PET/CT diagnosed all distant metastases correctly.

Conclusions: PSF-PET/CT produced images with higher lesion-to-background contrast than conventional PET/CT, which allowed improved detection of lymph node metastasis without compromising specificity, and showed comparable diagnostic value to MRI in local staging. PSF-PET/CT is likely to have a great value for initial staging in rectal cancer.

Keywords: Point spread function (PSF), 18F-FDG pet/ct, Pelvic MRI, Rectal cancer, Staging

* Correspondence: masatoshihotta@yahoo.co.jp
[1]Division of Nuclear Medicine, Department of Radiology, National Center for Global Health and Medicine, 1-21-1, Shinjuku-ku, Toyama, Tokyo 162-8655, Japan
Full list of author information is available at the end of the article

Background

Incidence of rectal cancer is relatively high and one of the major causes of cancer-related mortality worldwide [1]. Accurate initial staging is important for determining prognosis and treatment options in patients with rectal cancer [2–4]. While CT and MRI are commonly used for initial staging of rectal cancer, their diagnostic performance for N staging is not entirely satisfactory [5, 6]. Small lymph node metastases are common in rectal cancer, and these can be difficult to diagnose by CT and MRI, frequently resulting in false negatives which can lead to incorrect management decisions. In contrast, ^{18}F-FDG PET/CT has been shown to have high specificity for the diagnosis of lymph node (LN) metastasis in rectal cancer [7–10], as in addition to size criteria it evaluates glucose metabolism.

Recently, the point spread function (PSF) reconstruction technique has become commercially available for PET imaging [11, 12]. PSF reconstruction corrects photon mis-positioning (parallax effect) while gamma rays pass in the scintillation detectors at both non-oblique and oblique angles. This algorithm can improve the spatial resolution and signal-to-noise ratio of PET images [13, 14], leading to higher detection rates for small lesions. The latest PET scanners generally equipped with PSF reconstruction, which can be used only by changing its reconstruction algorithm, without additional image acquisition. ^{18}F-FDG PET/CT using PSF reconstruction has already been reported to improve the sensitivity of nodal staging for malignancies such as lung or breast cancer [15–17]. However, the utility of PSF for in rectal cancer has not been adequately clarified.

The aim of this study was to evaluate the effectiveness of ^{18}F-FDG PET/CT using PSF reconstruction for the initial staging in patients with rectal cancer, and compare it to both pelvic MRI and ^{18}F-FDG PET/CT using ordered subset expectation maximization (OSEM) reconstruction.

Methods

Patients

This retrospective study was approved by the Institutional Review Board of our hospital, and the need to obtain informed consent was waived. We included histologically proven rectal cancer patients who underwent ^{18}F-FDG PET/CT and pelvic MRI for their initial staging from November 2011 to August 2016. Exclusion criteria for this study were: patients with uncontrolled diabetes, and patients who were not indicated for surgery and therefore underwent preoperative radiation therapy or chemotherapy after PET evaluation.

Surgical protocol

The surgical protocol, including dissection area, followed the Japanese Society for Cancer of the Colon and Rectum (JSCCR) guidelines [18]. Patients with locally advanced lower rectal cancer had undergone pelvic sidewall dissection because of a greater probability of positive lateral lymph nodes [19]. Patients with upper rectal cancer showing possible lateral lymph node metastasis on preoperative imaging such as MRI, PET/CT, or enhanced-CT had undergone pelvic sidewall dissection, regardless of tumor location or T stage.

PET/CT examination

^{18}F-FDG was synthesized with an in-house cyclotron and automated synthesis system (F200; Sumitomo Heavy Industries, Shinagawa, Tokyo, Japan). PET/CT images were acquired 60 min after an intravenous injection of ^{18}F-FDG, fixed at 5.0 MBq/kg. Patients were instructed to urinate before scanning to reduce tracer accumulation in the bladder. All PET/CT images were obtained using a Discovery PET/CT 600 (GE Healthcare, Pewaukee, WI) with a multi-detector-row CT component (16 detectors). Scanning covered an area from the head to the mid-thigh. Low dose CT with shallow breathing was performed first and used for attenuation correction and image fusion. CT acquisition was performed with 120 kVp using an auto exposure control system, beam pitch of 0.938, slice thickness of 3.75 mm. Emission images were acquired in three-dimensional mode for 2.5 min per bed position. The 3D-OSEM reconstruction method (VUE point HD; GE Healthcare) was used both for (a) conventional PET (16 subsets; 3 iterations), and (b) PSF-PET [(16 subsets; 5 iterations) + PSF algorithm (Sharp IR, GE Healthcare)]. For both reconstructions, the matrix size was 192×192, resulting in a $3.65 \times 3.65 \times 3.65$ mm voxel size, and a 4 mm Gaussian filter was used.

MRI examination

MRI was performed with either a 1.5-T scanner (Avanto; Siemens Medical Systems, Erlangen, Germany) or a 3-T scanner (Verio; Siemens Medical Systems, Erlangen, Germany). The allocation of patients to both MRI scanners were performed randomly.

The following are imaging parameters for the acquired sequences, for the 1.5-T and the 3-T scanners, respectively. Axial T1-weighted images: repetition time (TR)/echo time (TE), 666/11 ms, matrix size, 192×320, slice thickness, 6 mm, intersection gap, 1.5 mm, number of excitations (NEX), 2, and field of view, 25×25 cm; TR/TE, 550/11 ms, matrix size, 256×320, slice thickness, 6 mm; intersection gap, 1.5 mm, NEX, 1, and field of view, 24×24 cm. Oblique (perpendicular to the tumoral axis) high resolution T2-weighted images: TR/TE, 5850/91 ms, matrix size 230×256, slice thickness, 3 mm, intersection gap, 0 mm, NEX, 1, and field of view, 20×20 cm; TR/TE, 5000/100 ms; matrix size 256×256, slice thickness, 3 mm, no gap, NEX, 1, and field of view, $18 \times$

18 cm. Axial diffusion-weighted images (DWI) were acquired using free breathing, single-shot acquisition, short tau inversion recovery (STIR)–echo planar imaging (EPI) sequence: TR/TE, 7600/75 ms, matrix size 79 × 128, slice thickness, 5 mm, no gap, NEX, 6, field of view, 36 × 36 cm, and b-value, 1000 s/mm^2; TR/TE, 9600/72 ms, matrix size 128 × 128, slice thickness, 5 mm, no gap, NEX, 5, field of view, 35 × 35 cm, and 1000 s/mm^2.

Image analysis

All PET/CT examinations were evaluated by consensus of two board-certified nuclear medicine physicians blind to clinical and pathological information. PSF and conventional PET/CT images were accessed independently. For N staging, lymph nodes that showed abnormal uptake compared to surrounding tissue were considered positive, regardless of size. For semi-quantitative analysis, a region of interest (ROI) was contoured over possible metastatic lymph nodes and maximum standard uptake values (SUVmax) were calculated. To measure background uptake, a circular ROI of 10 mm diameter was placed on the ascending aorta according to the CT image of the PET/CT. For both conventional PET/CT and PSF-PET/CT, a lesion-to-background (L/B) ratio was calculated from the values of the lymph node and background uptakes.

MRI images were anonymized and evaluated by consensus of two board-certified diagnostic radiologists. For N staging, lymph nodes greater than 8 mm in diameter, or that showed either irregular contour or mixed signal intensity in T2-weighted images were considered as metastasis [20, 21]. DWI was used for aiding in the detection of lymph nodes only, as DWI is not considered reliable for differentiating between benign and malignant lymph nodes with non-metastatic lymph nodes showing restricted diffusion [22, 23]. In both PET/CT and MRI, lymph nodes were evaluated on a per region basis: mesorectal, superior rectal, inferior mesenteric, internal iliac, and obturator. This anatomical grouping was based on the modified American Joint Committee on Cancer (AJCC) staging system [24], reported by Kim et al. [25]. For T staging, tumors that showed extended ^{18}F-FDG uptake or soft tissue density to surrounding mesorectal fat were considered as over T3 (T3-4). According to the AJCC staging system, tumors that invade perirectal tissue are classified as T3, and those that directly invade other organs are classified as T4. Metabolic tumor volumes (MTVs) were measured from ^{18}F-FDG PET images using the PET Edge tool (MIM software, Cleveland, OH), which creates boundary contours automatically detecting the steepest drop-off in SUV according to a gradient-based technique [26]. In MRI, tumors that showed invasion of mesorectal fat on T2-weighted images were considered as over T3 stage (T3-4).

These imaging findings for T and N staging were compared with histopathological analysis of the primary tumor and harvested lymph nodes. In addition, M staging was assessed in PET/CT and MRI, with the reference standard for metastasis set from the patient's clinical course and following scans including FDG PET/CT and contrast-enhanced CT.

Statistical analysis

Data are expressed as mean ± SD. Sensitivity, specificity, positive predictive value (PPV), negative predictive value (NPV), and accuracy values for T staging (T1-2 vs T3-4) and N staging were calculated for conventional PET/CT, PSF-PET/CT, and MRI (these values are expressed as means with 95% confidence intervals [CI]). The McNemar chi-square test was used to compare the sensitivity and specificity between PET/CT, PSF-PET/CT, and MRI. Wilcoxon signed-rank test was performed to compare SUVmax and L/B ratio of positive lymph nodes, and MTVs of the primary lesion between PSF and conventional PET. The relationship of SUVmax and L/B ratio between PSF and conventional PET was assessed by linear regression analysis. Kruskal-Wallis test was used for comparing the difference of MTVs among T stages, and receiver operating curve (ROC) analysis was performed to evaluate the diagnostic performance of MTVs to distinguish the T3-4 from T1-2 stages. Two-tailed p values < 0.05 were considered significant.

Results

Clinical data

Fifty-nine patients met the study inclusion criteria and, of these, 10 patients underwent radiation therapy or chemotherapy. No patient showed serum glucose concentrations > 150 mg/dL prior to ^{18}F-FDG administration. A final number of 49 patients were included in the analysis (Table 1). The median interval between PET/CT and MRI, between surgery and PET/CT, and between surgery and MRI were 4 (interquartile range: 2-8), 11 (7-23), and 17 (9-27) days, respectively. Twenty-one patients underwent MRI with the 3-T scanner, and 28 patients with the 1.5-T scanner.

Diagnostic performance for N staging

A total of 1200 LNs were resected by surgery, and 104 (8.7%) LNs were pathologically proven metastasis. On a per patient basis, 18 (36.7%) patients showed lymph nodal involvement. On a per region basis, the prevalence of lymph node metastasis was 15.5% (28/181) [mesorectal (n = 18/49), superior rectal (n = 3/49), inferior mesenteric (n = 2/45), internal iliac (n = 3/20), obturator (n = 2/18)]. The diagnostic performances for N staging on a per region basis are shown in Table 2. The sensitivity of PSF-PET/CT (78.6%) was higher than that of either

Table 1 Patients demographics

No. patients	49
Sex	M 34, F 15
Mean Age years (standard deviation)	66.8 (12.9)
Histological diagnosis	
Well differentiated adenocarcinoma	17
Moderately differentiated adenocarcinoma	29
Poorly differentiated adenocarcinoma	1
Mucinous adenocarcinoma	2
Pathological Stage (UICC)	
I	13
II	15
III	16
IV	5

M male, *F* female, *UICC* Union for International Cancer Control

conventional PET/CT (64.3%) or pelvic MRI (57.1%) but the differences were not statistically significant (PSF-PET vs conventional PET, *p* = 0.13; PSF-PET vs MRI, *p* = 0.07). PSF-PET/CT showed positive uptake for all the true positive lesions (*n* = 17) on conventional PET/CT. Metastasis in normal size lymph nodes was seen in 9/28 (32.1%) lesions. Of these, 4/9 (44.4%) and 1/9 (11.1%) were detected on PSF-PET/CT and conventional PET/CT, respectively. No significant differences were observed for specificity, PPV, NPV, or accuracy between the three methods. The average SUVmax and L/B ratios for visually positive regions are shown in Table 3. The increased percentages of SUVmax and L/B ratios by PSF reconstruction were 17% and 21%, respectively. The L/B

Table 2 Diagnostic performance of conventional PET/CT, PSF PET/CT, and pelvic MRI for nodal staging in patients with rectal cancer

	Conventional PET/CT	PSF-PET/CT	Pelvic MRI
Sensitivity, %	64.3 (0.51 to 0.73)	78.6 (0.65 to 0.88)	57.1 (0.42 to 0.69)
Specificity, %	96.7 (0.94 to 0.98)	95.4 (0.93 to 0.97)	93.5 (0.91 to 0.96)
Accuracy, %	91.7 (0.88 to 0.95)	92.8 (0.89 to 0.96)	87.8 (0.83 to 0.92)
PPV, %	78.3 (0.62 to 0.89)	75.9 (0.63 to 0.85)	61.5 (0.46 to 0.75)
NPV, %	93.7 (0.91 to 0.95)	96.1 (0.94 to 0.98)	92.3 (0.90 to 0.95)
Positive LR	19.6 (8.80 to 45.60)	17.2 (9.10 to 30.50)	8.7 (4.60 to 16.20)
Negative LR	0.37 (0.27 to 0.52)	0.23 (0.13 to 0.38)	0.46 (0.32 to 0.63)

The numbers in parentheses represent the 95% confidence interval
LR likelihood ratio, *NPV* negative predictive value, *PPV* positive predictive value, *PSF* point spread function

Table 3 Quantitative values of conventional PET/CT and PSF-PET/CT

	Conventional PET/CT	PSF-PET/CT	P value*
SUVmax	6.8 (5.0)	8.4 (7.0)	< 0.001
Background	2.3 (0.3)	2.2 (0.5)	0.32
L/B ratio	2.9 (1.8)	3.5 (2.3)	< 0.001

The numbers in parentheses represent the standard deviation. *Wilcoxon signed-rank test
L/B lesion to background, *PSF* point spread function, *SUV* standardized uptake value

ratio was significantly higher with PSF-PET/CT than with conventional PET/CT (*P* < 0.001). Linear regression analyses are shown in Fig. 1. An excellent correlation was found between quantitative measurements extracted from conventional PET/CT and PSF-PET/CT for SUVmax, and L/B ratios, with an r^2 value greater than 0.9. Similar results were found for SUVmax ratios. Figure 2 shows a representative case, comparing PSF-PET/CT, conventional PET/CT, and MRI.

Diagnostic performance for T and M staging

Pathological T staging of patients was as follows: T1 (*n* = 6, 12.2%), T2 (*n* = 10, 20.4%), T3 (*n* = 25, 51.0%), and T4 (*n* = 8, 16.3%). The diagnostic performances for visual differentiation of the T3-4 stage between conventional PET/CT, PSF-PET/CT, and MRI are presented on Table 4. Pelvic MRI showed higher sensitivity (70.0%) than that of PSF-PET/CT (57.6%) or conventional PET/CT (63.6%), but the differences were not statistically significant (pelvic MRI vs PSF-PET/CT, *p* = 0.29; pelvic MRI vs conventional PET/CT, *p* = 0.72). Figure 3 (a and b) shows MTVs of PSF-PET and conventional PET respectively, both showing significant differences (*p* < 0.001) among T stages. There were no significant differences for mean MTVs between PSF and conventional PET (PSF-PET: 33.9 ± 60.7, conventional PET33.7 ± 60.9, *p* = 0.57). Figure 3c shows the ROC analysis of PSF and conventional PET for determining T3-4. The AUC for PSF-PET was 0.837 and 0.839 for conventional PET, which showed no statistical difference (*p* = 0.91). When a cut-off value of MTVs was set at 18.1 mL in conventional PET, a sensitivity of 93.8% and specificity of 69.7% were obtained. This diagnostic value was as high as that of the MTVs of PSF-PET.

With regards to M staging, both PSF PET/CT and conventional PET/CT detected all distant metastasis [5/49 (10.2%) patients; 2 cases for lung, 1 case for liver, 1 case for para-aortic LNs, and 1 case for lung, liver, and bone metastasis], whereas pelvic MRI was not able to diagnose distant metastases because of its scanning range limitations.

Discussion

The purpose of this study was to investigate whether PSF-PET/CT improves diagnostic performance for initial

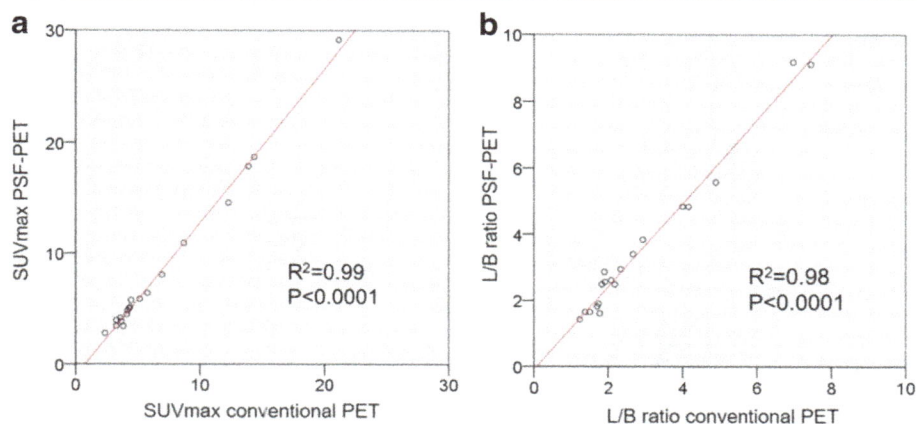

Fig. 1 Relationship between quantitative values obtained from conventional PET and point spread function (PSF) -PET, evaluated using linear regression analysis for maximum standardized uptake value (SUVmax) (**a**), and lesion to background (L/B) ratio (**b**)

staging of patients with rectal cancer, as compared to conventional PET/CT and pelvic MRI. For nodal staging, PSF-PET/CT provided higher sensitivity, without decreasing specificity, than conventional PET/CT and pelvic MRI. SUVmax and L/B ratio of PSF reconstruction were significantly higher than those of conventional OSEM reconstruction. For T staging, both PSF and conventional PET/CT provided similar diagnostic performance to pelvic MRI, in terms of discriminating stages T3-4 from T1-2.

When compared to conventional PET/CT for lymph node staging, PSF-PET/CT provided higher sensitivity than PET/CT. The increased L/B ratio can lead to the higher detectability of lymph node metastasis. This result was mostly an accordance with previous reports that examined PSF reconstruction for evaluating lymph node metastasis in malignancies including lung cancer [15, 16], breast cancer [17], and colorectal cancer [27]. However, the sensitivity improvement was relatively smaller than that in the lung and breast cancer studies. A possible explanation for this result is the use of a different

PSF reconstruction algorithm. We used the Sharp IR (GE healthcare) algorithm in this study, whilst the True X (Siemens Medical Systems, Erlangen, Germany) algorithm was used in the other two studies. While both algorithm increase SUVmax and L/B ratio, True X tends to overestimate SUVmax, especially in larger lesions, when compared to Sharp IR [28]. Indeed, the increased percentages of SUVmax and L/B ratio by PSF reconstruction were 17 and 21% for our study; and 48-66% for the lung and 27-67% for the breast studies using TrueX. This difference possibly influenced the detection of lymph node metastasis. Another possible reason for the differences in sensitivity between rectal and breast cancers could be anatomical features related to ^{18}F-FDG uptake. In the pelvis, physiological ^{18}F-FDG uptake in the small intestine, colon and bladder causes difficulties for distinguishing abnormal uptake adjacent to these organs [29]. In this study, all patients were instructed to urinate before scanning to reduce tracer accumulation in the bladder, but controlling physiological accumulation in the small intestine and colon remains challenging. In

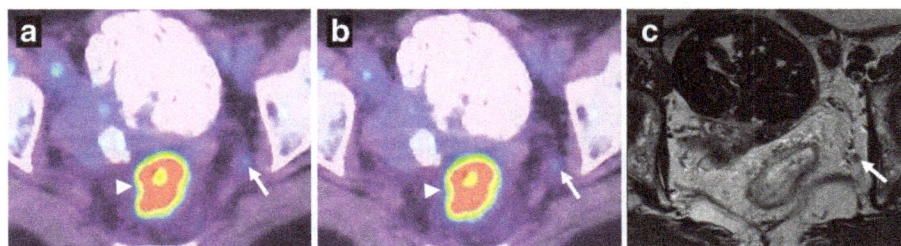

Fig. 2 A 83-year-old woman with rectal cancer. The rectal cancer (arrowhead) can be seen from ^{18}F-FDG uptake on both PSF-PET/CT (**a**) and conventional PET/CT (**b**) [images are scaled to the same maximum value]. A obturator lymph node (arrow) showed as ^{18}F-FDG avid compared to the surrounding tissue on PSF-PET/CT, and therefore considered a positive result. This lymph node was obscure on conventional PET/CT, and thus regarded as negative. This lymph node was 5 mm in diameter, and did not show mixed signal intensity nor irregular contour on the high resolution T2-weighted image (**c**), and therefore considered negative on MRI also. Subsequently, this lymph node was pathologically confirmed as containing metastasis

Table 4 Diagnostic performance of conventional PET/CT, PSF PET/CT, and pelvic MRI for differentiating T3-4 stage from T1-2 stage in patients with rectal cancer

	Conventional PET/CT	PSF-PET/CT	Pelvic MRI
Sensitivity, %	63.6 (0.45 to 0.80)	57.6 (0.39 to 0.74)	70.0 (0.51 to 0.84)
Specificity, %	93.8 (0.70 to 0.99)	93.8 (0.70 to 0.99)	81.2 (0.54 to 0.96)
Accuracy, %	73.5 (0.59 to 0.85)	69.4 (0.55 to 0.82)	73.5 (0.59 to 0.85)
PPV, %	95.5 (0.77 to 0.99)	95.0 (0.75 to 0.99)	88.8 (0.70 to 0.98)
NPV, %	55.6 (0.35 to 0.74)	51.7 (0.33 to 0.71)	56.5 (0.59 to 0.85)
Positive LR	10.2 (1.50 to 69.10)	9.2 (1.30 to 62.80)	3.7 (1.30 to 10.60)
Negative LR	0.38 (0.24 to 0.62)	0.45 (0.30 to 0.69)	0.37 (0.21 to 0.66)

The numbers in parentheses represent the 95% confidence interval

LR likelihood ratio, *NPV* negative predictive value, *PPV* positive predictive value, *PSF* point spread function

addition, various artifacts related to hip prosthesis, which are occasionally seen particularly in elderly patients, may lower small lesions detection [30, 31]. In such cases, PET/CT image quality may be improved with the use of metal artifact reduction algorithms [32].

In this study, the detection of small lymph node metastases using PSF-PET/CT was superior to that using conventional PET/CT and MRI. In rectal cancers, almost 60% of the lymph nodes involved are smaller than 5 mm in diameter, which is a major limitation for nodal staging using the size criteria alone [20]. Therefore, as in this study, MRI has shown to be limited for detection of metastasis in normal size lymph nodes, and a relative low specificity is an issue even if specificity can be improved by combining it with characteristic MRI imaging techniques such as DWI [10]. PSF reconstruction is known to increase apparent SUV compared to OSEM, especially in case of small lesions [33]. SUVmax calculated from PSF-PET/CT itself is known to be unreliable and is not recommended in assessing treatment response or multicenter trials [28, 34]. However, it can be very useful for

visually detecting small lymph node metastases, as evidenced by the higher L/B ratios in PSF-PET/CT than in conventional PET/CT seen in this study. Small lymph node commonly contains metastasis, not only in rectal cancers cases, but in other malignancies such as esophageal, gastric and uterine cervical cancers [35–37], with consequent lower lymph node metastasis detection rates. PSF PET/CT, which improves spatial resolution and small lesion detection, may also enhance the sensitivity of PET/CT for lymph node metastasis in such cancers.

The diagnostic ability of PSF and conventional PET/CT for T staging [T1-2 vs T3-4] was as high as that of MRI. It is important to distinguish T3-4 from T1-2 stages, as the former are considered advanced stages for which neoadjuvant therapy can be the first treatment option [38]. Higher MTVs were associated with more advanced T stages. Buijsen et al. [39] has reported that ^{18}F-FDG PET/CT based contours show the best correlation with the tumor dimension of surgically resected specimens in rectal cancer when compared to CT and MRI. This indicates that MTVs can correlate well with the actual tumor volume, which may

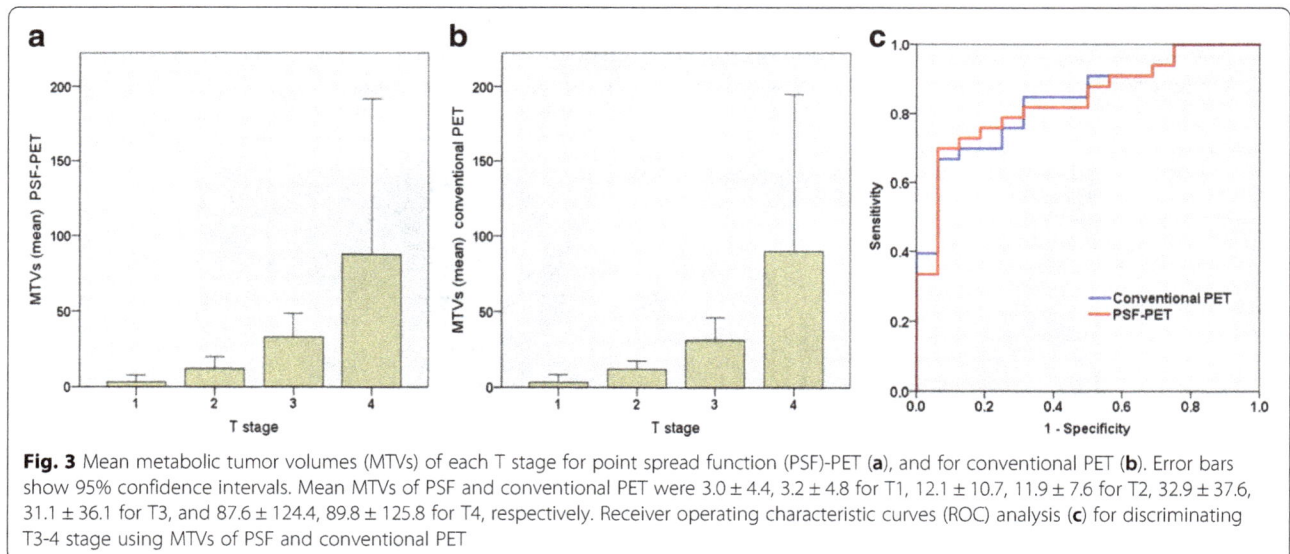

Fig. 3 Mean metabolic tumor volumes (MTVs) of each T stage for point spread function (PSF)-PET (**a**), and for conventional PET (**b**). Error bars show 95% confidence intervals. Mean MTVs of PSF and conventional PET were 3.0 ± 4.4, 3.2 ± 4.8 for T1, 12.1 ± 10.7, 11.9 ± 7.6 for T2, 32.9 ± 37.6, 31.1 ± 36.1 for T3, and 87.6 ± 124.4, 89.8 ± 125.8 for T4, respectively. Receiver operating characteristic curves (ROC) analysis (**c**) for discriminating T3-4 stage using MTVs of PSF and conventional PET

explain why MTVs yield high diagnostic performance for T staging. With regard to differences between PSF and conventional PET, there was no significant difference of MTVs for T staging. Previous reports described that MTVs calculated from PSF were smaller than that of conventional (OSEM reconstructed) PET, but this was not the case in the present study. Differences in PSF reconstruction algorithms and auto-segmentation software may possibly affect volume calculation [40, 41].

In this study, all distant metastasis including lung, liver, and bone were detected in PET/CT with or without PSF reconstruction. PET/CT reportedly enables accurate diagnosis for not only intrahepatic metastasis, but extrahepatic metastasis in colorectal cancer [42–45]. In this context, it would be advisable to perform ^{18}F-FDG PET/CT for rectal cancer staging, particularly in advanced cases. Not only for M staging, this study has shown that PET/CT (particularly PSF-PET/CT) can provide high diagnostic performance for N staging too, and that it has a diagnostic value comparable to MRI for T staging. Collectively, PSF PET/CT has potential to become a *one-stop shop* imaging solution for initial staging in rectal cancer.

There are limitations to this study. First, it was a single center study with a relatively small population and our findings need to be confirmed in a larger series. Second, highly advanced patients who were not indicated for operation and required neoadjuvant radiotherapy or chemotherapy were excluded, as pathological findings obtained from surgical operation were defined as the reference standard. However, as discussed above, PSF-PET/CT can provide a considerable impact on diagnosis of lymph node metastasis, which suggests that it could be useful for evaluation before neoadjuvant therapy as well. Thirdly, there was a difference in the iteration numbers between PSF-PET and conventional PET (PSF-PET: 5, conventional PET: 3). However, the PSF-PET iteration number in our study was adjusted to provide a clinically optimal image based on our institutional phantom study, and it has been previously reported that it is usually necessary to increase the number of iterations in order to obtain optimum image when PSF reconstruction is used [13]. In addition, other acquisition parameters including subset and matrix size, which has been reported to affect both the quality and quantitative values of PET images (particularly with PSF reconstruction) [46], were set to the same values for both PSF and conventional PET.

Conclusions

PSF-PET/CT has potential to provide superior sensitivity for lymph node staging in rectal cancer without reducing specificity compared with conventional PET/CT and pelvic MRI. As PET/CT can provide comparable diagnostic value to MRI for T staging and detect distant metastasis accurately, PSF-PET/CT is a promising methodology for increasing accuracy in staging rectal cancer.

Abbreviations
AJCC: American Joint Committee on Cancer; DWI: Diffusion-weighted images; EPI: Echo planar imaging; L/B: Lesion-to-background; LN: Lymph node; MTV: Metabolic tumor volume; NEX: Number of excitations; NPV: Negative predictive value; OSEM: Ordered subset expectation maximization; PPV: Positive predictive value; PSF: Point spread function; ROC: Receiver operating curve; ROI: Region of interest; STIR: Short tau inversion recovery; TE: Echo time; TR: Repetition time

Acknowledgements
Not applicable.

Funding
No funding.

Authors' contributions
MH contributed to the design, analysis and manuscript preparation and submission. RM contributed to the design, analysis and manuscript preparation. MH, RM, and HY are responsible for the study concepts and design. MH, RM, HY, GY, and SY performed the clinical studies. MH, RM, HY, GY, and SY performed the data analysis/interpretation. MH, RM, HY, GY, and SY did the manuscript preparation. MH, RM, HY, GY, and SY participated in the manuscript revision/review. All authors read and approved the final manuscript.

Competing interests
The authors declare that they have no competing interests.

Author details
[1]Division of Nuclear Medicine, Department of Radiology, National Center for Global Health and Medicine, 1-21-1, Shinjuku-ku, Toyama, Tokyo 162-8655, Japan. [2]Department of Surgery, National Center for Global Health and Medicine, 1-21-1, Shinjuku-ku, Toyama, Tokyo 162-8655, Japan.

References
1. Kang H, O'Connell JB, Leonardi MJ, Maggard MA, McGory ML, Ko CY. Rare tumors of the colon and rectum: a national review. Int J Color Dis. 2007;22:183–9.
2. Cohen AM, Tremiterra S, Candela F, Thaler HT, Sigurdson ER. Prognosis of node-positive colon cancer. Cancer. 1991;67:1859–61.
3. Engelen SM, Beets-Tan RG, Lahaye MJ, Kessels AG, Beets GL. Location of involved mesorectal and extramesorectal lymph nodes in patients with primary rectal cancer: preoperative assessment with MR imaging. Eur J Surg Oncol. 2008;34:776–81.
4. Harrison JC, Dean PJ, el-Zeky F, Vander Zwaag R. From dukes through Jass: pathological prognostic indicators in rectal cancer. Hum Pathol. 1994;25:498–505.
5. Li XT, Sun YS, Tang L, Cao K, Zhang XY. Evaluating local lymph node metastasis with magnetic resonance imaging, endoluminal ultrasound and computed tomography in rectal cancer: a meta-analysis. Color Dis. 2015;17:O129–35.
6. Bipat S, Glas AS, Slors FJ, Zwinderman AH, Bossuyt PM, Stoker J. Rectal cancer: local staging and assessment of lymph node involvement with endoluminal US, CT, and MR imaging–a meta-analysis. Radiology. 2004;232:773–83.
7. Abdel-Nabi H, Doerr RJ, Lamonica DM, Cronin VR, Galantowicz PJ, Carbone GM, et al. Staging of primary colorectal carcinomas with fluorine-18 fluorodeoxyglucose whole-body PET: correlation with histopathologic and CT findings. Radiology. 1998;206:755–60.

8. Kantorova I, Lipska L, Belohlavek O, Visokai V, Trubac M, Schneiderova M. Routine 18F-FDG PET preoperative staging of colorectal cancer: comparison with conventional staging and its impact on treatment decision making. J Nucl Med. 2003;44:1784–8.

9. Tsunoda Y, Ito M, Fujii H, Kuwano H, Saito N. Preoperative diagnosis of lymph node metastases of colorectal cancer by FDG-PET/CT. Jpn J Clin Oncol. 2008;38:347–53.

10. Kim DJ, Kim JH, Ryu YH, Jeon TJ, Yu JS, Chung JJ. Nodal staging of rectal cancer: high-resolution pelvic MRI versus 18F-FDGPET/CT. J Comput Assist Tomogr. 2011;35:531–4.

11. Panin VY, Kehren F, Michel C, Casey M. Fully 3-D PET reconstruction with system matrix derived from point source measurements. IEEE Trans Med Imaging. 2006;25:907–21.

12. Pichler BJ, Wehrl HF, Judenhofer MS. Latest advances in molecular imaging instrumentation. J Nucl Med. 2008;49(Suppl 2):5s–23s.

13. Akamatsu G, Ishikawa K, Mitsumoto K, Taniguchi T, Ohya N, Baba S, et al. Improvement in PET/CT image quality with a combination of point-spread function and time-of-flight in relation to reconstruction parameters. J Nucl Med. 2012;53:1716–22.

14. Andersen FL, Klausen TL, Loft A, Beyer T, Holm S. Clinical evaluation of PET image reconstruction using a spatial resolution model. Eur J Radiol. 2013;82:862–9.

15. Lasnon C, Hicks RJ, Beauregard JM, Milner A, Paciencia M, Guizard AV, et al. Impact of point spread function reconstruction on thoracic lymph node staging with 18F-FDG PET/CT in non-small cell lung cancer. Clin Nucl Med. 2012;37:971–6.

16. Ozawa Y, Hara M, Shibamoto Y, Tamaki T, Nishio M, Omi K. Utility of high-definition FDG-PET image reconstruction for lung cancer staging. Acta Radiol. 2013;54:916–20.

17. Bellevre D, Blanc Fournier C, Switsers O, Dugué AE, Levy C, Allouache D, et al. Staging the axilla in breast cancer patients with 18F-FDG PET: how small are the metastases that we can detect with new generation clinical PET systems? Eur J Nucl Med Mol Imaging. 2014;41:1103–12.

18. Watanabe T, Itabashi M, Shimada Y, Tanaka S, Ito Y, Ajioka Y, et al. Japanese Society for Cancer of the colon and Rectum (JSCCR) guidelines 2010 for the treatment of colorectal cancer. Int J Clin Oncol. 2012;17:1–29.

19. Sugihara K, Kobayashi H, Kato T, Mori T, Mochizuki H, Kameoka S, et al. Indication and benefit of pelvic sidewall dissection for rectal cancer. Dis Colon Rectum. 2006;49:1663–72.

20. Brown G, Richards CJ, Bourne MW, Newcombe RG, Radcliffe AG, Dallimore NS, et al. Morphologic predictors of lymph node status in rectal cancer with use of high-spatial-resolution MR imaging with histopathologic comparison. Radiology. 2003;227:371–7.

21. Kim JH, Beets GL, Kim MJ, Kessels AG, Beets-Tan RG. High-resolution MR imaging for nodal staging in rectal cancer: are there any criteria in addition to the size? Eur J Radiol. 2004;52:78–83.

22. Beets-Tan RG, Lambregts DM, Maas M, Bipat S, Barbaro B, Caseiro-Alves F, et al. Magnetic resonance imaging for the clinical management of rectal cancer patients: recommendations from the 2012 European Society of Gastrointestinal and Abdominal Radiology (ESGAR) consensus meeting. Eur Radiol. 2013;23:2522–31.

23. Heijnen LA, Lambregts DM, Mondal D, Martens MH, Riedl RG, Beets GL, et al. Diffusion-weighted MR imaging in primary rectal cancer staging demonstrates but does not characterise lymph nodes. Eur Radiol. 2013;23:3354–60.

24. Edge SB, Byrd DR, Compton CC, Fritz AG, Greene FL, Trotti A. AJCC cancer staging manual. 7th ed. Philadelphia: Lippincott-Raven; 2009.

25. Kim DJ, Chung JJ, Yu JS, Cho ES, Kim JH. Evaluation of lateral pelvic nodes in patients with advanced rectal cancer. AJR Am J Roentgenol. 2014;202:1245–55.

26. Werner-Wasik M, Nelson AD, Choi W, Arai Y, Faulhaber PF, Kang P, et al. What is the best way to contour lung tumors on PET scans? Multiobserver validation of a gradient-based method using a NSCLC digital PET phantom. Int J Radiat Oncol Biol Phys. 2012;82:1164–71.

27. Kawashima K, Kato K, Tomabechi M, Matsuo M, Otsuka K, Ishida K, et al. Clinical evaluation of (18)F-fludeoxyglucose positron emission tomography/CT using point spread function reconstruction for nodal staging of colorectal cancer. Br J Radiol. 2016;89:20150938.

28. Matheoud R, Ferrando O, Valzano S, Lizio D, Sacchetti G, Ciarmiello A, et al. Performance comparison of two resolution modeling PET reconstruction algorithms in terms of physical figures of merit used in quantitative imaging. Phys Med. 2015;31:468–75.

29. Subhas N, Patel PV, Pannu HK, Jacene HA, Fishman EK, Wahl RL. Imaging of pelvic malignancies with in-line FDG PET-CT: case examples and common pitfalls of FDG PET. Radiographics. 2005;25:1031–43.

30. Yu L, Li H, Mueller J, Kofler JM, Liu X, Primak AN, et al. Metal artifact reduction from reformatted projections for hip prostheses in multislice helical computed tomography: techniques and initial clinical results. Investig Radiol. 2009;44:691–6.

31. Goerres GW, Ziegler SI, Burger C, Berthold T, Von Schulthess GK, Buck A. Artifacts at PET and PET/CT caused by metallic hip prosthetic material. Radiology. 2003;226:577–84.

32. van der Vos CS, Arens AI, Hamill JJ, Hofmann C, Panin VY, Meeuwis AP, et al. Metal artifact reduction of CT scans to improve PET/CT. J Nucl Med. 2017; https://doi.org/10.2967/jnumed.117.191171.

33. Akamatsu G, Mitsumoto K, Taniguchi T, Tsutsui Y, Baba S, Sasaki M. Influences of point-spread function and time-of-flight reconstructions on standardized uptake value of lymph node metastases in FDG-PET. Eur J Radiol. 2014;83:226–30.

34. Boellaard R. Need for standardization of 18F-FDG PET/CT for treatment response assessments. J Nucl Med. 2011;52(Suppl 2):93s–100s.

35. Monig SP, Schroder W, Baldus SE, Holscher AH. Preoperative lymph-node staging in gastrointestinal cancer–correlation between size and tumor stage. Onkologie. 2002;25:342–4.

36. Yasuda K, Adachi Y, Shiraishi N, Yamaguchi K, Hirabayashi Y, Kitano S. Pattern of lymph node micrometastasis and prognosis of patients with colorectal cancer. Ann Surg Oncol. 2001;8:300–4.

37. Manfredi R, Mirk P, Maresca G, Margariti PA, Testa A, Zannoni GF, et al. Local-regional staging of endometrial carcinoma: role of MR imaging in surgical planning. Radiology. 2004;231:372–8.

38. Benson, AB, Venook AP, Cederquist L, Chan E, Chen YJ, Cooper HS, et al. NCCN Clinical Practice Guideline in Oncology, Rectal cancer, version 3.2017. National Comprehensive Cancer Network website. https://www.nccn.org/professionals/physician_gls/pdf/rectal.pdf. Accessed 14 Nov 2017.

39. Buijsen J, van den Bogaard J, Janssen MH, Bakers FC, Engelsman S, Öllers M, et al. FDG-PET provides the best correlation with the tumor specimen compared to MRI and CT in rectal cancer. Radiother Oncol. 2011;98:270–6.

40. Knausl B, Hirtl A, Dobrozemsky G, Bergmann H, Kletter K, Dudczak R, et al. PET based volume segmentation with emphasis on the iterative TrueX algorithm. Z Med Phys. 2012;22:29–39.

41. Foster B, Bagci U, Mansoor A, Xu Z, Mollura DJ. A review on segmentation of positron emission tomography images. Comput Biol Med. 2014;50:76–96.

42. Bipat S, van Leeuwen MS, Comans EF, Pijl ME, Bossuyt PM, Zwinderman AH, et al. Colorectal liver metastases: CT, MR imaging, and PET for diagnosis–meta-analysis. Radiology. 2005;237:123–31.

43. Kuehl H, Rosenbaum-Krumme S, Veit-Haibach P, Stergar H, Forsting M, Bockisch A, et al. Impact of whole-body imaging on treatment decision to radio-frequency ablation in patients with malignant liver tumors: comparison of [18F]fluorodeoxyglucose-PET/computed tomography, PET and computed tomography. Nucl Med Commun. 2008;29:599–606.

44. Georgakopoulos A, Pianou N, Kelekis N, Chatziioannou S. Impact of 18F-FDG PET/CT on therapeutic decisions in patients with colorectal cancer and liver metastases. Clin Imaging. 2013;37:536–41.

45. Kochhar R, Liong S, Manoharan P. The role of FDG PET/CT in patients with colorectal cancer metastases. Cancer Biomark. 2010;7:235–48.

46. Riegler G, Karanikas G, Rausch I, Hirtl A, El-Rabadi K, Marik W, et al. Influence of PET reconstruction technique and matrix size on qualitative and quantitative assessment of lung lesions on [18F]-FDG-PET: a prospective study in 37 cancer patients. Eur J Radiol. 2017;90:20–6.

13

^{18}F-FDG PET/CT response in a phase 1/2 trial of *nab*-paclitaxel plus gemcitabine for advanced pancreatic cancer

Ronald L. Korn[1*], Daniel D. Von Hoff[2], Mitesh J. Borad[3], Markus F. Renschler[4], Desmond McGovern[4], R. Curtis Bay[5] and Ramesh K. Ramanathan[3]

Abstract

Background: Positron emission tomography (PET) is poised to become a useful imaging modality in staging and evaluating therapeutic responses in patients with metastatic pancreatic cancer (mPC). This analysis from a phase 1/2 study examined the utility of early PET imaging in patients with mPC treated with *nab*-paclitaxel plus gemcitabine.

Methods: Tumors were measured by [^{18}F]2-fluoro-2-deoxyglucose PET/computed tomography (CT) in patients who received *nab*-paclitaxel 100 ($n = 13$), 125 ($n = 38$), or 150 ($n = 1$) mg/m^2 plus gemcitabine 1000 mg/m^2 on days 1, 8, and 15 of a 28-day cycle. Lesion metabolic activity was evaluated at baseline and 6 and 12 weeks postbaseline.

Results: Fifty-two patients had baseline and ≥1 follow-up PET scan. The median maximum standardized uptake values per pancreatic lesion in the *nab*-paclitaxel 100 mg/m^2 and 125 mg/m^2 cohorts were 5.1 and 6.5, respectively. Among patients who had a metabolic response by PET, those who received *nab*-paclitaxel 125 mg/m^2 had a 4-month survival advantage over those who received 100 mg/m^2. All patients in the *nab*-paclitaxel 125 mg/m^2 cohort experienced an early complete metabolic response (CMR; 34%) or partial metabolic response (PMR; 66%). In the *nab*-paclitaxel 125 mg/m^2 cohort, investigator-assessed objective response rates were 77% and 44% among patients with a CMR and PMR, respectively, with no correlation between PET and CT response (Spearman $r_s = 0.22$; $P = 0.193$). Patients in the *nab*-paclitaxel 125 mg/m^2 cohort with a CMR experienced a significantly longer overall survival vs those with a PMR (median, 23.0 vs 11.2 months; $P = 0.011$), and a significant correlation was found between best percentage change in tumor burden by PET and survival: for each 1% decrease in PET score, the risk of death decreased by 2%.

Conclusions: The majority of primary pancreatic tumors and their metastases were PET avid, and PET effectively measured changes in tumor metabolic activity at 6 and 12 weeks. These results support the antitumor activity of *nab*-paclitaxel 125 mg/m^2 plus gemcitabine 1000 mg/m^2 for treating mPC and the utility of PET for measuring treatment response. Treatment response by PET analysis may be considered when evaluating investigational agents in mPC.

Keywords: Pancreatic cancer, *nab*-Paclitaxel, Gemcitabine, Phase 1/2 clinical trial, Positron emission tomography

* Correspondence: rkorn@imagingendpoints.com
[1]Imaging Endpoints Core Lab, 9700 N 91st St, B-200, Scottsdale, AZ 85258, USA
Full list of author information is available at the end of the article

Background

The use of positron emission tomography (PET) with [^{18}F]2-fluoro-2-deoxyglucose as a tracer combined with computed tomography (^{18}F-FDG/CT) to evaluate tumors has increased in recent years because of its high sensitivity and specificity. Currently, ^{18}F-FDG/CT is used for diagnosing, initial staging, detecting recurrent disease, and evaluating response in various malignant tumors, including breast cancer, non-small cell lung cancer, colorectal cancer, esophageal cancer, head and neck cancer, cervical cancer, diffuse large B-cell lymphoma, and melanoma [1–10]. Primary pancreatic adenocarcinoma has also been shown to be FDG avid by PET/CT [11], and an association between metabolic response and survival has been demonstrated in patients with metastatic pancreatic cancer (mPC) [12], providing support for the feasibility of PET/CT for pancreatic tumors. Continued research may validate PET as a useful tool for measuring treatment response in this disease state.

The treatment of mPC is among the most challenging in clinical oncology, with a 5-year survival rate of only $\approx$ 3% [13, 14]. Since 1997, gemcitabine monotherapy has been a standard of care for treating mPC until recently, when the PRODIGE and MPACT trials demonstrated significant survival benefits with FOLFIRINOX (folinic acid, 5-fluorouracil, irinotecan, and oxaliplatin) and nab-paclitaxel plus gemcitabine, respectively, compared with gemcitabine monotherapy [15–17]. Based on the positive findings of the phase 3 MPACT trial, nab-paclitaxel plus gemcitabine was approved for the first-line treatment of mPC [17, 18]. Although these findings are encouraging, effective PC treatment remains a major challenge, and there is a need to identify those patients who are most likely to benefit from specific therapies.

At week 8 in the MPACT trial, $\approx$ 5 times more patients experienced a metabolic response by PET per criteria from the European Organisation for Research and Treatment of Cancer (EORTC) [19] than an objective response by CT per Response Evaluation Criteria In Solid Tumors (RECIST) [20, 21], and patients with a tumor response identified by either modality had a median overall survival (OS) of >10 months [12]. The initial findings on the utility of PET/CT to assess response with nab-paclitaxel plus gemcitabine in a phase 1/2 study of patients with mPC were previously reported [22]. The preliminary data demonstrated that a complete loss of FDG metabolic activity was associated with an improved OS with nab-paclitaxel plus gemcitabine [22]. Furthermore, assessment of treatment response by PET was more sensitive than by CT; for all patients, the median decrease in metabolic activity at 12 weeks was 79% (n = 55; by ^{18}F-FDG PET scan using EORTC criteria), whereas the overall response rate was 46% (n = 67; by CT scan using RECIST v1.0) [22]. Here we report the

final analysis of the PET/CT data from the phase 1/2 trial and a more detailed analysis of the ^{18}F-FDG PET/CT data in measuring efficacy outcomes in patients with mPC who received nab-paclitaxel 125 or 100 mg/m^2 plus gemcitabine.

Methods

This open-label study, consisting of a phase 1 dose-finding portion and an expanded phase 2 portion at the maximum tolerated dose, was conducted at 4 centers in the United States in accordance with the Declaration of Helsinki and Good Clinical Practice Guidelines of the International Conference on Harmonization. Written informed consent was obtained from all patients before they entered the study. Details of the patients and methods in this study were reported previously [22]. Briefly, patients aged ≥18 years who had histologically or cytologically confirmed mPC with measurable disease by CT scan, as defined by the RECIST v1.0 guidelines, and no previous treatment for metastatic disease received nab-paclitaxel (100, 125, or 150 mg/m^2) followed by gemcitabine (1000 mg/m^2)—both administered intravenously on days 1, 8, and 15 every 28 days. Sixty-seven patients were enrolled in the trial: 20, 44, and 3 patients received 100, 125, and 150 mg/m^2 nab-paclitaxel, respectively. The maximum tolerated dose was established as 125 mg/m^2 of nab-paclitaxel plus 1000 mg/m^2 of gemcitabine once a week for 3 weeks every 28 days, which was the dose and schedule used in the phase 3 MPACT trial [17, 22]. This regimen is also the US Food and Drug Administration–approved dose and schedule for the treatment of mPC according to the prescribing information [18].

^{18}F-FDG PET/CT acquisition and scan lesion evaluation

^{18}F-FDG PET/CT scans of target and nontarget lesions were taken at baseline and at 6 and/or 12 weeks postbaseline. Patients underwent at least a 4-h fast prior to each scan. Patients were injected with a mean 5.5 × 10^{11} mBq ^{18}F-FDG (range, 3.3 × 10^{11}–10.4 × 10^{11} mBq) based upon body mass 0.44 × 10^{10} to 1.5 × 10^{10} mBq/kg. All patients' fasting glucose values were within an acceptable range (< 200 mg/dL). The average uptake period was 66 min (range, 50 to 110 min; 88% of all scans were conducted at an uptake period of 50 to 85 min). Each patient also underwent a low-dose CT scan for attenuation correction followed by a whole-body (orbitomeatal line to mid thighs) PET emission scan. The PET images were acquired in 2D and 3D modes per site standards (2–5 min per bed position) and then iteratively reconstructed with z-axis postprocessing filtering and corrected for attenuation using the low-dose CT scan series.

Baseline

Target lesions were chosen based on size and location. No more than 5 lesions in any 1 organ system and no more than 10 lesions in total were chosen for analysis of standardized uptake values (SUVs). The maximum SUV (SUV_{max}) of all target lesions within a patient was then summed and served as a measure of tumor burden at the baseline time point, referred to as SUV_{max} Total. Note that SUV_{max} has been commonly used, particularly at the time this study was conducted, to evaluate tumor burden and change in tumor burden by PET [3–7, 12, 23]. Nontarget lesions were noted, and the anatomical location of both target and nontarget lesions was recorded.

Follow-up

Scans of target and nontarget lesions were performed at weeks 6 and 12 postbaseline. The SUV_{max} of all target lesions was then summed, and the total served as a measure of tumor burden for that particular scan (SUV_{max} Total). The images were then evaluated for the presence of new lesions on the ^{18}F-FDG PET/CT fused images as appropriate.

In addition to the confirmatory CT scans following the PET imaging at 6 and 12 weeks, contrast-enhanced diagnostic-quality spiral CT scans were performed separately at baseline and every 4 weeks to evaluate tumor response to therapy per RECIST. The diagnostic CT scans required the evaluation of the chest, abdomen, and pelvis using the kVp, mAs, and slice thickness ≤ 5 mm to perform lesion assessments according to RECIST guidelines. Comparisons of PET/CT and diagnostic-quality spiral CT scans as markers of efficacy at specific time points were not feasible because of the difference in timing of the scans.

Image analysis

De-identified images were interpreted by a single reader (RLK). Images were inspected for quality, body coverage, and dose infiltration at the injection site and for other factors that could have altered quantitative analysis. The images were interpreted to determine treatment response using the PET/CT and image-fusion ^{18}F-FDG PET/CT data sets. The locations of the metastatic lesions were noted, and SUVs were determined when appropriate. The SUV activity in normal tissue of the liver and mediastinum was recorded. ^{18}F-FDG activity was considered to indicate malignancy when the ^{18}F-FDG activity was focal, was greater than the background ^{18}F-FDG metabolism, and had a corresponding abnormality on CT. Target lesions were selected on baseline PET/CT scans without guidance from follow-up scans. Up to 5 lesions were selected for target lesion SUV_{max} analysis from visual inspection of the lesions with the greatest

FDG uptake. Both primary pancreatic and metastatic lesions were included. All other hypermetabolic tumor lesions were considered nontarget lesions. Subsequently, SUV_{max} measurements of the target lesions were assessed on follow-up PET/CT scans. In the case of resolved hypermetabolic activity, the target lesions were given an SUV_{max} value of 0. Nontarget lesions were followed qualitatively for 1) complete resolution of FDG activity, 2) significant increase of FDG uptake compared to baseline scans, or 3) neither resolution nor significant increase (ie, metabolically stable) of FDG activity. Finally, any FDG focus that was consistent with malignant uptake that was not present previously was declared a new lesion if, in the opinion of the reader, it was consistent with malignant uptake. In order to assign time-point response, the sum of the SUV_{max} for target lesions was used to assess interval change from baseline along with a determination of new lesion development and change in nontarget lesion FDG behavior for final response assignment (Table 1).

SUVs

Standardized uptake values were determined using an SUV function integrated into a GE Advantage Window Workstation. In order to obtain the SUV measurement, a 1.5-cm region of interest (ROI) was deposited on the image slice that had the most intense ^{18}F-FDG activity determined by visual inspection. By definition, an SUV is a reflection of the amount of ^{18}F-FDG activity in an ROI per the following formula:

$$SUV = [activity/mL \ tissue \ (decay\text{-}corrected)]/$$

$$(injected \ dose/body \ weight).$$

Calculation of % tumor response on ^{18}F-FDG PET/CT

The percentage of change in SUV activity was calculated using the following formula:

$$\%Change \ SUV_{max}Total = \frac{[SUV_{max}Total \ (current \ scan)] - SUV_{max}Total \ (baseline \ scan)]}{[SUV_{max}Total \ (baseline)]} \times 100$$

The metabolic response category on the follow-up scans was then determined based on the EORTC criteria for PET response (Table 1) [19].

Statistical analysis

The characteristics of the target lesions were analyzed using standard descriptive statistics. Statistical analyses were carried out using SPSS 19 software. The best ^{18}F-FDG PET/CT response rate for each patient, measured as the percentage of change in SUV_{max} Total at follow-up compared with baseline, was calculated and classified per EORTC criteria (Table 1); note that the more

Table 1 EORTC criteria for determining tumor response by PET [19]

Classification	Description
Progressive metabolic disease	• An increase in ^{18}F-FDG tumor SUV of >25% within the tumor region defined on the baseline scan • Visible increase in the extent of ^{18}F-FDG tumor uptake (>20% in the longest dimension) • The appearance of new ^{18}F-FDG uptake in metastatic lesions
Stable metabolic disease	• An increase in tumor ^{18}F-FDG SUV of <25% • A decrease of <15% and no visible increase in the extent of ^{18}F-FDG tumor uptake (>20% in the longest dimension)
Partial metabolic response[a]	• A decrease in tumor uptake of ^{18}F-FDG >25% after >1 cycle of treatment
Complete metabolic response	• Complete resolution of ^{18}F-FDG uptake within the tumor volume so that it is indistinguishable from surrounding normal tissue

EORTC European Organisation for Research and Treatment of Cancer, ^{18}*F-FDG* [^{18}F]2-fluoro-2-deoxyglucose, *PET* positron emission tomography, *SUV* standardized uptake value
[a]EORTC criteria also define a decrease in tumor uptake of ^{18}F-FDG of ≥15% to 25% after 1 cycle of treatment as a partial metabolic response; however, the more stringent 25% threshold was applied to all patients in this study

stringent threshold of a ≥ 25% decrease was always used to define partial response because even the first postbaseline scan was at week 6, which was considered to be >1 cycle of treatment (see Table).

The relationship between the best PET response and OS was tested, using a log-rank test, in the group with a complete metabolic response (CMR, defined in Table 1) vs the non-CMR group (all had a partial metabolic response [PMR]) in the *nab*-paclitaxel 125 mg/m^2 dose cohort. A Cox proportional hazards model was used to determine whether the best percentage of change in PET was associated with OS. A nonparametric rank-correlation test was used to determine whether a correlation existed between the best percentage of PET and radiographic (using CT) changes; the data were summarized by Spearman rank-correlation coefficient. The relationship of CT and PET response was also evaluated by comparing rates of objective response in patients who had a CMR vs a PMR (CT and PET responses evaluated as categorical variables). A *P* value ≤ 0.05 was considered statistically significant.

Results
Of the 67 enrolled patients, 61 had a baseline ^{18}F-FDG PET/CT scan, and 52 patients had both a baseline ^{18}F-FDG PET/CT scan and at least 1 follow-up ^{18}F-FDG PET/CT scan at 6 weeks, 12 weeks, or both. Of the 20 treated patients in the *nab*-paclitaxel 100 mg/m^2 cohort, 13 had a baseline and at least 1 follow-up ^{18}F-FDG PET/CT scan at 6 weeks, 12 weeks, or both. Of the 44 treated patients in the *nab*-paclitaxel 125 mg/m^2 cohort, 38 had a baseline and at least 1 follow-up ^{18}F-FDG PET/CT scan at 6 weeks, 12 weeks, or both. Lack of follow-up scans was primarily due to disease progression, patient choice, or logistical/monetary reasons. Of 13 patients in the *nab*-paclitaxel 100 mg/m^2 cohort who had at least 1 follow-up ^{18}F-FDG PET/CT scan, 12 had an ^{18}F-FDG PET/CT scan at 6 weeks, and 12 had an ^{18}F-FDG PET/CT scan at 12 weeks. Of 38 patients in the *nab*-paclitaxel 125 mg/m^2 cohort who had at least 1 follow-up ^{18}F-FDG

PET/CT scan, 37 had an ^{18}F-FDG PET/CT scan at 6 weeks, and 34 had an ^{18}F-FDG PET/CT scan at 12 weeks. The median age of all patients was 61 years and of those in the *nab*-paclitaxel 100 and 125 mg/m^2 cohorts was 57 and 61 years, respectively (Table 2).

Distribution of lesions on ^{18}F-FDG PET/CT
The distribution and baseline SUV$_{max}$ of lesions from patients enrolled in this study are summarized in Table 3. Among all patients, primary pancreatic (*n* = 43) lesions were the most common target lesions examined. The mean SUV$_{max}$ of pancreatic lesions was 6.9 (median, 6.4; range, 1.5–17.5). The most common sites of metastases were liver (*n* = 37), with an average SUV$_{max}$ of 7.6 (median, 6.6; range, 2.2–15.7); peritoneum (*n* = 28), with an average SUV$_{max}$ of 5.9 (median, 5.3; range, 0.6–20.7); and mediastinal lymph nodes (*n* = 18), with an average SUV$_{max}$ of 4.5 (median, 4.0; range, 1.5–11.3). These findings were generally consistent between the 2 dose cohorts, with liver and peritoneum being the most common sites of metastases. Metastatic lesions were identified by PET/CT in most anatomical sites, with the exception of the brain and kidney. This distribution of involved sites is consistent with the known spread of PC metastasis by both lymphatic and hematogeneous routes.

Individual lesion analysis
A total of 42 and 154 lesions were evaluated on the ^{18}F-FDG PET/CT scans for patients in the *nab*-paclitaxel 100 and 125 mg/m^2 cohorts, respectively. The median numbers of target lesions per patient to be scanned by ^{18}F-FDG PET/CT at baseline were 3.0 and 4.0 in patients in the *nab*-paclitaxel 100 and 125 mg/m^2 cohorts, respectively. The best PET responses from baseline in patients in the *nab*-paclitaxel 100 and 125 mg/m^2 cohorts are shown in Fig. 1. Among patients in the *nab*-paclitaxel 100 mg/m^2 cohort, the median SUV$_{max}$ per lesion was 5.1 (quartiles 1–3 range, 3.4–11.2). Among patients in the *nab*-paclitaxel 125 mg/m^2 cohort, the median SUV$_{max}$ per lesion was 6.5 (quartiles 1–3 range, 3.9–9.5).

Table 2 Selected baseline patient characteristics for patients with a baseline and ≥1 follow-up PET scan

Characteristic	nab-Paclitaxel Dose[a]		
	100 mg/m^2 (n = 13)	125 mg/m^2 (n = 38)	All dose levels (n = 52)
Age, median (range), years	57.0 (30–79)	61.0 (28–76)	61.0 (28–79)
Male sex, n (%)	7 (54)	17 (45)	24 (46)
ECOG PS, n (%)			
0	6 (46)	21 (55)	28 (54)
1	7 (54)	17 (45)	24 (46)
CA 19–9 at baseline, median (range), units/mL	n = 12 1220.1 (16.8–180,062.0)	n = 37 880.8 (1.1–96,990.0)	n = 50 1062.6 (1.1–180,062.0)

[a]1 patient received nab-paclitaxel 150 mg/m^2 and their baseline characteristics are included in the "All dose levels" column

CA 19–9 carbohydrate antigen 19–9, ECOG PS Eastern Cooperative Oncology Group performance status, PET positron emission tomography

^{18}F-FDG PET/CT metabolic response

A summary of the ^{18}F-FDG response by dose cohort is presented in Table 4. Of the 52 evaluable patients, 17 (33%) had an EORTC-defined CMR, 32 (62%) had a PMR, and 3 (6%) had stable metabolic disease. No patients had progressive disease based on PET during this testing interval up to 12 weeks. Patients in the nab-paclitaxel 100 mg/m^2 cohort (n = 13) experienced an EORTC-defined CMR (3 [23%]), a PMR (7 [54%]), or stable metabolic disease (3 [23%]). Patients in the nab-paclitaxel 125 mg/m^2 cohort

(n = 38) had either an EORTC-defined CMR (13 [34%]) or a PMR (25 [66%]).

Among patients in the nab-paclitaxel 100 mg/m^2 cohort with a follow-up ^{18}F-FDG PET/CT scan at 6 and 12 weeks (n = 11), 6 (55%) had a decrease, 4 (36%) had an increase, and 1 (9%) had no change (either no change or change <1%) in SUV$_{max}$ from week 6 to week 12. Among patients in the nab-paclitaxel 125 mg/m^2 cohort with a follow-up ^{18}F-FDG PET/CT scan at 6 and 12 weeks (n = 33), 19 (58%) had a decrease, 7 (21%) had

Table 3 Lesions at baseline[a]

Lesion Location	nab-Paclitaxel 100 mg/m^2 (n = 13) n (%)	nab-Paclitaxel 125 mg/m^2 (n = 38) n (%)	All dose levels (n = 51) n (%)	Baseline SUV$_{max}$ Mean (St Dev)	Median
Pancreas	11 (85)	32 (84)	43 (84)	6.9 (3.6)	6.4
Liver	8 (62)	29 (76)	37 (73)	7.6 (3.4)	6.6
Peritoneum	4 (31)	24 (63)	28 (55)	5.9 (3.9)	5.3
Mediastinal nodes	3 (23)	15 (39)	18 (35)	4.5 (2.9)	4.0
Lung	3 (23)	11 (29)	14 (27)	2.6 (3.0)	2.1
Pelvic nodes	2 (15)	7 (18)	9 (18)	6.8 (2.7)	7.6
Hilar nodes	2 (15)	7 (18)	9 (18)	3.8 (1.8)	4.1
Neck nodes	1 (8)	5 (13)	6 (12)	6.7 (4.8)	5.1
Omentum/mesentery	1 (8)	5 (13)	6 (12)	6.8 (2.2)	6.6
Pleura	4 (31)	2 (5)	6 (12)	2.8 (2.0)	1.8
Bone	1 (8)	2 (5)	3 (6)	5.0 (1.4)	4.2
Adrenal glands	0	3 (8)	3 (6)	2.7 (1.4)	2.1
Spleen	0	2 (5)	2 (4)	3.1 (0.3)	3.1
Skin	2 (15)	0	2 (4)	5.9 (1.8)	5.9
Muscle	0	2 (5)	2 (4)	5.3 (1.1)	5.3
Other	0	0	0	Not Applicable	
Brain	0	0	0	Not Applicable	
Kidneys	0	0	0	Not Applicable	

[a]Based on a nominal alpha of .05 (2-tailed) and using Fisher exact tests, the 2 groups differed significantly on number of lesions in only 1 site: the pleura (P = 0.031)

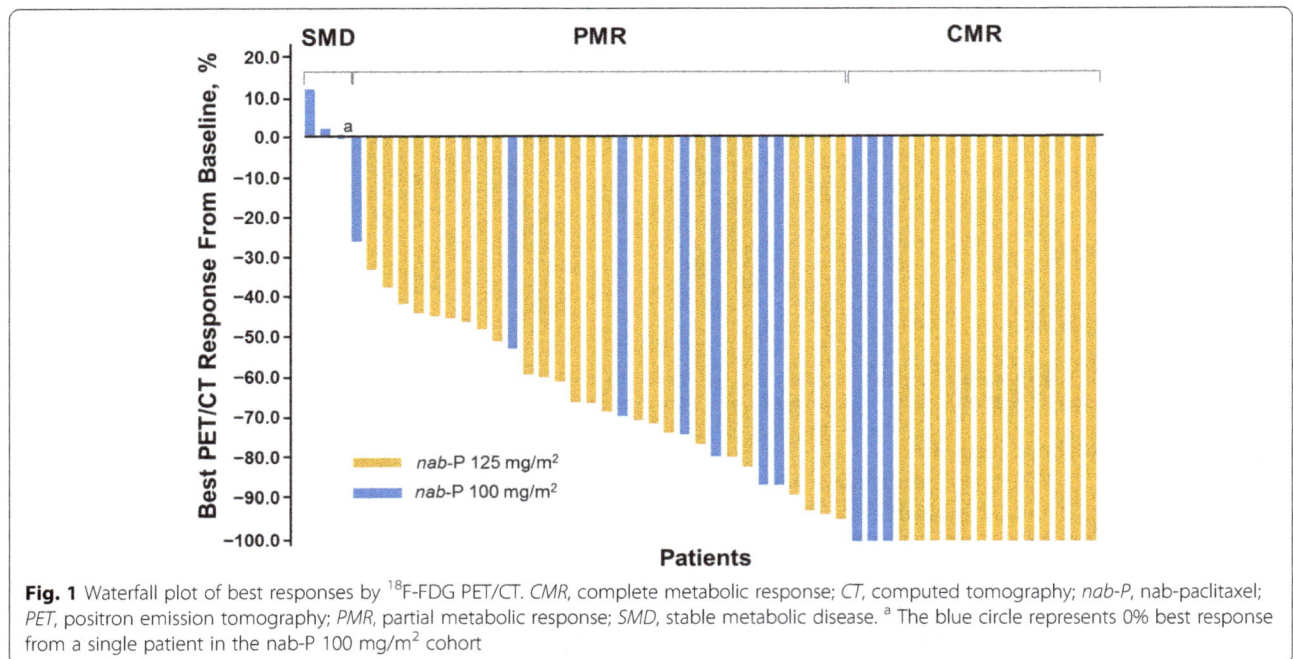

Fig. 1 Waterfall plot of best responses by ^{18}F-FDG PET/CT. *CMR*, complete metabolic response; *CT*, computed tomography; *nab-P*, nab-paclitaxel; *PET*, positron emission tomography; *PMR*, partial metabolic response; *SMD*, stable metabolic disease. [a] The blue circle represents 0% best response from a single patient in the nab-P 100 mg/m^2 cohort

an increase, and 7 (21%) had no change (either no change or change <1%) in SUV_{max} from week 6 to week 12.

^{18}F-FDG PET/CT response and median overall survival

Among patients who achieved a CMR or PMR by PET, a survival difference of ≈ 4 months was observed in favor of the *nab*-paclitaxel 125 mg/m^2 cohort vs the 100 mg/m^2 cohort (median, 15.6 vs 11.4 months, respectively; Table 5). In the *nab*-paclitaxel 125 mg/m^2 cohort, the OS in patients with a CMR was significantly longer than that of patients with a PMR (median, 23.0 vs 11.2 months; $P = 0.011$; Fig. 2). Within this cohort, a significant correlation was observed between best percentage of change in tumor burden by PET, evaluated as a continuous variable, and OS; namely, for each 1% decrease in PET SUV, the risk of death decreased by 2% (hazard ratio 0.98; 95% CI, 0.965–0.995; $P = 0.010$).

Radiographic response by CT scan and relationship with PET

Among patients in the *nab*-paclitaxel 125 mg/m^2 cohort, the investigator-assessed objective CT response rates by

diagnostic (spiral) CT per RECIST v1.0 were 77% in patients with a CMR vs 44% in patients with a PMR (both evaluated as categorical variables; $P = 0.053$); 21 of 38 patients had a partial response, and 8 of 38 patients had stable disease for ≥16 weeks by CT scan. The every-4-week response rates (per CT) over 28 weeks are reported in Table 6. The median time to best response by CT, as determined by the investigator, was 2.7 months collectively in patients in both the *nab*-paclitaxel 125 and 100 mg/m^2 cohorts (Fig. 3). No significant correlation was observed between best percentage of change in tumor burden by ^{18}F-FDG PET/CT and radiographic measurement by CT scan (Spearman analysis; $r_s = 0.22$; $P = 0.193$).

Discussion

The current study from a phase 1/2 trial provides evidence that pancreatic tumors and their associated

Table 4 ^{18}F-FDG PET/CT best response

nab-Paclitaxel Dose Cohort[a], n (%)	CMR	PMR	SMD	PMD
100 mg/m^2 (*n* = 13)	3 (23)	7 (54)	3 (23)	0
125 mg/m^2 (*n* = 38)	13 (34)	25 (66)	0	0

[a]1 patient received *nab*-paclitaxel 150 mg/m^2 and their best response by ^{18}F-FDG PET/CT was CMR

CMR complete metabolic response, *CT* computed tomography, ^{18}F-FDG [^{18}F]2-fluoro-2-deoxyglucose, *PET* positron emission tomography, *PMD* progressive metabolic disease, *PMR* partial metabolic response, *SMD* stable metabolic disease

Table 5 Overall survival by *nab*-paclitaxel cohort and response

	nab-Paclitaxel Dose	
	100 mg/m^2	125 mg/m^2
All PET-evaluable patients, n	13	38
Median OS, months	10.9	15.6
Patients with a CMR or PMR, n	10	38
Median OS, months	11.4	15.6
All patients, n	20	44
Median OS, months	9.3	12.2[a]

[a]Data previously published [22]

CMR complete metabolic response, *OS* overall survival, *PET* positron emission tomography, *PMR* partial metabolic response

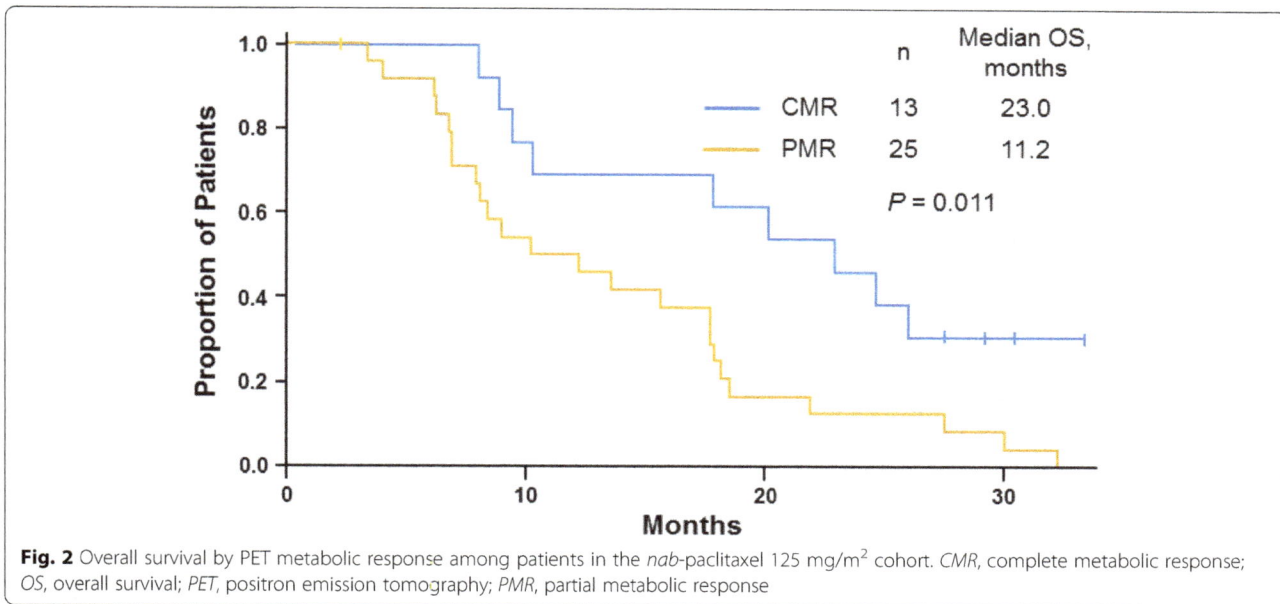

Fig. 2 Overall survival by PET metabolic response among patients in the *nab*-paclitaxel 125 mg/m^2 cohort. *CMR*, complete metabolic response; *OS*, overall survival; *PET*, positron emission tomography; *PMR*, partial metabolic response

metastases are hypermetabolic. ^{18}F-FDG PET/CT is a useful tool for monitoring treatment response, changes in tumor metabolic activity, and predicting survival in this disease setting.

The results described here support the previously reported survival benefit and antitumor activity of the *nab*-paclitaxel 125 mg/m^2 plus gemcitabine 1000 mg/m^2 regimen for treating mPC [17, 22]. The CMR and PMR rates were numerically higher in patients in the *nab*-paclitaxel 125 mg/m^2 cohort than in those in the *nab*-paclitaxel 100 mg/m^2 cohort (34% vs 23% and 66% vs 54%, respectively). Furthermore, a survival difference favoring the 125 vs the 100 mg/m^2 *nab*-paclitaxel group was observed in both the PET-evaluable population (> 4-month survival benefit for 125 vs 100 mg/m^2 [median, 15.6 vs 10.9 months, respectively]) and the all-evaluable population (≈ 3-month survival benefit [median, 12.2 vs 9.3 months, respectively) [22]. The longer survival in patients treated with *nab*-paclitaxel 125 mg/m^2, despite a similar or even higher baseline SUV_{max}, suggests a greater

Table 6 Every-4-week spiral CT tumor response rates in the 125 mg/m^2 *nab*-paclitaxel cohort over 28 weeks

Week	Patients (responders/evaluable), n/N	Response Rate, %
4	4/38	11
8	9/38	24
12	12/37	32
16	14/32	44
20	10/28	36
24	10/21	48
28	9/17	53

CT computed tomography

clinical benefit with the 125 mg/m^2 dose than with the 100 mg/m^2 dose. Additionally, the high metabolic response rates observed in the PET-evaluable cohorts (100% and 77% in the 125 and 100 mg/m^2 *nab*-paclitaxel dose cohorts, respectively) may reflect the previously published relatively high radiological response rates observed in this study (48% and 45% in the 125 and 100 mg/m^2 *nab*-paclitaxel dose cohorts, respectively [22]).

In this study, ^{18}F-FDG PET/CT responses at 6 or 12 weeks predicted survival among patients in the *nab*-paclitaxel 125 mg/m^2 cohort. The OS in patients in this cohort who had a CMR was significantly longer than that of patients who had a PMR (median, 23.0 vs 11.2 months, respectively; *P* = 0.011)—an observation that is consistent with our previous report for all patients with a CMR vs those without a CMR (median, 20.1 vs 10.3 months, respectively; *P* = 0.01) [22]. In addition, a significant correlation was found between the best percentage of change in PET score—evaluated as a continuous variable—and survival. These findings agree with the findings of a phase 1 study of patients with advanced PC that reported a significant correlation between improved OS and a decreased metabolic activity via PET in hepatic metastases [24]. That study, by Beatty and colleagues, underscores the utility of PET in analyses involving immunotherapies, in which radiological methods by CT could be complicated by inflammation. The validation of correlating a change in metabolic activity with survival strongly supports the clinical utility of PET analysis.

The analysis of change in SUV_{max} from week 6 to week 12 is informative of the dynamics of tumor metabolic response to therapy. This analysis suggests that

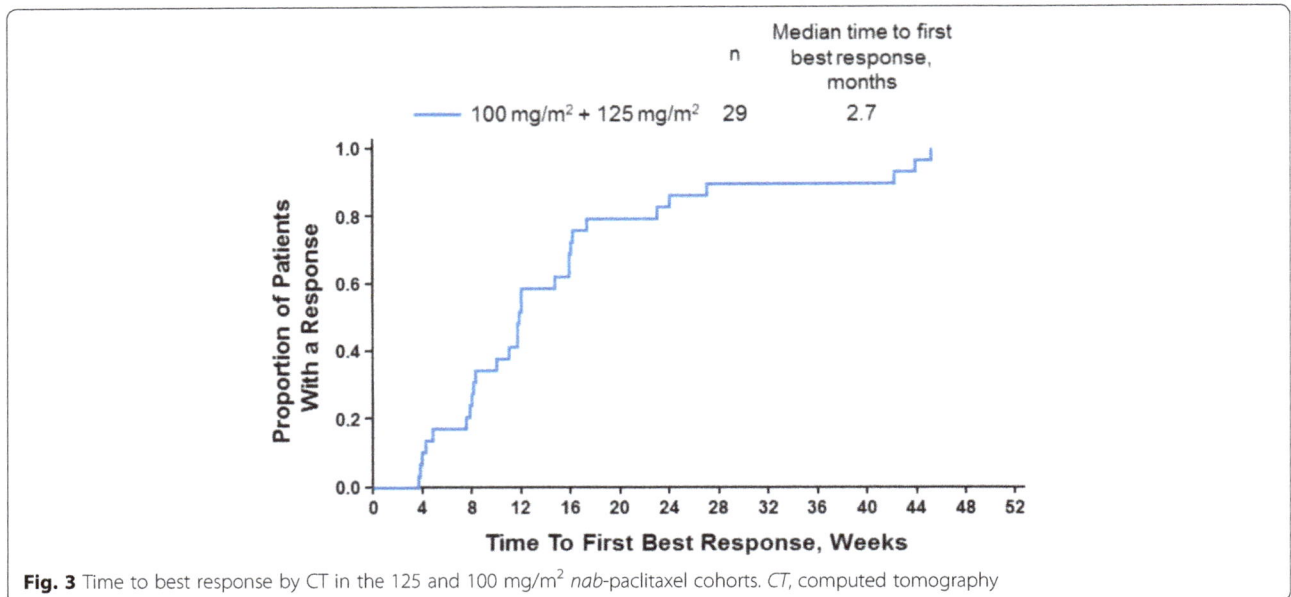

Fig. 3 Time to best response by CT in the 125 and 100 mg/m² *nab*-paclitaxel cohorts. *CT*, computed tomography

when patients experience a metabolic response following treatment with *nab*-paclitaxel 125 mg/m² plus gemcitabine 1000 mg/m², that response is unlikely to be reversed over a 6-week period. Determining the clinical activity of a particular treatment regimen at an early time point could inform the physician about whether to continue the current therapy or to switch to a different therapeutic option. Early assessment of clinical activity is particularly important given the recent interest in developing treatment plans for patients with mPC. In a study of neoadjuvant human epidermal growth factor receptor 2–positive breast cancer, metabolic responses determined by ^{18}FDG PET/CT were evident at 2 weeks post-treatment, and a significant correlation (R^2 = 0.81) was observed between the change in SUV_{max} at weeks 2 and 6 [5]. At weeks 2 and 6, the metabolic response rates (CMR plus PMR) of the primary tumor were 72% and 60%, respectively. Reductions in tumor metabolic activity reflected treatment outcome—the reduction in SUV_{max} at both 2 and 6 weeks was significantly greater in those with a pathological complete response (pCR) vs those without a pCR (P = 0.02 at both time points). Similarly, in a study of patients with previously treated non-small cell lung cancer, patients with a PMR 14 days after erlotinib treatment (26% of PET-evaluable patients) had a longer OS compared with patients without a metabolic response (P = .03) [23].

Previously, a controversy existed among oncologists regarding the usefulness of ^{18}F-FDG PET/CT for measuring tumor response in the mPC setting because of the perceived lack of sufficient FDG uptake in pancreatic lesions and the increased expense associated with the procedure. The current analysis confirms that primary pancreatic tumors and their metastases are PET avid and that ^{18}F-FDG-PET/CT is useful for monitoring their metabolic activity in this setting. Although the combined/hybrid device is more expensive than CT alone, it has the advantage of providing both functions as stand-alone examinations. This allows for improved staging and monitoring of disease progression and, thus, for potentially improved treatment plans. Furthermore, our data suggest that ^{18}F-FDG PET/CT is a valuable adjunct for assessing treatment response and can predict clinical outcomes in patients treated with *nab*-paclitaxel plus gemcitabine, particularly in patients who received the indicated dose and schedule.

Although the use of ^{18}F-FDG PET/CT in the mPC setting is promising, our study had some limitations. First, the number of patients evaluated by ^{18}F-FDG PET/CT was relatively small, and not all trial participants underwent PET/CT imaging because of either patient or physician discretion. Another limitation of the analysis was that 15 patients (6 in the *nab*-paclitaxel 125 mg/m² cohort) had PET scans only at baseline. Although this limitation could have had some effect on the overall correlation of PET responses with survival, it is unlikely that all of the patients would have had a CMR if a follow-up PET scan had been performed. Such a result would not negate the important observation of the long survival durations in patients who experienced a CMR.

The PET results of the phase 1/2 study presented here agree with those of the phase 3 MPACT trial in that PET appeared to be a more sensitive modality than spiral CT for measuring treatment response [12]. Both data sets support the notion that a metabolic response by PET is associated with longer survival. It is important to point out that these were distinct studies that differed in design and conduct, as reflected by the different median baseline SUV_{max} values (6.5 in this study and 4.6 in the phase 3 trial; both among patients in the *nab*-paclitaxel 125 mg/m^2 plus gemcitabine cohorts); thus, a direct comparison cannot be made.

Conclusions

The results of this study support the idea that metastatic and primary pancreatic lesions are FDG avid and that ^{18}F-FDG PET/CT in mPC is a useful tool for monitoring treatment response in patients treated with *nab*-paclitaxel plus gemcitabine, particularly at the indicated dose and schedule. The metabolic response rates observed in this study using PET/CT support the activity of the *nab*-paclitaxel 125 mg/m^2 plus gemcitabine 1000 mg/m^2 combination regimen for treating mPC. The significant correlation between the decrease in metabolic activity, as evident by FDG uptake, and decreased risk of death highlights the clinical utility of PET and suggests that this modality may be useful in predicting the success of experimental regimens. The median OS of 23.0 months in the CMR group deserves further evaluation in subsequent studies.

Abbreviations

^{18}F-FDG: [^{18}F]2-fluoro-2-deoxyglucose; CA 19–9: Carbohydrate antigen 19–9; CMR: Complete metabolic response; CT: Computed tomography; ECOG PS: Eastern Cooperative Oncology Group performance status; EORTC: European Organisation for Research and Treatment of Cancer; FOLFIRINOX: Folinic acid, 5-fluorouracil, irinotecan, and oxaliplatin; mPC: Metastatic pancreatic cancer; *nab*-P: *nab*-paclitaxel; OS: Overall survival; pCR: Pathological complete response; PET: Positron emission tomography; PMD: Progressive metabolic disease; PMR: Partial metabolic response; RECIST: Response Evaluation Criteria In Solid Tumors; ROI: Region of interest; SMD: Stable metabolic disease; SUV: Standardized uptake values; SUV_{max}: Maximum standardized uptake values; SUV_{max} Total: Standardized uptake values of all target lesions

Acknowledgements
Medical writing assistance was provided by Aaron Runkle, PhD, MediTech Media, Ltd. Biostatistical support was provided by Helen Liu and Xiaobin Yuan, Celgene Corporation. The authors are fully responsible for all content and editorial decisions related to this manuscript.

Funding
A research grant from the Stand Up To Cancer (SU2C) Dream Team to Dr. Daniel D. Von Hoff provided support for the translational studies. This study was supported by Celgene Corporation, Summit, NJ.

Authors' contributions
All authors read and approved the final manuscript.

Competing interests
RLK: research funding: Celgene; DDVH: consultant or advisory role, honoraria, and research funding: Celgene; MJB: nothing to disclose; RCB: consultant: Celgene; DM: employment: Celgene; MFR: employment: Celgene; RKR: consultant or advisory role, honoraria, and research funding: Celgene. The manuscript has not been submitted for publication nor is it under consideration for publication elsewhere.

Author details
^{1}Imaging Endpoints Core Lab, 9700 N 91st St, B-200, Scottsdale, AZ 85258, USA. ^{2}Translational Genomics Research Institute and HonorHealth, 445 North Fifth St, Suite 600, Phoenix, AZ 85004, USA. ^{3}Mayo Clinic, 13400 E Shea Blvd, Scottsdale, AZ 85259, USA. ^{4}Celgene Corporation, 86 Morris Ave, Summit, NJ 07901, USA. ^{5}Department of Interdisciplinary Health Sciences, A. T. Still University, 5850 E Still Circle, Mesa, AZ 85206, USA.

References

1. Koers K, Francken AB, Haanen JB, Woerdeman LA, van der Hage JA. Vemurafenib as neoadjuvant treatment for unresectable regional metastatic melanoma. J Clin Oncol. 2013;31:e251–3.
2. Li J, Xiao Y. Application of FDG-PET/CT in radiation oncology. Front Oncol. 2013;3:80.
3. McArthur GA, Puzanov I, Amaravadi R, Ribas A, Chapman P, Kim KB, et al. Marked, homogeneous, and early [18F]fluorodeoxyglucose-positron emission tomography responses to vemurafenib in BRAF-mutant advanced melanoma. J Clin Oncol. 2012;30:1628–34.
4. Qiao W, Zhao J, Xing Y, Wang C, Wang T. Predictive value of [^{18}F]fluoro-2-deoxy-D-glucose positron emission tomography for clinical outcome in patients with relapsed/refractory diffuse large B-cell lymphoma prior to and after autologous stem cell transplant. Leuk Lymphoma. 2014;55:276–82.
5. Gebhart G, Gamez C, Holmes E, Robles J, Garcia C, Cortes M, et al. ^{18}F-FDG PET/CT for early prediction of response to neoadjuvant lapatinib, trastuzumab, and their combination in HER2-positive breast cancer: results from neo-ALTTO. J Nucl Med. 2013;54:1862–8.
6. van Gool MH, Aukema TS, Schaake EE, Rijna H, Codrington HE, Valdés Olmos RA, et al. ^{18}F-fluorodeoxyglucose positron emission tomography versus computed tomography in predicting histopathological response to epidermal growth factor receptor-tyrosine kinase inhibitor treatment in resectable non-small cell lung cancer. Ann Surg Oncol. 2014;21:2831–7.
7. Engelmann BE, Loft A, Kjaer A, Nielsen HJ, Gerds TA, Benzon EV, et al. Positron emission tomography/computed tomography and biomarkers for early treatment response evaluation in metastatic colon cancer. Oncologist. 2014;19:164–72.
8. Teyton P, Metges JP, Atmani A, Jestin-Le Tallec V, Volant A, Visvikis D, et al. Use of positron emission tomography in surgery follow-up of esophageal cancer. J Gastrointest Surg. 2009;13:451–8.
9. Prestwich RJ, Subesinghe M, Gilbert A, Chowdhury FU, Sen M, Scarsbrook AF. Delayed response assessment with FDG-PET-CT following (chemo) radiotherapy for locally advanced head and neck squamous cell carcinoma. Clin Radiol. 2012;67:966–75.
10. Yu L, Jia C, Wang X, Lu P, Tian M, Wang W, et al. Evaluation of ^{18}F-FDG PET/CT in early-stage cervical carcinoma. Am J Med Sci. 2011;341:96–100.
11. Reske SN, Grillenberger KG, Glatting G, Port M, Hildebrandt M, Gansauge F, et al. Overexpression of glucose transporter 1 and increased FDG uptake in pancreatic carcinoma. J Nucl Med. 1997;38:1344–8.
12. Ramanathan RK, Goldstein D, Korn RL, Arena F, Moore M, Siena S, et al. Positron emission tomography response evaluation from a randomized phase III trial of weekly nab-paclitaxel plus gemcitabine versus gemcitabine alone for patients with metastatic adenocarcinoma of the pancreas. Ann Oncol. 2016;27:648–53.
13. Cancer Facts and Figures 2017. American Cancer Society. https://www.cancer.org/content/dam/cancer-org/research/cancer-facts-and-statistics/annual-cancer-facts-and-figures/2016/cancer-facts-and-figures-2016.pdf. 2017. Accessed 10 Feb 2017.
14. SEER Stat Fact Sheets: Pancreas Cancer. Surveillance, Epidemiology, and End Results Program. http://seer.cancer.gov/statfacts/html/pancreas.html 2017. Accessed 10 Feb 2017.

15. Conroy T, Desseigne F, Ychou M, Bouche O, Guimbaud R, Becouarn Y, et al. FOLFIRINOX versus gemcitabine for metastatic pancreatic cancer. N Engl J Med. 2011;364:1817–25.

16. Goldstein D, El-Maraghi RH, Hammel P, Heinemann V, Kunzmann V, Sastre J, et al. nab-Paclitaxel plus gemcitabine for metastatic pancreatic cancer: long-term survival from a phase III trial. J Natl Cancer Inst. 2015. doi 10.1093/jnci/dju413.

17. Von Hoff DD, Ervin T, Arena FP, Chiorean EG, Infante J, Moore M, et al. Increased survival in pancreatic cancer with nab-paclitaxel plus gemcitabine. N Engl J Med. 2013;369:1691–703.

18. Celgene Corporation. Abraxane for injectable suspension (paclitaxel protein-bound particles for injectable suspension) (albumin-bound): Summit, NJ: Celgene Corporation; 2015.

19. Young H, Baum R, Cremerius U, Herholz K, Hoekstra O, Lammertsma AA, et al. Measurement of clinical and subclinical tumour response using [^{18}F]-fluorodeoxyglucose and positron emission tomography: review and 1999 EORTC recommendations. European Organization for Research and Treatment of Cancer (EORTC) PET Study Group. Eur J Cancer. 1999;35:1773–82.

20. Therasse P, Arbuck SG, Eisenhauer EA, Wanders J, Kaplan RS, Rubinstein L, et al. New guidelines to evaluate the response to treatment in solid tumors. European Organization for Research and Treatment of Cancer, National Cancer Institute of the United States, National Cancer Institute of Canada. J Natl Cancer Inst. 2000;92:205–16.

21. Therasse P, European Organisation for Research and Treatment of Cancer Data Center. Evaluation of response: new and standard criteria. Ann Oncol. 2002;13(Suppl 4):127–9.

22. Von Hoff DD, Ramanathan RK, Borad MJ, Laheru DA, Smith LS, Wood TE, et al. Gemcitabine plus nab-paclitaxel is an active regimen in patients with advanced pancreatic cancer: a phase I/II trial. J Clin Oncol. 2011;29:4548–54.

23. Mileshkin L, Hicks RJ, Hughes BG, Mitchell PL, Charu V, Gitlitz BJ, et al. Changes in 18F-fluorodeoxyglucose and 18F-fluorodeoxythymidine positron emission tomography imaging in patients with non-small cell lung cancer treated with erlotinib. Clin Cancer Res. 2011;17:3304–15.

24. Beatty GL, Torigian DA, Chiorean EG, Saboury B, Brothers A, Alavi A, et al. A phase I study of an agonist CD40 monoclonal antibody (CP-870,893) in combination with gemcitabine in patients with advanced pancreatic ductal adenocarcinoma. Clin Cancer Res. 2013;19:6286–95.

14

CT texture analysis: a potential tool for prediction of survival in patients with metastatic clear cell carcinoma treated with sunitinib

Masoom A. Haider[1]*, Alireza Vosough[2], Farzad Khalvati[1], Alexander Kiss[3], Balaji Ganeshan[4] and Georg A. Bjarnason[5]

Abstract

Background: To assess CT texture based quantitative imaging biomarkers in the prediction of progression free survival (PFS) and overall survival (OS) in patients with clear cell renal cell carcinoma undergoing treatment with Sunitinib.

Methods: In this retrospective study, measurable lesions of 40 patients were selected based on RECIST criteria on standard contrast enhanced CT before and 2 months after treatment with Sunitinib. CT Texture analysis was performed using TexRAD research software (TexRAD Ltd, Cambridge, UK). Using a Cox regression model, correlation of texture parameters with measured time to progression and overall survival were assessed. Evaluation of combined International Metastatic Renal-Cell Carcinoma Database Consortium Model (IMDC) score with texture parameters was also performed.

Results: Size normalized standard deviation (nSD) alone at baseline and follow-up after treatment was a predictor of OS (Hazard ratio (HR) = 0.01 and 0.02; 95% confidence intervals (CI): 0.00 – 0.29 and 0.00 – 0.39; $p = 0.01$ and 0.01). Entropy following treatment and entropy change before and after treatment were both significant predictors of OS (HR = 2.68 and 87.77; 95% CI = 1.14 – 6.29 and 1.26 – 6115.69; $p = 0.02$ and $p = 0.04$). nSD was also a predictor of PFS at baseline and follow-up (HR = 0.01 and 0.01: 95% CI: 0.00 – 0.31 and 0.001 – 0.22; $p = 0.01$ and $p = 0.003$). When nSD at baseline or at follow-up was combined with IMDC, it improved the association with OS and PFS compared to IMDC alone.

Conclusion: Size normalized standard deviation from CT at baseline and follow-up scans is correlated with OS and PFS in clear cell renal cell carcinoma treated with Sunitinib.

Keywords: Prediction of outcome, Metastatic clear cell carcinoma, Quantitative imaging biomarkers, CT image features, CT texture analysis

Background

Multi-targeted tyrosine kinase inhibitor (TKI) therapy with Sunitinib is a standard treatment of metastatic clear cell renal cell carcinoma (RCC). Non-imaging related clinical prognostic factors have been identified for patients receiving targeted therapy and introduced into treatment guidelines and used to stratify patients on clinical trials [1]. This clinical prognostic model and the associated factors are described in the International Metastatic Renal-Cell Carcinoma Database Consortium Model (IMDC), which is used most commonly [2].

It is well known that enhancement features of RCC can change on contrast enhanced CT in patients receiving TKI's such as Sunitinib and this is not always reflected in an early change in the size of tumors thus limiting the application of RECIST criteria [3]. Multiple alternative response criteria which combine size and enhancement change such as Choi, modified Choi and Morphology Attenuation, Size and Structure (MASS) criteria have demonstrated a predictive ability by combining size and enhancement criteria to predict progression free survival (PFS) in patients with metastatic RCC [4–8].

* Correspondence: masoom.haider@sunnybrook.ca
[1]Department of Medical Imaging, Sunnybrook Health Sciences Center, University of Toronto, Rm AG-46, 2075 Bayview Ave, Toronto, Onatrio M4N 3M5, Canada
Full list of author information is available at the end of the article

Intratumoral heterogeneity is a recognized feature of cancer behavior and in particular, therapeutic resistance [9]. Analysis of tumor heterogeneity using CT texture analysis has shown promise as a prognostic and predictive measure in RCC. A previous study by Goh et al. showed that CT texture analysis reflecting tumor heterogeneity is an independent factor associated with PFS and has the potential to be used as a predictive imaging biomarker of response of metastatic RCC of various histologic types [10]. A more recent study has also included a variety of RCC histologies and confirmed potential prognostic value of CT texture features in assessment of the primary tumor site and outcome [11]. There have been other studies on the prognostic value of CT texture features for different types of cancer including breast [12] lung [13], hepatic metastatic colorectal cancer [14], pancreatic cancer [15] as well as reproducibility of CT texture parameters [16]. To our knowledge, a study specifically reviewing the potential prognostic and predictive value of texture features in a pure clear cell RCC cohort and evaluating this in the light of the IMDC prognostic score has not been performed.

The purpose of this study was to assess CT texture analysis based Quantitative Imaging Biomarkers (QIB's) in the prediction of PFS and Overall Survival (OS) in patients with clear cell RCC undergoing treatment with Sunitinib.

Methods

Patients

The institutional research ethics board approved this retrospective single institution study and waived the requirement for informed consent.

Patients with metastatic clear cell carcinoma who received the TKI Sunitinib as first or second line therapy at our institution between December 2005 and March 2010 were identified from institutional renal cancer database. An attempt was made to optimize the activity of Sunitinib by treating each patient to toxicity using individualized dose and schedule [17]. An IMDC prognostic score was assigned to each patient at baseline.

Patients were included if they were TKI naïve and had received Sunitinib as the first or second line treatment for metastatic clear cell carcinoma. Patients were excluded if: their baseline contrast enhanced CT was not performed within 6 weeks before the start of treatment; both their baseline and followup CT were not performed with contrast enhancement; they did not have measurable disease at baseline as defined by RECIST 1.1.

From a total of 172 patients who were identified in the institution database, 132 patients were excluded with 40 patients left for analysis. The most common reasons for exclusion was lack of availability for the pre-treatment or first follow-up scan, typically due to imaging being performed at another institution.

CT examination

All patients underwent contrast enhanced CT examination of their chest, abdomen and pelvis (GE Lightspeed Plus or GE Lightspeed VCT) following injection of 100 ml of an iodinated contrast agent (Omnipaque 300, Iohexol, GE Healthcare, Princeton, NJ, USA) at a rate of 3 ml/s via an automated injector.

Images of the thorax were analyzed in arterial phase (25-s delay) and images of the abdomen and pelvis were analyzed in portal venous phase (70-s delay) with the following acquisition parameters: 120 kV; auto mA and Smart mA (angular and z-axis modulation); pitch 0.75:1 and 0.9:1; 20 mm collimation, 5 mm slice thickness and 40 mm collimation reconstructed; scan field of view (FOV) 50 cm and display FOV adjusted to patient size; matrix: 512x512 (pixel spacing: 0.933 mm). Region of interest (ROI) was drawn by a radiologist with 6 years of experience of reporting abdominal CT who was blinded to the clinical outcome. Each ROI was drawn on the slice through the largest diameter of the tumor site.

CT Texture Analysis

Target lesions were selected according to RECIST, version 1.1 (maximum of five target lesions, maximum of two lesions per organ). If the patient had not had resection of primary tumor, it was included as a measurable tumor and used for analysis. RECIST 1.1 criteria were used to identify disease progression, which was confirmed using subsequent imaging. Using RECIST 1.1, initial response after two cycles of treatment was evaluated. CT texture analysis of the lesions was performed using TexRAD commercial research software (TexRAD Ltd, www.texrad.com, part of Feedback Plc, Cambridge, UK) by drawing a ROI around the peripheral margin of the selected lesions used for RECIST. Metastases/primary lesions less than 1 cm in maximal diameter were not included in the analysis. Air, streak artifacts and dense calcifications were excluded from the regions of interest. CT texture analysis comprised a filtration-histogram technique where the filtration step extracted and enhanced (amplified) features using a band-pass Laplacian of Gaussian spatial scale filter [18]. Quantification was done using different histogram based statistical parameters in the selected region of interest in CT images after the application of the band-pass filter at intermediate scale which was chosen to mimic the scale used by Goh et al. [10].

Histogram based statistical parameters comprised of mean positive pixel intensity (the average value of the positive pixels within the ROI), standard deviation (SD), skewness (symmetry of the pixel intensity distribution), kurtosis (pointiness of the pixel intensity distribution), and entropy which represents irregularity or complexity of pixel intensity in space. These are all first-order statistical features except for entropy which is a second-order statistical feature. A newer secondary histogram parameter derived from the above parameters, size normalized standard deviation (nSD), was also evaluated. This was done as it is known that SD estimate can be affected by the size (meaning the number of pixels) specifically in case of small tumors which may need correction or normalization [18] (Eq. 1).

nSD of a given ROI is calculated as follows:

$$nSD = \frac{Ln(SD)}{Ln(N)} \tag{1}$$

where SD is the standard deviation of ROI (i.e., tumor) and N is the total number of pixels in the ROI.

These parameters were recorded for each lesion in baseline CT images and the first follow-up CT images after treatment with Sunitinib. Percentage change (*PerC*) of the CT texture parameters before and after treatment were calculated (Eq. 2).

$$PerC = \frac{(\text{Parameter post treatment}) - (\text{Parameter pre-treatment})}{(\text{Parameter pre- treatment})} \times 100 \tag{2}$$

As the value of Kurtosis can vary from −3 to +3, to negate division by 0 when calculating the percentage change, we added 3, i.e. [((Kurtosis post treatment +3) - (Kurtosis pre-treatment +3))/(Kurtosis pre-treatment +3)] × 100. In case of Skewness, in order to avoid dividing by 0, only change (not the percentage change) was used, i.e. Skewness post treatment − Skewness pre-treatment.

Statistical Analysis

For statistical analysis, average texture measurements of all measured lesions in each patient at baseline CT and the first follow-up CT performed about 2 months after the start of treatment, the percentage change from baseline value as well as the percentage change in lesion size based on RECIST 1.1 criteria, which measures the amount of lesion size reduction, were used. PFS was defined as the time from the date of baseline CT to the date of disease progression based on RECIST response criteria. A Cox proportional hazards survival model was performed to determine if any parameter was predictors of OS or PFS. No adjustments for multiple testing were carried out as these analyses are considered exploratory and their results will serve to enhance future larger studies. All statistical analysis was performed using SAS Version 9.3 (SAS Institute, Cary, NC, USA).

The International Metastatic Renal-Cell Carcinoma Database Consortium Model (IMDC) allocates patient to three prognostic groups (good, intermediate and poor) based on the degree of anemia, thrombocytosis, neutrophilia, and hypercalcemia, as well as the Karnofski performance status <80%, and <1 year from diagnosis to treatment. To assess whether any of the CT texture parameters adds to IMDC in prediction of PFS and OS, we ran 2 variable Cox proportional hazards regression models and assessed model fit using −2 log likelihood (−2LL) statistics. For addition of one variable to IMDC, a change of greater than 3.84 (the critical value associated with one degree of freedom for a chi-square statistic) would indicate a significant model improvement. We could not explore models with 3 or more variables due to limitations in sample size. A P value of less than 0.05 was considered to indicate statistical significance.

Results

The cohort consisted of 35 men and 5 women with a mean age of 60 years (range of 34–76 years). All the patients had clear cell carcinoma. 34 patients received Sunitinib as first line therapy and 6 patients received Sunitinib as the second line treatment after being treated with a non-TKI drug (e.g. interferon). A total of 87 target lesions were analyzed. These lesions were scattered across different locations as listed in Table 1.

The baseline contrast enhanced CT of the patients included in the analysis was performed within 6 weeks before the start of treatment (mean was 12.8 day pre-treatment) and their followup CT was performed with contrast enhancement (mean followup time was 67.5 days). Six of 40 patients had progressed during the study period with a PFS of 60 days (range: 64–171 days). The length of followup was up to 22.8 months following baseline CT or until death whichever sooner. The significance of each texture

Table 1 Tumor Sites

Tumor Site	Number of lesions
Lymph node	15
Lung	14
Primary	10
Bone	10
Liver	8
Peritoneum	6
Adrenal	4
Mediastinal Lymph Nodes	4
Nephrectomy bed	4
Other kidney	3
Hilar Lymph Nodes	3
Pleura	1
IVC Thrombus	1
Muscle	1
Spleen	1
Omentum	1
Psoas major muscle	1
Total	87

parameter in prediction of OS and PFS is summarized in Tables 2 and 3, respectively.

Overall survival

Size normalized standard deviation (nSD) prior to treatment with Sunitinib was a significant predictor for OS ($p = 0.01$) such that higher nSD before treatment predicted for increased survival (positive correlation) (HR = 0.01, 95% CI = 0.00 − 0.29). In addition, nSD following treatment with Sunitinib was found to be significant in predicting OS ($p = 0.01$) such that higher nSD after treatment was associated with a lower hazard of death or higher survival (positive correlation) (HR = 0.02, 95% CI = 0.001 − 0.39). Entropy following treatment and entropy change both were significant predictors of OS such that higher entropy following treatment or entropy change predicted decreased survival (negative correlation) ($p = 0.02$, HR = 2.68, 95% CI = 1.14 − 6.29 and $p = 0.04$, HR = 87.77, 95% CI = 1.26 − 6115.69, respectively) (Table 2).

Progression free survival

With regards to PFS, nSD prior to treatment with Sunitinib was a significant predictor ($p = 0.01$) such that higher nSD before treatment was related to increased PFS (positive

Table 2 Imaging parameters as predictors of OS

Variable	P-value	Hazard ratio	95% CI
Mean positive pixel intensity prior to treatment	0.34	1.01	0.98 − 1.05
Mean positive pixel intensity following treatment	0.77	1.00	0.99 − 1.02
SD prior to treatment	0.24	0.98	0.96 − 1.01
SD following treatment	0.46	0.99	0.98 − 1.01
Entropy prior to treatment	0.27	1.74	0.65 − 4.68
Entropy following treatment	**0.02**	**2.68**	**1.14 − 6.29**
nSD prior to treatment	**0.01**	**0.01**	**0.00 − 0.29**
nSD following treatment	**0.01**	**0.02**	**0.001 − 0.39**
Kurtosis prior to treatment	0.26	1.24	0.85 − 1.82
Kurtosis following treatment	0.78	1.03	0.81 − 1.32
Skewness prior to treatment	0.15	2.02	0.77 − 5.30
Skewness following treatment	0.30	1.47	0.70 − 3.09
Percent change in size	**0.02**	**0.97**	**0.94 − 0.99**
Mean pixel intensity Change	0.37	0.99	0.98 − 1.01
SD Change	0.80	1.14	0.42 − 3.09
Entropy Change	**0.04**	**87.77**	**1.26 − 6115.69**
nSD Change	0.39	0.18	0.004 − 8.56
Kurtosis Change	0.46	0.66	0.21 − 2.02
Skewness Change	0.98	0.99	0.60 − 1.65

Entries in bold were significant
Abbreviations: SD standard deviation, *nSD* size normalized standard deviation
OS overall survival

Table 3 Imaging parameters as predictors of PFS

Variable	P-value	Hazard ratio	95% CI
Mean positive pixel intensity prior to treatment	0.61	1.01	0.98 − 1.04
Mean positive pixel intensity following treatment	0.72	1.00	0.99 − 1.02
SD prior to treatment	0.71	0.99	0.97 − 1.02
SD following treatment	0.33	0.99	0.97 − 1.01
Entropy prior to treatment	0.25	1.84	0.64 − 5.32
Entropy following treatment	0.08	2.23	0.91 − 5.49
nSD prior to treatment	**0.01**	**0.01**	**0.000 − 0.31**
nSD following treatment	**0.003**	**0.01**	**0.001 − 0.22**
Kurtosis prior to treatment	0.21	1.28	0.87 − 1.87
Kurtosis following treatment	0.34	1.12	0.89 − 1.41
Skewness prior to treatment	0.32	1.66	0.62 − 4.41
Skewness following treatment	0.65	1.20	0.55 − 2.61
Percent change in size	0.14	0.98	0.96 − 1.01
Mean pixel intensity change	0.36	0.99	0.98 − 1.01
SD change	0.51	0.70	0.25 − 2.02
Entropy change	0.21	15.12	0.21 − 1096.9
nSD change	0.06	0.02	0.00 − 1.21
Kurtosis change	0.92	1.06	0.37 − 3.04
Skewness change	0.81	0.94	0.56 − 1.58

Entries in bold were significant
Abbreviations: SD standard deviation, *nSD* size normalized standard deviation, *PFS* progression free survival

correlation) (HR = 0.01, 95% CI = 0.00 − 0.31). Moreover, nSD following treatment with Sunitinib was found to be significant in predicting PFS ($p = 0.003$) such that higher nSD after treatment leads to lower hazard of death or increased PFS (positive correlation) (HR = 0.01, 95% CI = 0.00 − 0.22). Neither entropy following treatment nor entropy change was significant predictor of PFS (Table 3).

The lesion's size change (percentage change, in terms of reduction, in sum of the lesions' size in each patient prior to and following treatment with Sunitinib) demonstrated a significant relation to OS (positive correlation) ($p = 0.02$), (HR = 0.97, 95% CI = 0.94 − 1.00), while size change was not a significant predictor of PFS.

Imaging variables combined with IMDC

To analyze the added predictive value of imaging variables to IMDC, we started with a baseline Cox proportion hazards model that only included the IMDC and then added each of the imaging variables found to be significant in the univariate survival analyses for OS or PFS. The baseline model with IMDC alone was significantly related to OS and had a −2 log likelihood statistic of 181.3. Therefore, to see an improved fit in any of the two-variable models tested, this statistic would have to change by a minimum of 3.84 (a 1° of freedom change for a chi-square statistic). This means that any value of 177.5 or less indicated a significant improvement in model fit. This improvement was seen for all two-variable models tested, however the ones that contained nSD prior to treatment and nSD following treatment showed the greatest improvement in fit. For both of these models, IMDC was no longer significant. Therefore, these variables (i.e., nSD prior to and following treatment) were seen as stronger predictors of survival in a model that included IMDC. The ability of each texture parameter to add to IMDC model in the prediction of OS is summarized in Table 4.

For PFS models, the baseline model with IMDC alone was not significantly related to PFS and had a −2 log likelihood statistic of 174.4. Therefore to see an improved fit in any of the two-variable models tested, this statistic would have to change by a minimum of 3.84 (a 1° of freedom change for a chi-square statistic). This means that any value of 170.6 or less indicated a significant improvement in model fit. This improvement was only seen for the 2 variable models that contained nSD prior to treatment and nSD following treatment. For both of these models, the nSD variables significantly improved the model in predicting PFS whereas in neither model IMDC was significant. Therefore, these variables were seen as stronger predictors of survival in a model that included IMDC. The ability of each texture parameter to improve IMDC model in the prediction of PFS is summarized in Table 5.

When added, the lesion size (percentage change in sum of the largest diameter of the lesions' size prior to and post treatment) did not make a significant improvement to IMDC in prediction of OS. Finally, separate univariate Cox proportional hazards models

Table 4 Imaging variables combined with IMDC to see if they improve on the prediction of OS

Model	IMDC	IMDC Combined Model	Fit statistic value (−2LL)
Baseline model with IMDC alone	**Significant**		**181.3**
IMDC + Entropy following treatment	**Not Significant**	**Significant**	**176.4**
IMDC + nSD prior to treatment	**Not significant**	**Significant**	**176.1**
IMDC + nSD following treatment	**Not significant**	**Significant**	**175.3**
IMDC + percent change in lesion size	Not significant	Not significant	177.8
IMDC + Entropy change	Not significant	Not significant	177.4

Entries in bold were significant
Abbreviations: nSD size normalized standard deviation, *IMDC* International Metastatic Renal-Cell Carcinoma Database Consortium Model, *OS* overall survival

Table 5 Imaging variables combined with IMDC to see if they improve on prediction of the PFS

Model	IMDC	IMDC Combined Model	Fit statistic value (−2LL)
Baseline model with IMDC alone	Not significant		174.4
IMDC + nSD pre treatment	**Not significant**	**Significant**	**169.3**
IMDC + nSD post treatment	**Not significant**	**Significant**	**165.9**

Entries in bold were significant
Abbreviations: nSD = size normalized standard deviation, *IMDC* International Metastatic Renal-Cell Carcinoma Database Consortium Model, *PFS* progression free survival

were run, one for percent change in size, the other for nSD prior to treatment, to compare the two variables. nSD prior to treatment was found to be a better predictor of OS ($p = 0.01$ versus 0.02) with HR = 0.01, 95% CI = 0.00 − 0.29).

Examples of CT images demonstrating the appearance of lesions in patients with varying outcomes (OS and PFS) are presented in Fig. 1 and Table 6. The Kaplan-Meier plots for significant parameters for OS and PFS are shown in Figs. 2 and 3.

Discussion

In this study, we demonstrate that texture related CT QIB's are predictive of OS and PFS in metastatic RCC treated with Sunitinib. This study is different from prior studies including the ones done by Goh et al. [10] and Lubner et al. [11] in that the population is limited to patients with clear cell RCC and that it assesses the imaging features in combination with the IMDC prognostic model for RCC patients treated with targeted therapy [1]. This is clinically relevant as one of the proposed uses of QIB's for personalized medicine is the selection of optimal drug therapies. In the context of clear cell RCC, there are more than one potential first line TKI's. Thus, it is important to know the baseline characteristic in the context of single histologic tumor type with the standard first line agent as a monotherapy. We have shown that size normalized standard deviation at baseline and follow-up, tumor size change, entropy at initial follow-up, and entropy change before and after treatment are potentially useful QIB's.

In addition, the study in Goh et al. [10] only looks at PFS while in this paper, both OS and PFS are studied. Furthermore, we limited our cohort to clear cell carcinoma only and a single TKI drug while Goh et al. [10] includes multiple TKI's and multiple tumor types. Thus, the cohort used in this study would be more reflective to be used as a benchmark of baseline Sunitinib activity to compare new TKI's in drug trials. The study by Lubner et al. [11] includes a variety of RCC subtypes and does

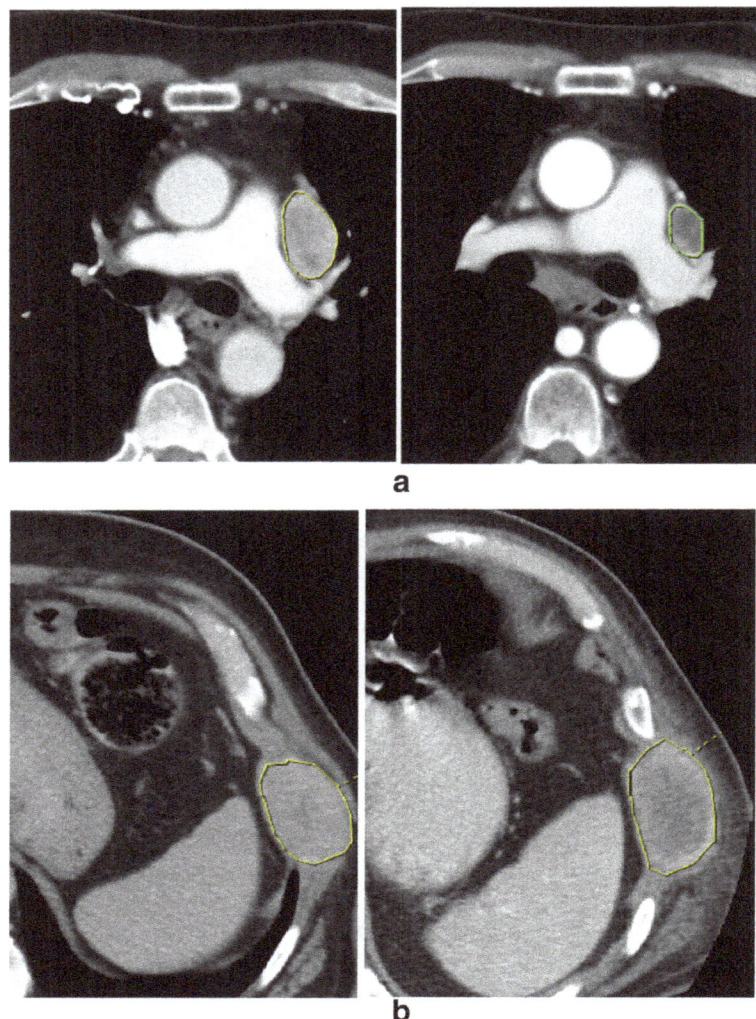

Fig. 1 Baseline CT in patients with metastatic clear cell renal cell carcinoma and intermediate IMDC score (Left: prior to treatment, Right: following the treatment). **a** 72-year-old man: OS and PFS in this patient was 1074 and 1063 days, respectively with a baseline nSD = 0.66. Although the tumor remains heterogeneous in appearance there is response by RECIST criteria. **b** 40-year-old man: OS and PFS in this patient were poor at 159 and 113 days, respectively with a lower baseline nSD of 0.54. The tumor is slightly larger but stable by RECIST criteria. The list of significant parameters for 2 cases is shown in Table 6 below. As it can be seen from the table, higher nSD prior to and following treatment and higher percent change in lesion size (i.e., higher size reduction) were associated with higher survival; and higher entropy following treatment and entropy change predicted decreased survival. It should be noted that for PFS, only nSD prior to and following treatment were statistically significant parameters

not specify what drugs used for patient treatment and focuses more on prediction of histologic features.

CT texture features and IMDS

Given that the IMDC prognostic model is well established in RCC patients, we have demonstrated the potential additional value of nSD to further improve prediction of OS and PFS when added to IMDC. In our study, nSD measured in CT images acquired before and after treatment were added to IMDC model. The entropy change prior to and following the treatment and percentage change in the sum of the largest diameter of

Table 6 The list of significant parameters (with median values) for 2 cases shown in Fig. 1

	OS	PFS	Entropy following treatment	nSD prior to treatment	nSD following treatment	Percent change in size	Entropy Change
Median	729	358	4.76	0.58	0.56	7.65	−0.036
A	1074	1063	4.57	0.66	0.88	33	−0.119
B	159	113	4.79	0.54	0.55	−1	−0.002

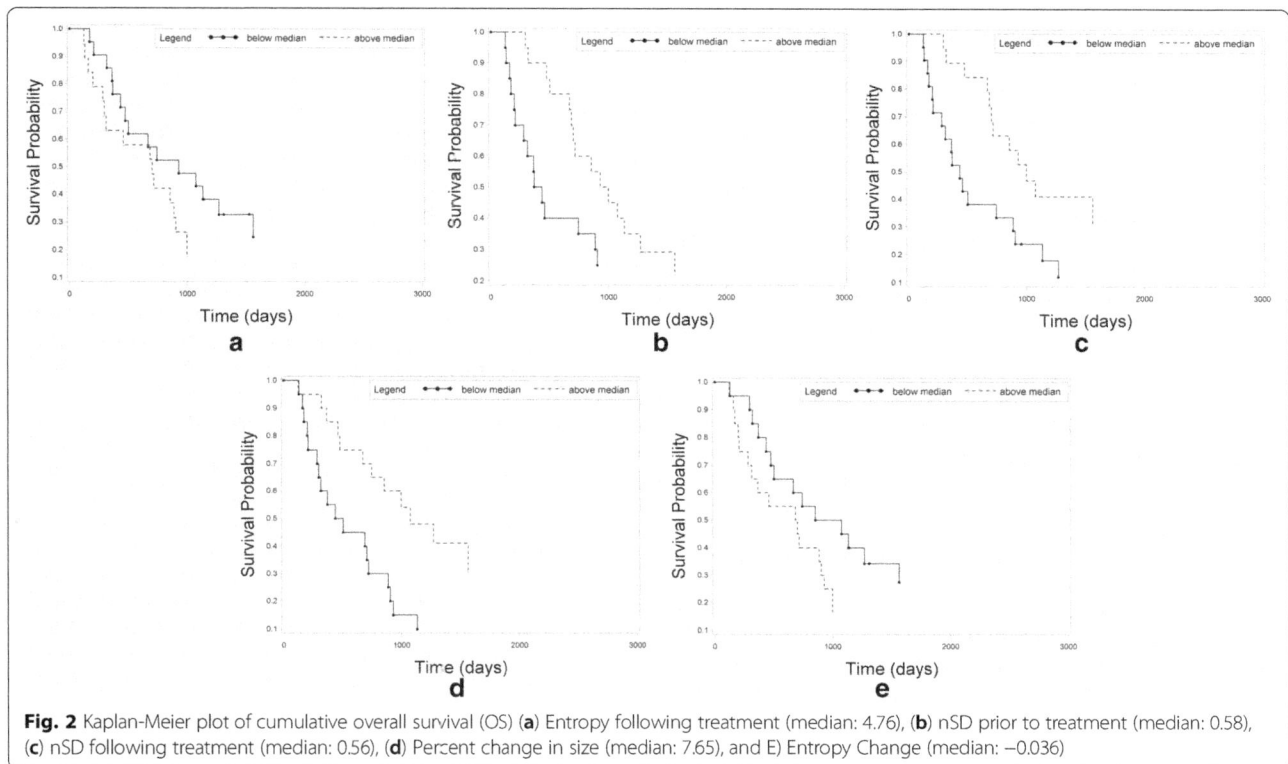

Fig. 2 Kaplan-Meier plot of cumulative overall survival (OS) (**a**) Entropy following treatment (median: 4.76), (**b**) nSD prior to treatment (median: 0.58), (**c**) nSD following treatment (median: 0.56), (**d**) Percent change in size (median: 7.65), and E) Entropy Change (median: −0.036)

the lesions size prior to and post treatment did not make a significant improvement to IMDC in the prediction of OS. In a model comparing size and nSD prior to treatment, the latter was a better predictor of OS.

CT texture features and RECIST criteria

The fact that early size change measured by RECIST is correlated with OS but not PFS is interesting. This discrepancy might be explained by the fact that PFS is reflective of the time course of a single drug as patients would not switch to a second line TKI unless they progressed while OS includes a course of therapy which may include second line and third line TKI's. Thus, the early size change on Sunitinib could be reflective of overall responsiveness to the TKI's family including second and third line therapies. RECIST is a very intuitive QIB. In contrast, the visual correlate of nSD may not be intuitive and this may be a barrier to adoption. Therefore, further study is required to investigate the visual patterns of QIBs such as nSD and their histologic correlates to make them more meaningful to the clinicians so that they are not considered as the output of a black box. A preliminary study has been done in this regard by Miles et al. [18] however, further work is required.

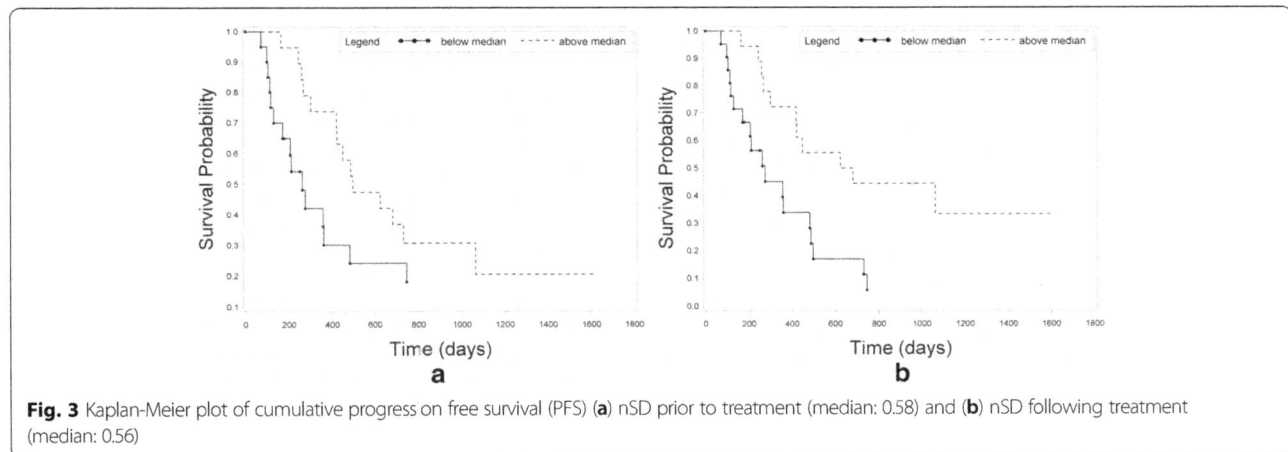

Fig. 3 Kaplan-Meier plot of cumulative progress on free survival (PFS) (**a**) nSD prior to treatment (median: 0.58) and (**b**) nSD following treatment (median: 0.56)

For example, it is possible that nSD, by combining the number of voxels in a ROI and standard deviation, is combining both size and variation into a single biomarker and thus, providing value by not wholly dispensing with size as a QIB.

Incorporation of new imaging response criteria such as changes in attenuation, morphology and structure into new classifications (Choi, modified Choi and Morphology, Attenuation, Size, and Structure (MASS) criteria) [4, 8] to assess response to antiangiogenic therapies provides more accurate assessment of tumor response to the targeted therapies, but has some limitations. These criteria require follow-up imaging and are not in themselves QIB's, however, they are intuitive and pragmatic. Further research into the optimal approach and use of these measures in personalized medicine is required.

Study limitations

Our study has limitations. In particular, we note that the small sample size did not allow for multiple testing correction for the large number of QIB's tested. This means that the results for this study remain hypothesis generating and further prospective validation will be required as with other similar studies published to date. In addition, this study was retrospective, raising potential selection biases. For example, patients who had a decline in renal function and did not have contrast on their follow-up were excluded from this analysis.

Clinical value

Of clinical interest is the value of baseline nSD both as a predictive and prognostic parameter and its potential additive value to the IMDC score at baseline. This opens the door to prospective validation with the aim to define a predictive biomarker for optimal drug selection initially without having to wait for a follow-up scan using a practical and low cost standard of care test, a simple contrast enhanced CT.

Conclusion

In conclusion, size normalized standard deviation is a quantitative imaging biomarker texture feature that in patients with metastatic clear cell carcinoma may add to the IMDC score in prediction of therapy response and overall survival. Further validation of this biomarker in prospective trials is required.

Abbreviations

CI: Confidence interval; HR: Hazard ratio; IMDC: International Metastatic Renal-Cell Carcinoma Database Consortium Model; nSD: normalized standard deviation; OS: Overall survival; PerC: Percentage change; PFS: Progression free survival; QIB: Quantitative imaging biomarker; RCC: Renal cell carcinoma; ROI: Region of interest; SD: Standard deviation; TKI: Multi-targeted tyrosine kinase inhibitor

Acknowledgements
Not applicable.

Funding
This research has been supported by Ontario Institute for Cancer Research (OICR).

Authors' contributions
MAH, AV, FK, AK, BG, and GAB contributed to the design and implementation of the concept. MAH, AV, and GAB contributed in collecting and reviewing the data. MAH, FK, and AK contributed to the design and implementation of quantitative feature extraction modules. AK contributed to the statistical analysis of the data. All authors contributed to the writing and reviewing of the paper. All authors read and approved the final manuscript.

Competing interests
B. Ganeshan is a director, part-time employee and shareholder of Feedback Plc (Cambridge, UK), a company that develops and commercializes the TexRAD texture analysis research software analysis described in this manuscript. The remaining authors declare that they have no competing interests.

Author details
[1]Department of Medical Imaging, Sunnybrook Health Sciences Center, University of Toronto, Rm AG-46, 2075 Bayview Ave, Toronto, Onatrio M4N 3M5, Canada. [2]Department of Radiology, North Bristol NHS Trust, Southmead Hospital, Bristol, UK. [3]Sunnybrook Health Sciences Center, Toronto, Canada. [4]Institute of Nuclear Medicine, University College London, London, UK. [5]Sunnybrook Odette Cancer Centre, Division of medical Oncology, University of Toronto, Toronto, ON, Canada.

References
1. National Comprehensive Cancer Network-Kidney Cancer 3. 2016.
2. Heng DYC, Xie W, Regan MM, Harshman LC, Bjarnason GA, Vaishampayan UN, et al. External validation and comparison with other models of the international metastatic renal-cell carcinoma database consortium prognostic model: a population-based study. Lancet Oncol. 2013;14(2):141–8.
3. Griffin N, Gore ME, Sohaib SA. Imaging in metastatic renal cell carcinoma. AJR Am J Roentgenol. 2007;189(2):360–70.
4. van der Veldt AAM, Meijerink MR, van den Eertwegh AJM, Haanen JBAG, Boven E. Choi response criteria for early prediction of clinical outcome in patients with metastatic renal cell cancer treated with sunitinib. Br J Cancer. 2010;102(5):803–9.
5. Schmidt N, Hess V, Zumbrunn T, Rothermundt C, Bongartz G, Potthast S. Choi response criteria for prediction of survival in patients with metastatic renal cell carcinoma treated with anti-angiogenic therapies. Eur Radiol. 2013;23(3):632–9.
6. Thian Y, Gutzeit A, Koh D-M, Fisher R, Lote H, Larkin J, et al. Revised choi imaging criteria correlate with clinical outcomes in patients with metastatic renal cell carcinoma treated with sunitinib. Radiology. 2014;273(2):132702.
7. Kinkel K, Helbich TH, Esserman LJ, Barclay J, Schwerin EH, Sickles EA, et al. Dynamic high-spatial-resolution MR imaging of suspicious breast lesions: diagnostic criteria and interobserver variability. AJR Am J Roentgenol. 2000;175(1):35–43.
8. Smith AD, Shah SN, Rini BI, Lieber ML, Remer EM. Morphology, Attenuation, Size, and Structure (MASS) criteria: Assessing response and predicting clinical outcome in metastatic renal cell carcinoma on antiangiogenic targeted therapy. Am J Roentgenol. 2010;194(6):1470–8.
9. Marusyk A, Almendro V, Polyak K. Intra-tumour heterogeneity: a looking glass for cancer? Nat Rev Cancer. 2012;12(5):323–34.

CT texture analysis: a potential tool for prediction of survival in patients with metastatic clear cell carcinoma...

127

10. Goh V, Ganeshan B, Nathan P, Juttla JK, Vinayan A, Miles KA. Assessment of response to tyrosine kinase inhibitors in metastatic renal cell cancer: CT texture as a predictive biomarker. Radiology. 2011;261(1):165–71.

11. Lubner MG, Stabo N, Abel EJ, Munoz Del Rio A, Pickhardt PJ. CT textural analysis of large primary renal cell carcinomas: pretreatment tumor heterogeneity correlates with histologic findings anc clinical outcomes. Am J Roentgenol. 2016;207(1):96–105.

12. Zhu Y, Li H, Guo W, Drukker K, Lan L, Giger ML, et al. Deciphering genomic underpinnings of quantitative MRI-based radiomic phenotypes of invasive breast carcinoma. Nat Sci Reports. 2015;5:17787.

13. Coroller TP, Grossmann P, Hou Y, Rios Velazquez E, Leijenaar RTH, Hermann G, et al. CT based radiomic signature CT-based radiomic signature predicts distant metastasis in lung adenocarcinoma. Radiother Oncol. 2015. [cited 2016 Apr 29];114:345–50. Available from: http://dx.doi.org/ 10.1016/j.radonc.2015.02.015.

14. Lubner MG, Stabo N, Lubner SJ, del Rio AM, Song C, Halberg RB, et al. CT textural analysis of hepatic metastatic colorectal cancer: pre-treatment tumor heterogeneity correlates with pathology and clinical outcomes. Abdom Imaging. Springer US; 2015 Oct 13 [cited 2016 May 3];40(7):2331–7. Available from: http://link.springer.com/10.1007/s00261-015-0438-4.

15. Campbell D. CT Textural Analysis (CTTA) of Metastatic Treatmenti-Resistant Pancreatic Adenocarcinoma (PDAC): Identifying Biomarkers for Genetic Instability and Overall Survival [Internet]. The University of Arizona College of Medicine; 2016 [cited 2017 Jan 5]. Available from: http://hdl.handle.net/10150/603564.

16. Zhao B, Tan Y, Tsai W-Y, Qi J, Xie C, Lu L, et al. Reproducibility of radiomics for deciphering tumor phenotype with imaging. Nat Sci Reports [Internet]. 2016 [cited 2016 Apr 29];6:23428. Available from: http://doi.org/10.1038/srep23428.

17. Bjarnason GA, Khalil B, Hudson JM, Williams R, Milot LM, Atri M, et al. Outcomes in patients with metastatic renal cell cancer treated with individualized sunitinib therapy: correlation with dynamic microbubble ultrasound data and review of the literature. Urol Oncol Semin Orig Investig. 2014;32(4):480–7. Available from: http://dx.doi.org/10.1016/j.urolonc.2015.03.003.

18. Miles KA, Ganeshan B, Hayball MP. CT texture analysis using the filtration-histogram method: what do the measurements mean? Cancer Imaging. 2013;13(3):400–6.

15

3.0T MRI for long-term observation of lung nodules post cryoablation

Jing Li, Jinrong Qu, Hongkai Zhang, Yingshu Wang, Lin Zheng, Xiang Geng, Yan Zhao and Hailiang Li* ⓘ

Abstract

Background: The purpose of this study was to use serial magnetic resonance imaging (MRI) examinations to observe changes in malignant lung tumors over time post-cryoablation.

Methods: The study protocol was approved by Institutional Review Board, and written informed consent was obtained from each participant in accordance with the Declaration of Helsinki. Patients with primary or metastatic lung tumors eligible for cryoablation were included in this prospective study. Cryoablation was performed according to standard procedures. Unenhanced and dynamic contrast-enhanced MRI scans were performed pre-cryoablation and at 1 day, 1 week, and 3-, 6-, and 12 months after cryoablation. At each time point, the signal intensity of the ablated zone on both T_1WI and T_2WI images, and volume and characteristics of the ablation zone were examined, and changes over time analyzed.

Results: A total of 26 nodules in 23 patients were included in the study. The mean patient age was 53.7 ± 13.6 years, and 57.7% were males. Ablation zone volume increased to 1 week after the procedure, and then returned to baseline by 3 months. Cavitation post-cryoablation was found in 34.6% (9/26) of the nodules 1 month after treatment. Two types of time-signal intensity curves post-cryoablation were found: a straight line representing no definite enhancement from 1-day to 1-month, and an inflow curve representing mild delayed enhancement from month 3 to month 12. Local progression was associated with an incomplete hypointense rim around the ablation zone and absence of cavitation post-treatment.

Conclusions: Characteristic changes are present on MRI after cryoablation of lung tumors. A complete hypointense rim and cavitation may be signs of adequate treatment and that local tumor progression is less likely.

Keywords: Lung cancer, Magnetic resonance imaging, Percutaneous cryotherapy

Background

Lung cancer is the most common cancer worldwide, and is the leading cause of cancer-related death in both men and women [1]. Surgical resection is the standard treatment for early-stage patients. However, patients with advanced stage disease and those with significant comorbidities may not be eligible for surgery. Metastases is the second most common pulmonary malignancy, and resectability depends on many factors [2]. Nonsurgical candidates are usually managed with systemic chemotherapy; however, side effects can be severe and not all tumors respond to chemotherapy [3–5].

* Correspondence: cjr.lihailiang@vip.163.com
Department of Radiology, the Affiliated Cancer Hospital of Zhengzhou University, Henan Cancer Hospital, 127 Dongming Road, Jinshui District, Zhengzhou, Henan Province 450008, China

Cryoablation of a tumor can reduce its size, or completely eliminate it, and can thus alleviate symptoms and improve survival [1, 6]. Cryosurgery is commonly used for the treatment of prostate and liver tumors [7, 8]. Although percutaneous cryoablation of tumors in the thorax was first reported in 2005 [9], and it has been shown to be safe and effective for lung tumors [3, 5, 10], it is still not widely used for lung malignancies [11]. No tissue is removed during cryoablation; thus, imaging is necessary to determine if the extent of ablation is adequate, and to determine how the lesion has responded to the treatment. Imaging studies are mainly utilized for intra-operative guidance, and there is only 1 report on application of computed tomography (CT) for determination of the ablated zone and the examination of serial post-ablative changes [12]. While the study showed that

CT was useful for examining changes following cryoablation, the large radiation dose from multiple CT scans cannot be ignored.

Magnetic resonance imaging (MRI) has advanced such that artifacts due to breathing and heart function can be reduced or eliminated, and MRI is frequently used for the diagnosis of thoracic disease [13, 14]. MRI has been shown to clearly reflect changes in the ablation zone after radiofrequency ablation of liver lesions [15]. Unlike CT, MRI is not associated with ionizing radiation. However, there is currently only 1 report of MR-guided cryoablation for lung cancer [16], and data of long-term changes of the ablation zone using MRI are not available.

We hypothesized that MRI can identify changes in the ablation zone after radiofrequency ablation of lung tumors, and thus may be useful for monitoring treatment effectiveness. Thus, the purpose of this study was to use serial MRI examinations to observe changes in malignant lung tumors over time post-cryoablation, and correlate these changes with the effects of treatment.

Methods

Patients

The study protocol was approved by Institutional Review Board, and written informed consent was obtained from each participant in accordance with the Declaration of Helsinki.

This prospective study included patients with primary or metastatic lung cancer who received cryoablation from December 2013 to December 2015. Malignancy was diagnosed by a tissue specimen obtained via percutaneous or transbronchial lung biopsy, or clinical changes in the nodule such as rapid enlargement or glucose uptake on positron emission tomography (PET/CT). Other inclusion criteria were 1) newly diagnosed and had received no prior treatment; 2) were judged able to tolerate general anesthesia and the cryoablation procedure; 3) had a single nodule in the target lobe; 4) nodule size <4 cm and no invasion into the adjacent structure; and 5) can complete the entire MRI scanning plan. Patients were excluded if 1) they had more than 1 tumor in the target lobe or had received prior therapy; 2) image quality was too poor to meet diagnostic requirements; 3) significant comorbidities or vital organ failure were present; and 4) nodule size >4 cm, or invasion into mediastinal structures, chest wall, segmental bronchi, vessels, or nerves.

During the post ablation follow-up period, progression was diagnosed by biopsy only if the patient was able to tolerate the procedure, or changes in the nodule such as rapid enlargement or increased glucose uptake were identified on positron emission tomography (PET/CT).

Cryoablation protocol

Cryoablation was performed under general anesthesia and CT guidance. All procedures were performed with a percutaneous cryoablation device utilizing 1.7 mm diameter cryoprobe and an Ar-He cryosurgery unit (CryoHit type; Galil Medical, Yokneam, Israel). The target lung nodule was identified, and a 3-dimensional (3D) treatment plan was designed based on 16 slice helical CT images (Light Speed; GE Medical Systems, Milwaukee, WI). The criteria for effective treatment were an ice hockey puck zone 1 cm or more from the edge of the target nodule, and the frozen range after 1 single procedure covered more than 80% of the lesion. The needle interval was set to 2 cm when using 2 needles so that the ice ball produced by each needle slightly overlapped and formed a seamless large frozen ball. The number of needles used depended on the size of the tumor.

After the skin was prepped and draped, 1% lidocaine was injected subcutaneous from the skin to the pleura. A 21-gauge guide needle was inserted along the planned optimized path using scout CT images. The needle position was confirmed in the targeting area by repeat CT scanning, then the 17-gauge stainless steel cryoablation probes consisting of an external sheath and inner-guide needle was inserted. The guide needle was removed after confirming the position, and the cryoprobe was introduced through the external sheath. The needle always penetrated the tumor, and the tip of the needle was placed at the far end of the lesion. Freeze-thaw cycles were then performed. A single cycle consisted of a 10 min freezing period in which the local temperature decreased to minus 170 °C due to argon gas rapid expansion, and a 2-min re-warming period in which the local temperature increased to plus 20 °C as a result of helium rapid expansion. Generally, a single procedure consisted of 2 freeze-thaw cycles; however, in the case of large tumors multiple cycles were performed.

MRI scanning program and parameters

All patients received chest unenhanced and dynamic enhanced MR scans pre-cryoablation, and at 1 day, 1 week, and 1, 3, 6, and 12 months after the procedure. Scanning was done with a 3.0T MR scanner (SignaHDx; GE Healthcare, Waukesha, WI), using a TORSO coil. Patients were in the supine position, foot ahead. Imaging was performed from the apex to the top of the diaphragm, including the target lung nodule. Six different sequences were used, and the sequences and parameters are summarized in Additional file 1: Table S1.

Image analysis

The size of the ablation zone was measured in 3 dimensions on each imaging study. In prior studies, the post-ablation zone was characterized by regional ground-glass opacity on CT images [2, 12, 17]. As MRI characteristics of the ablation zone for pulmonary nodules are not available, we referred to studies of MRI characteristics after cryoablation for liver tumors [18, 19]. The ablation zone was defined as an area of high signal intensity on both T1WI and T2WI images, and no enhancement, which histologically represents the region of coagulative necrosis. Tumor volume (lesion length × lesion width × lesion height)/2) was recorded for each ablation zone. Each diameter was measured 3 times by an independent radiologist, and the average value was used for further calculations.

All MRI images at each time point were analyzed by 2 radiologists with more than 5 years of MRI diagnostic experience. Analyses were done independently and blindly. If there were inconsistencies at the final review of all of the analysis, a third highly qualified radiologist with more than 10 years of MRI diagnostic experience reviewed the imaging studies and made the final determination.

Signal intensity of the ablation zone on T_1WI and T_2WI images were observed carefully, and changing characteristics and time-signal intensity changes were recorded. There are no standard criteria or quantitative parameters of T_1WI and T_2WI sequences for evaluating lung nodule post-cryoablation. However, a 5-point grading scale method has been proven to be effective and reliable for subjectively evaluating image quality, and to compare different technologies in tumor diagnosis [20, 21]. Thus, we applied a 5-point grading scale ranging from 1 (low) to 5 (high) on both T_1WI and T_2WI images for scoring signal intensity of the ablation zone. The scoring criteria were: On T_1WI images, lung parenchyma background was scored as 1 point, muscle signals as 3 points, fat tissue signal intensity as 5 points, signal intensity between lung parenchyma and muscle as 2 points, between muscle and fat tissues as 4 points (Fig. 1a). On T_2WI images, lung parenchyma background was scored as 1 point, muscle signals as 3 points, water-like high signal intensity as 5 points, signals between parenchyma and muscles as 2 points, and between muscle and water as 4 points (Fig. 1b). The ablation zone on T_1WI and T_2WI images at 1-day post-cryotherapy often showed heterogeneous signal intensity. When this occurred, the scores were determined by the dominant signals at the largest part of the ablation zone. Accompanying signs were also observed, including inflammation, atelectasis, and pleural effusion. Inflammation was identified as a large flake appearance with blurred margins, slightly high T_1WI and T_2WI signals with bronchial low signal intensity inside, and marked enhancement and blood vessels penetrating signs. Atelectasis was identified as a reduced wedge shape of a segment or lobe, slightly high signal intensity on T_1WI and T_2WI images without a bronchial low signal intensity inside, and significantly enhanced with a clear and straight border. Pleural effusion was identified by a crescent or ribbon-like intra-thoracic water-like signal intensity.

Dynamic enhanced sequences, including mask phase, were transmitted to a Work Station 4.5, and processed by the SER software package. A region of interest (ROI) was placed in the aorta, and in the largest cross-section of the ablation zone on the same slice. Time-signal intensity curves were automatically generated.

Statistical analysis

Mean and standard deviation were computed for age, nodule volume, T_1WI, and T_2WI, and age range was reported as well. Categorical variables were summarized as frequency and percentage. Inter-rater reliability for T_1WI and T_2WI analysis was examined by weighted Kappa. Five levels of agreement were defined according to the Kappa statistic: poor ($\kappa < 0.2$), fair ($0.2 \leq \kappa < 0.4$), moderate ($0.4 \leq \kappa < 0.6$), good ($0.6 \leq \kappa < 0.8$), and very good ($0.8 \leq \kappa \leq 1.00$). Nodule volume at various time points were presented as a box plot: 1st quartile (top of the box), median (line shown in box), 3rd quartile (bottom of the box). Data on nodule volume were examined by Friedman's test, while the time trends of T_1WI and T_2WI signal intensity were presented as line charts and examined using a linear mixed model. If the time effect was significant, post-hoc tests were implemented using Bonferroni's correction method. To compare differences in T_1WI and T_2WI signal intensity between patients with and without local tumor progression, the Mann-Whitney U test was also performed. A value of $p < 0.05$ was considered statistical significant; the significance level was adjusted to 0.002 (0.05/21) if post-hoc tests were required. All statistical analyses were performed with PASW statistical software (version 21.0, IBM Corp., Armonk, NY, USA).

Results
Patients
Data of 26 nodules from 23 patients were used for the analysis (Table 1). The mean patient age was 53.7 ± 13.6 (range: 25–78) years, and 57.7% were males. Of the 23 patients, 12 were lost to follow-up at 18 months, and another 5 were lost at 24 months.

Volume change characteristics
Changes in nodule volume through the study period are illustrated in Fig. 1a. The volume was increased at post-procedure day 1, then became smaller gradually at 1 week and 1 month, and then reduced in size to the baseline value at 3 months and remained at that size until the 12th month examination.

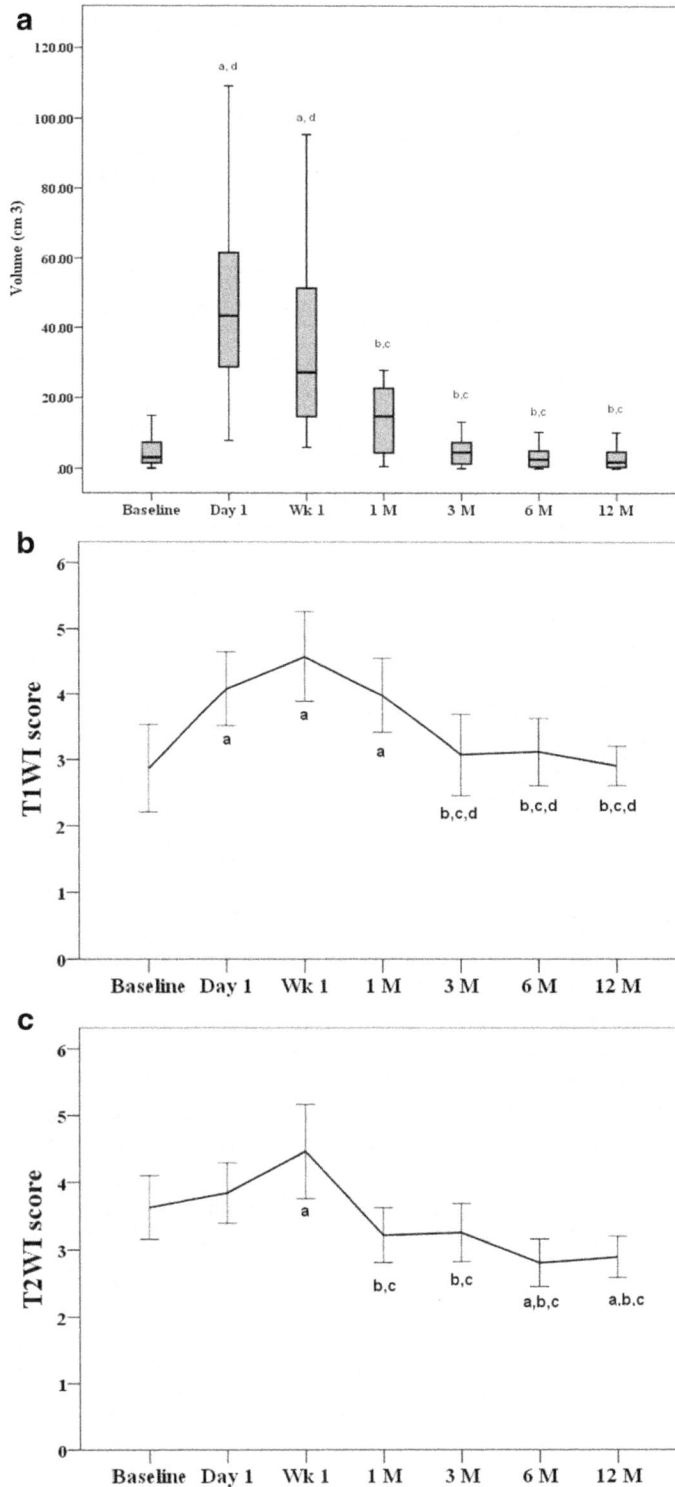

Fig. 1 Changes in volume (**a**) and T_1WI (**b**) and T_2WI score (**c**) during the study period ($n = 26$ nodules). Nodule volume data are presented as a box plot: 1st quartile (top of the box), median (line shown in box), 3rd quartile (bottom of the box), and examined Friedman's test. T_1WI and T_2WI data are presented as mean ± standard deviation, and tested by linear mixed model. Letters denote significant difference between the given time and baseline[a], day 1[b], week 1[c], or 1 month [d] ($p < 0.002$). Volume (cm^3)

Table 1 Characteristics of 26 nodules in 23 patients

Age, years		53.7 ± 13.6 (25–78)
Gender	Female	11 (42.3)
	Male	15 (57.7)
Metastasis	No	11 (42.3)
	Yes	15 (57.7)
Histological type	Adenocarcinoma	22 (84.6)
	Squamous cell carcinoma	4 (15.4)
Local progression	No	20 (76.9)
	Yes	6 (23.1)

Age reported as mean ± standard deviation with (range); other data reported as number (percentage)

Cavity formation

Other MRI findings such as cavitation and complications are summarized in Table 2. Cavitation post-cryoablation was found in 34.6% (9/26) of the nodules 1 month after treatment, but no further cavitation was noted as time progressed. Six of the 9 cases of cavitation were resolved at 3 months, and the others were resolved by 6 months. Interestingly, none of the patients with cavitation post-cryoablation developed local tumor progression.

Consolidation, atelectasis, and pneumothorax were found in 42.3%, 30.8%, and 26.9% of nodules 1 day after the treatment, respectively. No consolidation or atelectasis was observed after 3 months, and pneumothoraces were resolved by 1 month.

Changes of signal intensity

The inter-rater reliability with regard to observation of T_1WI and T_2WI signal intensity are reported in Table 3. Regardless of time, the inter-rater reliability of T_1WI and T_2WI were good or very good, except that T_2WI measured at month 6 only achieved moderate reliability. Changes in T_1WI and T_2WI are illustrated in Fig. 1b and c. The T_1WI score increased from 2.87 at baseline to the peak of 4.58 at week 1, then declined to around 3 after 3 months (Fig. 1b). A similar trend was found for T_2WI, except the T_2WI score significantly decreased to 3.2 at 1 month, and then leveled off to around 2.9 at 6 months (Fig. 1c).

Enhancement characteristics

Lung nodules exhibited different enhancement characteristics pre-cryoablation. The majority (73.1%, 19/26) exhibited moderate persistent enhancement, and the time-intensity curve was plateau (type II). However, there were 2 types of time-signal intensity curves post-cryoablation: a straight line representing no definite enhancement from 1-day to 1-month, and an inflow curve representing mild delayed enhancement from month 3 to month 12 (Fig. 2). Images of a progressive lesion are shown in Fig. 3.

Local tumor progression

At 12 months after treatment, 4 nodules showed local tumor progression. At 18 months after treatment, and additional 2 nodules developed local progression. A difference in T_1WI signal intensity between patients with and without local tumor progression was found; however, the difference was no longer statistically significant after 1 week. A difference in T_2WI signal intensity was also noted after treatment, but the difference became none significant at 6 months. At 3 months after treatment the ablation zone in 22.7% (5/22) of nodules remain round or nodule-like in the non-progression group, and at 12 months 77.3% (17/22) of ablation zones had streaks and or a patch shape.

Of 6 patients that developed local tumor progression, 4 were male and adenocarcinoma was the histological type in 4 cases. Complications like consolidation, atelectasis, and pneumothorax occurred within 1 week to 3 months after treatment (Table 4). Two patients received treatment with embedded ^{125}I particles, 2 a second cyroablation, and 2 local radiotherapy. The ablation zone in the 6 patients with progression showed an incomplete ring at 1 week and 3 months on T_1WI and T_2WI images, suggesting that this finding early post-cryoablation may be an indicator for progression.

Discussion

A number of studies have shown that cryoablation is an effective treatment for primary lung tumors and

Table 2 MRI findings and complications (26 nodules)

	Post-cryoablation cavitation	Time-intensity curve type[a]	Consolidation	Atelectasis	Pneumothorax
Baseline	0	Vary	0	0	0
Day 1	0	1	42.3% (11/26)	30.8% (8/26)	26.9% (7/26)
Week 1	0	1	26.9% (7/26)	7.7% (2/26)	3.8% (1/26)
Month 1	34.6% (9/26)	1	7.7% (2/26)	3.8% (1/26)	0
Month 3	11.5% (3/26)	2	0	0	0
Month 6	0	2	0	0	0
Month 12	0	2	0	0	0

[a]Two classifications of time-intensity curve: 1, no definite enhancement as a straight line; 2, mild delayed enhancement as an inflow curve

Table 3 Inter-rater reliability for T_1WI and T_2WI

	T_1WI		T_2WI	
Time	Weighted Kappa	95% CI	Weighted Kappa	95% CI
Baseline	0.943	(0.831–1.000)	0.824	(0.593–1.000)
Day 1	0.750	(0.446–1.000)	0.800	(0.533–1.000)
Week 1	0.878	(0.706–1.000)	1.000	(1.000–1.000)
Month 1	0.930	(0.794–1.000)	0.885	(0.665–1.000)
Month 3	0.875	(0.704–1.000)	0.898	(0.702–1.000)
Month 6	0.829	(0.595–1.000)	0.500	(0.076–0.924)
Month 12	1.000	(1.000–1.000)	0.776	(0.357–1.000)

CI confidence interval

pulmonary metastasis [3, 4, 22]. However, familiarity with the post-procedural findings, and the ability to discriminate them from local progression, is critically important.

Our study showed there are characteristic changes of lung nodules after cryotherapy. There is an early increase in volume of the ablated zone that peaks at 1 day after the procedure, remains consistent to 1 week, and then gradually declines to the baseline size at 3 months. The volume increase at 1 day is secondary to ice ball formation and acute lung changes in the target region. However, the reason why the signal is heterogeneous at 1 day post-cryoablation is not clear. Heterogeneous signals can reflect post-cryoablation complications; a high signal on T_1WI and T_2WI images can be due to alveolar hemorrhage, which is suggestive of small vessel rupture, whereas a low signal in the outer periphery may be the result of alveolar wall collapse and small bronchi rupture. In an animal study, Romaneehsen et al. [23] showed that a volume decrease at 1 week after cryoablation was associated with a reduction or disappearance of a low signal region in the outer periphery, which is suggestive that tissue repair begins in the outer region. A signal increase in the core of the ablated zone has been shown by animal experiments to be secondary to coagulation necrosis [23, 24]. This findings has also been found in radiofrequency ablation in the liver [15].

The persistent initial volume increase is secondary to the mobilization of macrophages and neutrophils into the cryoablation zone as part of the post-cryoablation immunologic cascade, which leads to tumor lysis and ensuing tissue repair [24]. Subsequently, as the concentration of cellular debris, macrophages, and neutrophils decreases, there is steady reduction in the volume of the cryoablation zone [24], as noted in our study. It is unclear why there is an increase of T_2WI signal intensity in the ablated zone at 1-month post-cryoablation, as there is no relevant literature on the topic. It may secondary to stromal hyperplasia, which is abundant in newly developing small vessels and new fibrous tissue, thus

reflecting tissue repair [6, 24]. The continuous decrease of signal intensity on T_1WI and T_2WI images in the ablated zone from 3 months onward may represent repair and fibrosis.

In our study, at 1 day, 1- week, and 1 month post-cryoablation, the ablated zone showed no enhancement, which may be due to complex changes related to cell necrosis [15, 23]. From 3 months onward mild enhancement was note in nodules that did not develop local progression. This is consistent with CT findings of lung nodules post-ablation [6, 12].

The local progression rate in our study during a 12-month follow-up period was lower than that reported by Liu et al. [16] and Inoue et al. [10] Most nodules (73.7%) in our study had a diameter < 30 mm, and approximately 30% had a diameter of 30–40 mm; thus, they were relatively small. The low progression rate in this study may due to the limited sample size, size of the nodules, or the histological cancer types.

The presence of hypointense rim as a "ring" appears to be critically important, as suggested from study of radiofrequency ablation [25]. In this study, the hypointense rim was present at 1-week and 1-month post-cryoablation, and was a complete rim in 84.6% of nodules and incomplete in 15.4%. Although statistical comparative analysis in the progression group could not be performed due to the small sample size, all cases with local progression exhibited an incomplete ring at the ablation zone at 1 week and 3 months on T_1WI and T_2WI images, suggesting that this finding early post-cryoablation may be an indicator for progression.

Studies of radiofrequency ablation indicate the presence of cavitation is a very important predictor of prognosis [6, 12]. We found cavitation in approximately 30% of nodules after treatment, which is similar to the 35% reported by Ito et al. [26], but lower than the 53% reported by Chaudhry et al. [12]. The spectrum of pulmonary nodules in our study was similar to that of the study by Ito et al., but different from that of Chaudhry et al. who only included patients with stage I non-small

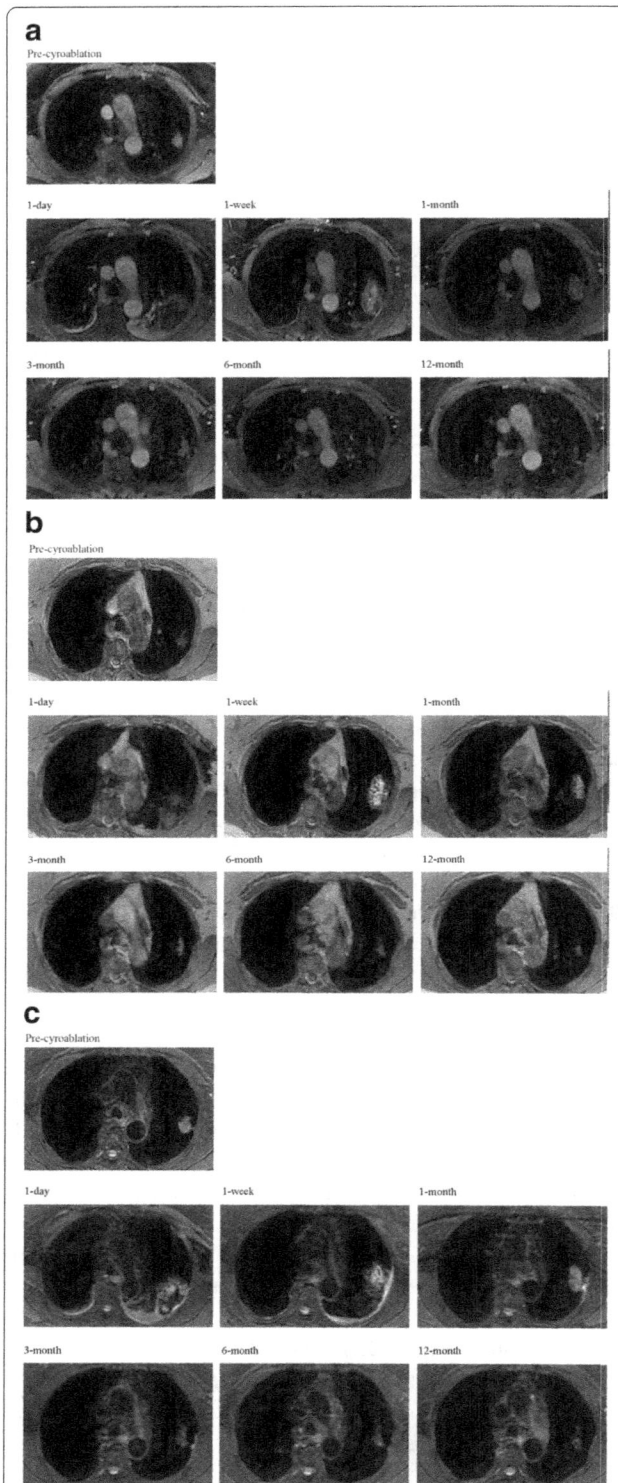

Fig. 2 Post-contrast images of venous phase (**a**), T$_1$WI (**b**), and T$_2$WI (**c**) of a non-progressive lesion. At the early stage (1 day, 1-month and 3-month), there was no definite enhancement in the ablation zone; later, mild enhancement was noted. Similarly, at the early stage the time-signal curve was a straight line type, and later became an inflow type

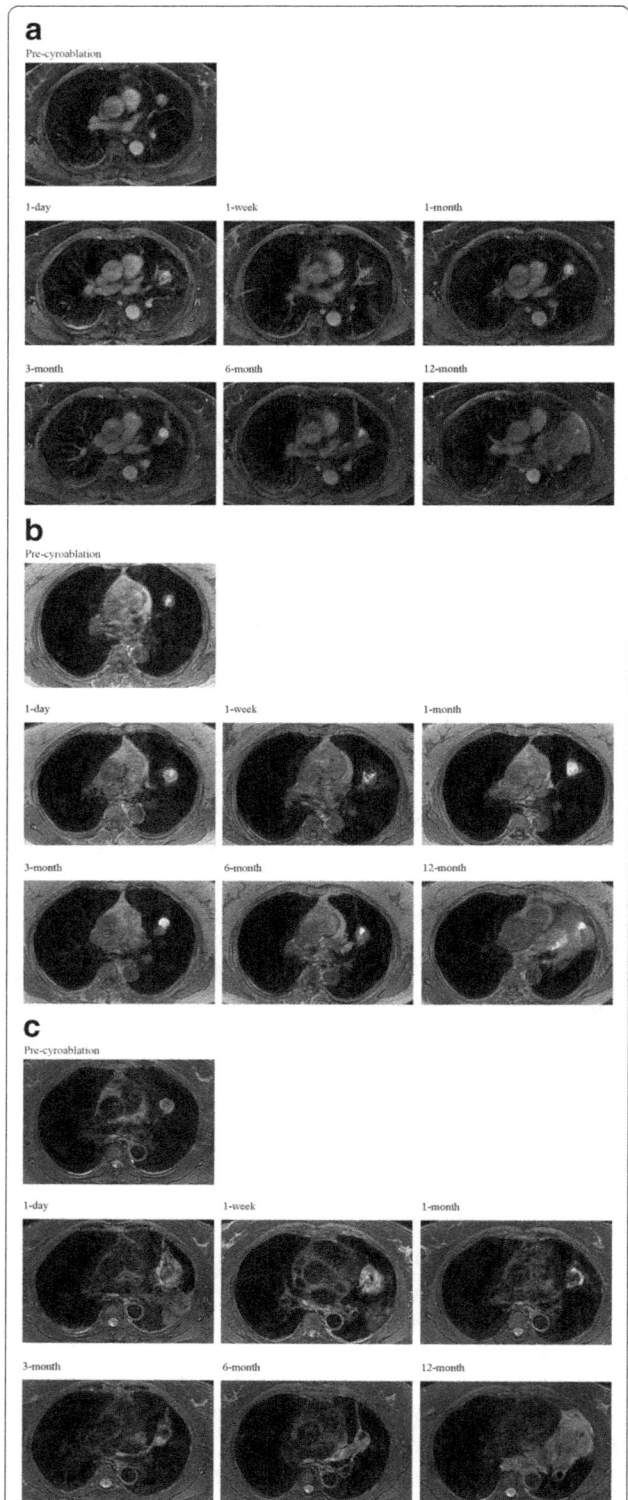

Fig. 3 Post-contrast images of venous phase (**a**), T$_1$WI (**b**), and T$_2$WI (**c**) of a progressive lesion. Progression was noted at 3 months postoperatively. Images obtained at 1 week and 1 month postoperatively showed an unclear and incomplete hypointense rim, especially the T$_2$WI images

Table 4 Characteristics of 6 patients with local tumor progression

	Patient 1	Patient 2	Patient 3	Patient 4	Patient 5	Patient 6
Age, years	25	57	62	56	55	57
Gender	M	F	M	M	F	M
Number of treated nodules	1	1	1	1	1	1
Histological type	AD	SCC	AD	AD	AD	SCC
Metastasis	Y	N	Y	Y	N	N
Volume, cm^3						
Baseline	1.46	14.91	5.66	1.52	0.25	4.20
Day 1	29.71	51.89	124.71	29.74	46.37	35.34
Week 1	16.09	47.05	95.47	22.46	26.04	26.84
Month 1	7.15	23.25	27.84	8.54	20.39	9.98
Month 3	1.37	7.95	8.72	1.37	5.92	7.30
Month 6	0.52	5.83	N/A	1.82	4.54	3.56
Month 12	0.46	4.83	N/A	N/A	N/A	N/A
T1WI						
Baseline	2	2	3	3	2	2
Day 1	4	5	4	4	5	5
Week 1	5	5	5	5	5	5
Month 1	4	5	4	4	4	5
Month 3	4	3	3	3	3	3
Month 6	4	3	N/A	3	3	3
Month 12	3	3	N/A	N/A	N/A	N/A
T2WI						
Baseline	4	4	4	4	3	4
Day 1	4	4	4	4	4	4
Week 1	5	5	5	5	5	5
Month 1	3	3	3	3	3	3
Month 3	3	4	4	4	4	4
Month 6	3	3	N/A	3	3	3
Month 12	3	3	N/A	N/A	N/A	N/A
Post-cryoablation cavitation	N	N	N	N	N	N
Consolidation						
Baseline	N	N	N	N	N	N
Day 1	Y	Y	Y	Y	Y	Y
Week 1	Y	Y	Y	Y	Y	Y
Month 1	N	Y	Y	Y	Y	Y
Month 3	N	N	Y	Y	Y	N
Month 6	N	N	N/A	N	N	N
Month 12	N	N	N/A	N/A	N/A	N/A
Atelectasis						
Baseline	N	N	N	N	N	N
Day 1	Y	Y	Y	Y	Y	Y
Week 1	Y	Y	Y	Y	Y	Y
Month 1	N	Y	Y	Y	Y	Y
Month 3	N	N	Y	N	N	N

Table 4 Characteristics of 6 patients with local tumor progression *(Continued)*

	Patient 1	Patient 2	Patient 3	Patient 4	Patient 5	Patient 6
Month 6	N	N	N/A	N	N	N
Month 12	N	N	N/A	N/A	N/A	N/A
Pneumothorax						
Baseline	N	N	N	N	N	N
Day 1	N	Y	Y	Y	Y	N
Week 1	N	N	Y	N	Y	N
Month 1	N	N	N	N	N	N
Month 3	N	N	N	N	N	N
Month 6	N	N	N/A	N	N	N
Month 12	N	N	N/A	N/A	N/A	N/A

AD adenocarcinoma, *N* no, *N/A* not available, *SC* squamous cell carcinoma, *Y* yes

cell lung cancer. None of the patients who developed tumor progression had evidence of cavitation, suggesting that cavitation may predict a good clinical outcome. In our study, the ablated zone in approximately 77% of patients without local progression eventually developed streaks and a patch shape, and the other cases remained round or nodule shaped. Chaudhry et al. [12] found that shape change in the ablated occurred up to 6 months after treatment, and then remains stable to 12 months after cryoablation.

While the current study focused on MRI changes, other studies examined CT and PET/CT for the evaluation of nodules post ablation. Abtin et al. [6] examined CT, PET, and dual-modality imaging with combined PET and CT (PET/CT) for their value in identifying partial ablation, tumor recurrence, and progression in lung nodules treated with RFA. The authors divided post ablation into 3 periods: early (up to 1 week), intermediate (> 1 week to 2 months), and late (> 2 months). Imaging features that were suggestive of residual or recurrent disease included 1) increasing contrast agent uptake in the ablation zone (>180 s on dynamic images), nodular enhancement >10 mm, central enhancement >15 HU, and enhancement greater than baseline any time after ablation; 2) growth of the ablation zone after 3 months as compared with baseline, peripheral nodular growth, and change from ground-glass opacity to solid opacity; 3) increased metabolic activity beyond 2 months, residual activity centrally or at the ablated tumor, and development of nodular activity.

There are limitations to what we consider a preliminary study. The sample size was small, the nodules were extremely heterogeneous, i.e., they were both primary and metastatic cancer and the histological type varied, and because of patients lost to follow-up only data up to 12 months could be analyzed. We could not correlate MRI findings with histopathological changes as performing repeat biopsies solely for the purposes of research is

not ethical. We did not examine DWI sequence data and ADC values, which have been proven a reliable for the diagnosis of pulmonary nodules [2, 27], and evaluation of therapeutic response [21, 28]. These examinations were not performed because there were artifacts on DWI images at 1 day and 1 week post-cryoablation, and putting the ROI in the correct place was difficult due to cavity formation. The method of evaluating the effect of cryoablation, tissue changes, and local residual tumor and local tumor progression was subjective, and was based on CT observations of lung tumors and MRI observations of liver tumors, changes to lung tumors that have been cryoablated identified by MRI may not correspond. Positron emission thermography (PET)-CT may have provided greater value and more objective data with respect to examining serial changes in the tumors. However, PET is not generally covered by insurance (only 7 patients in the current study received PET-CT as part of their initial work-up), and our budget did not allow for us to perform the procedure on all patients, and there is the concern of ionizing radiation with repeated CT scanning. We did not compare MRI and CT data, as study has evaluated the value of CT, MRI, and histological examination after cryoablation of renal tumors and concluded that MRI is superior to CT [29].

Conclusions

The results of this study showed there are characteristic changes that can be identified on MRI after cryoablation of lung tumors. A complete hypointense rim at 1 week and 1 month post-cryoablation, and cavitation in the ablation zone at 1 month post-cryoablation may be signs of adequate treatment and that local tumor progression is less likely. Though we consider this a preliminary study, the results suggest that MRI may be a good method to follow the results of cryoablation of lung tumors.

Acknowledgements
None

Funding
National Natural and Science Fund of China (NO. 81372370).

Authors' contributions
JL: manuscript preparation, literature research, and data analysis. JQ: study concepts; definition of intellectual content, literature research, study design, manuscript editing and data analysis. HZ: data acquisition. YW: data acquisition. LZ: clinical studies. XG: clinical studies. YZ: statistical analysis. HL: guarantor of integrity of the entire study, manuscript review, study concepts, definition of intellectual content, literature research, and data analysis. All authors read and approved the final manuscript.

Competing interests
The authors declare that they have no competing interests.

References
1. Tomic R, Podgaetz E, Andrade RS, Dincer HE. Cryotechnology in diagnosing and treating lung diseases. J Bronchology Interv Pulmonol. 2015;22:76–84.
2. Davidson RS, Nwogu CE, Brentjens MJ, Anderson TM. The surgical management of pulmonary metastasis: current concepts. Surg Oncol. 2001;10:35–42.
3. Yamauchi Y, Izumi Y, Kawamura M, Nakatsuka S, Yashiro H, Tsukada N, Inoue M, Asakura K, Nomori H. Percutaneous cryoablation of pulmonary metastases from colorectal cancer. PLoS One. 2011;6:e27086.
4. Macbeth F, Russell C, Treasure T. Cryotherapy for lung metastases: a justifiable procedure? J Thorac Oncol. 2015;10:e120–1.
5. Kawamura M, Izumi Y, Tsukada N, Asakura K, Sugiura H, Yashiro H, Nakano K, Nakatsuka S, Kuribayashi S, Kobayashi K. Percutaneous cryoablation of small pulmonary malignant tumors under computed tomographic guidance with local anesthesia for nonsurgical candidates. J Thorac Cardiovasc Surg. 2006; 131:1007–13.
6. Abtin FG, Eradat J, Gutierrez AJ, Lee C, Fishbein MC, Suh RD. Radiofrequency ablation of lung tumors: imaging features of the post ablation zone. Radiographics. 2012;32:947–69.
7. Bahn DK, Lee F, Badalament R, Kumar A, Greski J, Chernick M. Targeted cryoablation of the prostate: 7-year outcomes in the primary treatment of prostate cancer. Urology. 2002;60:3–11.
8. Lee FT Jr, Mahvi DM, Chosy SG, Onik GM, Wong WS, Littrup PJ, Scanlan KA. Hepatic cryosurgery with intraoperative US guidance. Radiology. 1997;202: 624–32.
9. Wang H, Littrup PJ, Duan Y, Zhang Y, Feng H, Nie Z. Thoracic masses treated with percutaneous cryotherapy: initial experience with more than 200 procedures. Radiology. 2005;235:289–98.
10. Inoue M, Nakatsuka S, Yashiro H, et al. Percutaneous cryoablation of lung tumors: feasibility and safety. J Vasc Interv Radiol. 2012;23:295–302.
11. Dupuy DE, Zagoria RJ, Akerley W, Mayo-Smith WW, Kavanagh PV, Safran H. Percutaneous radiofrequency ablation of malignancies in the lung. AJR Am J Roentgenol. 2000;174:57–9.
12. Chaudhry A, Grechushkin V, Hoshmand M, Kim CW, Pena A, Huston B, Chaya Y, Bilfinger T, Moore W. Characteristic CT findings after percutaneous cryoablation treatment of malignant lung nodules. Medicine (Baltimore). 2015;94:e16.
13. NH L, Hung CM, Liu KY, Chen TB, Huang YH. Diagnosed chest lesion on diffusion-weighted magnetic resonance images using apparent diffusion coefficients. J Xray Sci Technol. 2016;24:133–43.
14. Souza CA. MRI of the chest: review of imaging strategies. Radiol Bras. 2015; 48(V-VI)
15. Onishi H, Matsushita M, Murakami T, et al. MR appearances of radiofrequency thermal ablation region: histopathologic correlation with dog liver models and an autopsy case. Acad Rad ol. 2004;11:1180–9.
16. Liu S, Ren R, Liu M, Lv Y, Li B, Li CMR. Imaging-guided percutaneous cryotherapy for lung tumors: initial experience. J Vasc Interv Radiol. 2014;25: 1456–62.
17. Goldberg SN, Gazelle GS, Compton CC, McLoud TC. Radiofrequency tissue ablation in the rabbit lung: efficacy and complications. Acad Radiol. 1995;2: 776–84.
18. Rong G, Bai W, Dong Z, et al. Long-term outcomes of percutaneous cryoablation for patients with hepatocellular carcinoma within Milan criteria. PLoS One. 2015;10:e0123065.
19. Niu LZ, Li JL, Percutaneous XKC. Cryoablation for liver cancer. J Clin Transl Hepatol. 2014;2:182–8.
20. Heye T, Sommer G, Miedinger D, Bremerich J, Bieri O. Ultrafast 3D balanced steady-state free precession MRI of the lung: assessment of anatomic details in comparison to low-dose CT. J Magn Reson Imaging. 2015;42:602–9.
21. Park HJ, Kim SH, Jang KM, Lim S, Kang TW, Park HC, Choi D. Added value of diffusion-weighted MRI for evaluating viable tumor of hepatocellular carcinomas treated with radiotherapy in patients with chronic liver disease. AJR Am J Roentgenol. 2014;202:92–101.
22. de Baere T, Tselikas L, Woodrum D, Abtin F, Littrup P, Deschamps F, Suh R, Aoun HD, Callstrom M. Evaluating cryoablation of metastatic lung tumors in patients–safety and efficacy: the ECLIPSE trial–interim analysis at 1 year. J Thorac Oncol. 2015;10:1468–74.
23. Romaneehsen B, Anders M, Röhrl B, Hengstler JG, Schiffer I, Neugebauer B, Teichmann E, Schreiber WG, Thelen M. Cryotherapy of malignant tumors: studies with MRI in an animal experiment and comparison with morphological changes. Rofo. 2001;173:632–8.
24. Chu KF, Dupuy DE. Thermal ablation of tumours: biological mechanisms and advances in therapy. Nat Rev Cancer. 2014;14:199–208.
25. Suh RD, Wallace AB, Sheehan RE, Heinze SB, Goldin JG. Unresectable pulmonary malignancies: CT-guided percutaneous radiofrequency ablation-preliminary results. Radiology. 2003;229:821–9.
26. Ito N, Nakatsuka S, Inoue M, Yashiro H, Oguro S, Izumi Y, Kawamura M, Nomori H, Kuribayashi S. Computed tomographic appearance of lung tumors treated with percutaneous cryoablation. J Vasc Interv Radiol. 2012; 23:1043–52.
27. Koyama H, Ohno Y, Seki S, Nishio M, Yoshikawa T, Matsumoto S, Maniwa Y, Itoh T, Nishimura Y, Sugimura K. Value of diffusion-weighted MR imaging using various parameters for assessment and characterization of solitary pulmonary nodules. Eur J Radiol. 2015;84:509–15.
28. Ludwig JM, Camacho JC, Kokabi N, Xing M, Kim HS. The role of diffusion-weighted imaging (DWI) in locoregional therapy outcome prediction and response assessment for hepatocellular carcinoma (HCC): the new era of functional imaging biomarkers. Diagnostics (Basel). 2015;5:546–63.
29. Nielsen TK, Østraat Ø, Graumann O, Pedersen BG, Andersen G, Høyer S, Borre M. Computed tomography perfusion, magnetic resonance imaging, and histopathological findings after laparoscopic renal cryoablation: an in vivo pig model. Technol Cancer Res Treat. 2017;16:406–13.

16

Crizotinib Associated Renal Cysts [CARCs]: incidence and patterns of evolution

Laird B Cameron[1], Damian H S Jiang[2], Kate Moodie[2], Catherine Mitchell[3], Benjamin Solomon[4] and Bimal Kumar Parameswaran[2*]

Abstract

Background: Novel therapeutic agents recently introduced for the treatment of cancer have several unusual side effects. An increased incidence of renal cystic lesions, often with features concerning for malignancy or infection, has been reported in patients with anaplastic lymphoma kinase (ALK) - rearranged advanced non-small cell lung cancer (NSCLC) treated with Crizotinib. Many of these lesions undergo spontaneous resolution despite developing complex features on imaging. We assess the incidence and patterns of evolution of Crizotinib Associated Renal Cysts [CARCs] at our institute and provide histopathology correlation of their benign nature.

Methods: A retrospective analysis of renal lesions in computerised tomography (CT) scans of 35 patients with advanced *ALK*-rearranged NSCLC who had been prescribed crizotinib at our institution was performed by three radiologists, who analysed the evolution of these lesions, particularly for pre-defined significant and complex changes.

Results: Of 26 patients eligible for this analysis, 4 (15%) had cysts at baseline that remained stable on crizotinib treatment while 11(42%) developed significant change in 28 renal cysts. Commonest pattern of cyst evolution was enlargement from baseline followed by spontaneous regression (17/28 lesions) while other patterns noted were stable lesions, regression from baseline and ongoing enlargement. The median maximum size reached was 23 mm (range 9 – 67 mm) after a median of 178 days (160 to 1342) on crizotinib. Complex change occurred in 12 cysts, in 7/26 (27%) patients and within 60 days of starting Crizotinib in 10 cysts. Imaging features were falsely concerning for malignancy or abscess in 4/26 patients.

Conclusion: Most CARCs resolve spontaneously, or have a benign evolution despite enlargement and other features concerning for malignancy or infection on imaging. This unusual manifestation of chemotherapy should be recognised, particularly by radiologists, so that inappropriate treatment decisions are avoided.

Keywords: Crizotinib, Renal cyst, Spontaneous resolution, CT, Non-small cell lung cancer, Anaplastic lymphoma kinase

Background

Anaplastic Lymphoma Kinase (*ALK*) gene rearrangements were first identified in NSCLC in 2007 [1] and subsequently found to be present in approximately 4% of patients with NSCLC [2]. Crizotinib (Xalkori, Pfizer; PF0234066), a tyrosine kinase inhibitor with efficacy against ALK [3], c-MET [4] and ROS1 [5] kinase, has demonstrated superior efficacy over chemotherapy in the first line systemic treatment of advanced ALK-

rearranged NSCLC and represents standard of care for this patient population [6]. With observed median progression free survival (PFS) of 10.9 months and further benefit gained in some cases by continuing crizotinib beyond progression [7], many patients remain on this treatment for years. CT scans performed regularly to monitor disease response also reveal crizotinib related toxicities. Complex renal cysts were reported as a rare complication of crizotinib therapy during clinical trials, initially with an incidence of 4% [8], and more recently, of up to 22% [9, 10]. These cysts have even been noted to invade extrarenal spaces and in a minority, these complex masses can be symptomatic with flank pain

---

* Correspondence: drbimalkumar@yahoo.com
[2]Department of Cancer Imaging, Peter MacCallum Cancer Centre, Grattan Street, Melbourne, Australia
Full list of author information is available at the end of the article

[10]. Complex renal lesions arising while on crizotinib therapy can regress without intervention, regardless of whether crizotinib therapy is ceased [9, 11]. We performed a retrospective analysis of the incidence and pattern of evolution of all renal lesions in CT in lung cancer patients who received crizotinib at our centre.

Methods

Patients with advanced *ALK*-rearranged NSCLC who had been prescribed crizotinib at our institution were identified via the institutional Thoracic Malignancies Cohort database that commenced data collection in July 2012. The cohort included patients on clinical trial and those receiving crizotinib via a special access scheme with Pfizer. The collection of data for our retrospective study was conducted under an ethics approved protocol: the Peter MacCallum Cancer Centre thoracic malignancies cohort study (Peter MacCallum Cancer Centre Human Research Ethics Committee project 11/88) to which patients gave consent to allowing their clinical data and tissue biopsies to be used for future research. To be included in our study, patients needed to have been recruited to the cohort prior to July 2014, have been on crizotinib therapy for at least 2 months, had intravenous contrast enhanced Computed Tomography (IVCECT) prior to commencement of crizotinib therapy and regular follow up IVCECTs, with all scans covering the renal region completely. Patients whose baseline or most follow up CT scans were suboptimal (from lack of IV contrast or movement artefacts affecting assessment of kidneys), those who had proven renal metastases at baseline and those who had interventional procedures on kidneys other than biopsy while on crizotinib were excluded from this analysis. Patients whose baseline scan was [18]FDG PET/CT scan without IV contrast were included in our study only if the CT component of the PET scan unequivocally showed the renal lesion identified in the subsequent IVCECT. The presence, size, number and morphology of all renal lesions were analysed at baseline and in all CT scans performed while on crizotinib by three radiologists [DJ, KM and BP], obtaining consensus regarding lesion description and morphology as described later. Whilst the vast majority of scans were performed in-house, with sub-millimetre axial helical CT acquisition [Siemens Definition AS+, Siemens AG, Germany], images of the renal region available for review on the image archiving system were the standard 5 mm thick axial and coronal reconstructions.

Renal lesions were included if they were at least 4 mm and were able to be assessed in at least two consecutive scans. They were considered as cysts if they were well defined and showed fluid attenuation [less than 20 HU]. As the CT scans were performed to stage lung cancer, the renal region was covered in most cases only in the portal venous phase, technically not permitting accurate classification of renal lesions by Bosniak criteria. Renal cysts were considered complex if they demonstrated poorly defined margins, density higher than simple fluid (for lesions larger than 1 cm), septae or solid or mixed cystic and solid appearance. Significant renal cystic change was defined as an increase or decrease in size of the cyst by more than 3 mm, or development of any of the complex features mentioned above. Additional patient, malignancy and treatment related information was extracted from the prospective cohort database and collected on retrospective review of clinical records.

Results

Thirty five patients with NSCLC received crizotinib therapy at our centre in the defined 4 year period. Nine of these patients were excluded from our study; 6 due to suboptimal imaging, 1 due to biopsy proven renal metastases on baseline scan, 1 due to nephrostomy while on treatment and 1 due to an insufficient period of treatment with crizotinib. Of the remaining 26 patients, 10 (38%) remained on crizotinib at our data collection cut-off and only one patient discontinued therapy due to complex renal cyst formation. Patient, tumour and treatment characteristics are presented in Table 1.

Eleven of 26 (42%) patients had no cysts as per our criteria at baseline or in the study period [8 had no cysts at all; 3 had cysts smaller than 4 mm]. 4 of 26 (15%) had cysts at baseline that remained stable on crizotinib treatment. 1 of these patients had a cyst that was complex (due to high density content) at baseline. The remaining 11 (42%) developed a significant change in renal cysts as per our study criteria in a total of 28 renal lesions.

Table 1 Patient, tumour and treatment characteristics (*N* = 26)

Age (median, range)	52 (34-66)
Sex (Female)	42%
Ethnicity	Asian 31%, Caucasian 69%
Smoking status	Never 58%, light (<10-pyHx) 15%, heavy (>10pyHx) 27%
Diagnosis	Stage IV 96%, confirmed Adenocarcinoma 96%. ALK FISH rearranged: 92%.
Crizotinib provision	Trial: 69%, Access scheme: 31%
Crizotinib duration (median, range weeks)	58 (22-240)
Crizotinib as line of treatment	1st 34%, 2nd 31%, 3rd 27%, 4th 0%, 5th 8%.
Best radiological response	PD 0%, SD 12%, PR 73%, CR 15%

PD progressive disease, *SD* stable disease, *PR* partial response, *CR* complete response

Radiologically significant renal cyst changes

Eight of the 11 patients with significant change in the renal lesions had more than 1 lesion, with as many as 5 in 1 patient. The evolution in size of the 28 cysts varied greatly between and within patients as demonstrated in Table 2 and Fig. 1. Interestingly, all patients who had more than one cyst showed a mixed pattern of cyst evolution Among them, these 11 patients had 20 cysts at baseline that subsequently showed significant changes; 8 new CARCs were noted in four patients during the study period.

Size

Nineteen of the 28 lesions in these 11 patients had a significant growth of renal cysts by our definition (Table 2). In these growing lesions, the median maximum size reached was 23 mm (range 9 – 67 mm) after a median of 178 days (160 to 1342) on crizotinib. The median maximum increase in cyst size from baseline was 10 mm (range 4-52 mm) which corresponded to a median percentage increase in size of 63% (range 40 to 347). 95% (18/19) grew by more than 50%. The median rate of growth was 18 mm/year.

The most common pattern of evolution of the renal cysts was enlargement from baseline followed by spontaneous regression (17/28 lesions), either partially (13/17 lesions) or completely (4/17 lesions), with residual mild cortical scarring (Fig. 2). New cysts developed in 4 patients; 3 of these patients had other pre-existing lesions that were enlarging when new lesions arose. Although *de novo* cysts did arise and significantly evolve, all 11 patients in whom significant renal cystic change occurred had at least 1 renal cyst at baseline. Eleven other patients

without any cysts at baseline did not go on to develop renal cysts.

Less common patterns of evolution of renal lesions noted concurrently in patients with significantly changing cysts were stable cysts (7 lesions in 5 patients), regression of cysts existing at baseline (2 lesions in 2 patients; 1 with partial and the other with complete regression), and ongoing enlargement. 2 patients showed ongoing enlargement of renal cysts at the end of our study period. 1 patient had a cyst that continued to enlarge at data cutoff, from 6 mm to 27 mm (Fig. 3) over 45 months on treatment. A new cyst that developed in another patient 2 months after start of crizotinib also continued to enlarge, reaching 49 mm on imaging 2 months later, shortly before the patient died due to disease progression.

Complexity

The development of complex features, as defined above, apart from simple changes in size, occurred in 12 cysts, affecting 7/26 (27%) patients overall (Table 3). The median (range) time on crizotinib to development of initial and most complex changes were 172 (0 to 380) days and 199 (130 to 380) days respectively. In 10 cysts, the most complex changes were seen within 60 days of onset. The earliest development of new complex features was seen after 51 days on crizotinib. Bosniak classification was not applied but development of lesions with septations or mixed cystic and solid appearances were noted to be the two most common patterns of complex change in CARCs. Psoas muscle or abdominal wall invasion was seen in 2 lesions in one patient (Table 3). In 4/26 patients, the imaging features of the lesions were concerning for malignant change or abscess and 2 of these

Table 2 Cyst evolution in patients with significant renal cystic change (N = 11): PR - partial regression

Patient #	Duration of crizotinib (days)	No: of Cysts during study period	Mixed pattern of evolution of lesions	New cysts	Enlarged from baseline			Stable during study period	Regressed from baseline
					Then regressed		Ongoing enlargement		
					CR	PR			
1	280	2	Y	0	1			1	
2	1344	1	N	0		1			
3	678	2	Y	0	1				1; CR
4	126	5	Y	4	(+4)	1			
5	686	4	Y	0	1			2	1; PR
6	150	3	Y	0		1		2	
7	547	1	N	0		1			
8	1109	4	Y	1	2 (+1)			1	
9	160	2	Y	1			(1)	1	
10	1477	1	N	0			1		
11	1456	3	Y	2	1(+2)				
Median age 48 years; 45% F; 64% Asian	Median 678	28		4/11 patients	13/28 cysts	4/28 cysts	2/28 cysts	7/28 cysts	2/28 cysts

CR complete regression, (+) new lesion

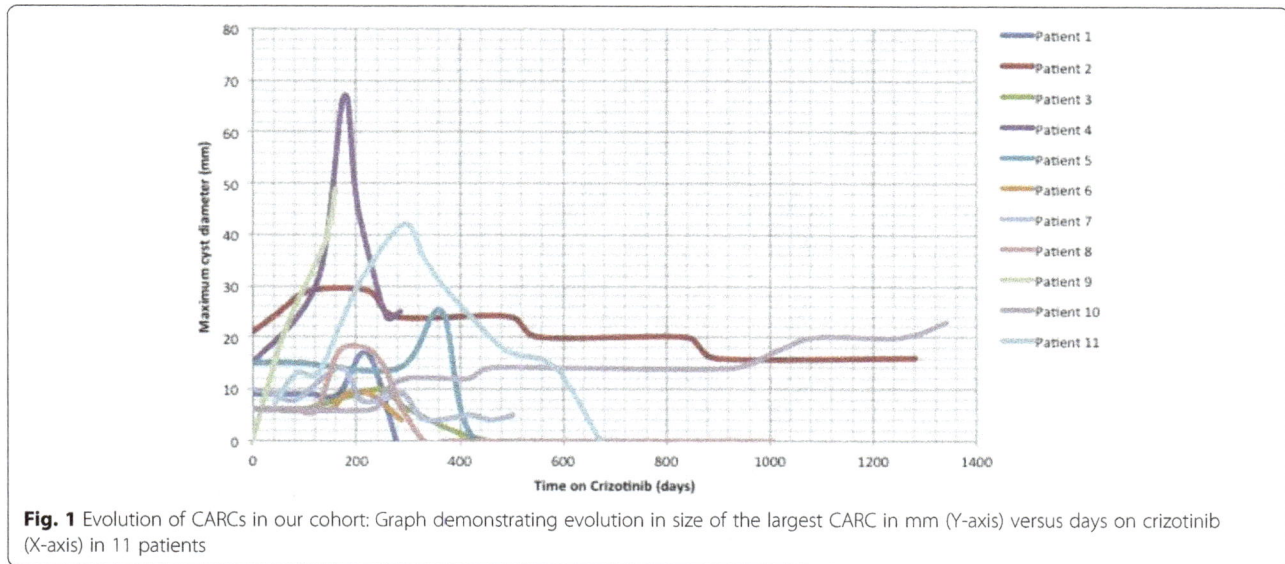

Fig. 1 Evolution of CARCs in our cohort: Graph demonstrating evolution in size of the largest CARC in mm (Y-axis) versus days on crizotinib (X-axis) in 11 patients

patients (Figs. 4 and 5) developed flank pain. Subsequent CT guided biopsy and diagnostic aspiration of few millilitres of cyst contents in these 2 patients (from psoas lesion in one patient and from the renal lesion in the other) revealed benign histology, with both samples showing xanthogranulomatous inflammation. The biopsies showed degenerate cellular debris, fibrosis and a mixed inflammatory infiltrate, including lymphocytes, neutrophils and numerous macrophages, many with foamy cytoplasm. No residual cyst wall was identified, no micro-organisms were seen or cultured, and no malignant cells were present. Both patients had resolution of cystic changes, one after cessation of crizotinib (Fig. 4) and the other despite ongoing treatment with crizotinib (Fig. 5).

Correlation between evolution of renal cysts and disease response/ renal function

Of the 11 patients with significant renal cystic change, 2 had progressive disease and 9 had continued response (2

complete, 7 partial) at the time of maximum cystic change. There was no apparent association between cyst evolution and renal impairment. The median (range) serum Creatinine was 78 (57 to 92) µmol/L at commencement of Crizotinib and 79 (61 to 106) µmol/L at the time of maximum cystic change. Urinalysis was performed on 5 patients at the time of maximum cystic change and all results were normal.

Discussion

In the general population, renal cysts are thought to be acquired lesions that evolve from diverticula in distal convoluted and collecting renal tubules [12]. The prevalence of CT detected simple cysts increases with age and has been estimated at 27.5% in 40-60 year olds; 49% in those 60-80 years and 60.6% in those above 80 [13]. The natural history of simple renal cysts is to slowly enlarge, with reported average size increase and rate of enlargement of 1.6 mm and 3.9% per year,

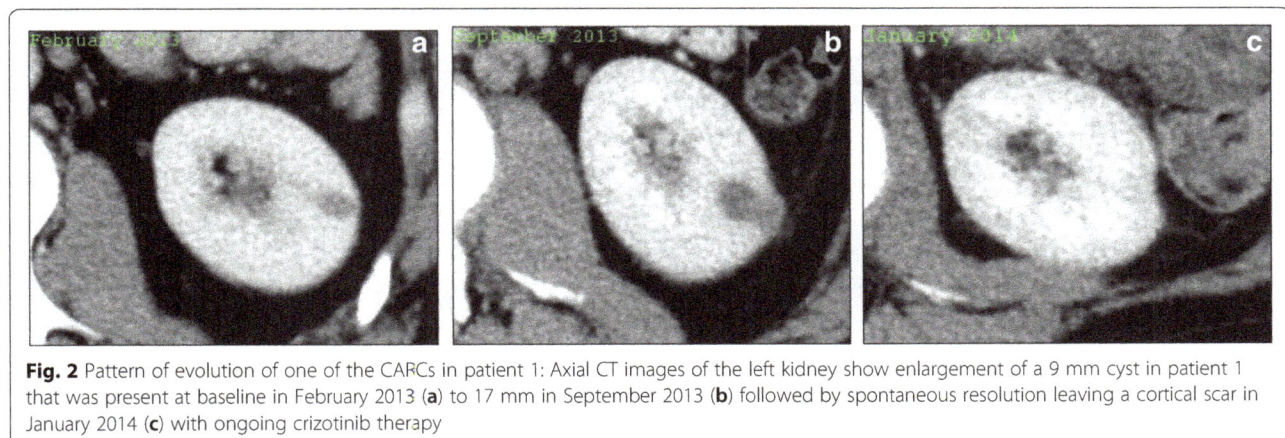

Fig. 2 Pattern of evolution of one of the CARCs in patient 1: Axial CT images of the left kidney show enlargement of a 9 mm cyst in patient 1 that was present at baseline in February 2013 (**a**) to 17 mm in September 2013 (**b**) followed by spontaneous resolution leaving a cortical scar in January 2014 (**c**) with ongoing crizotinib therapy

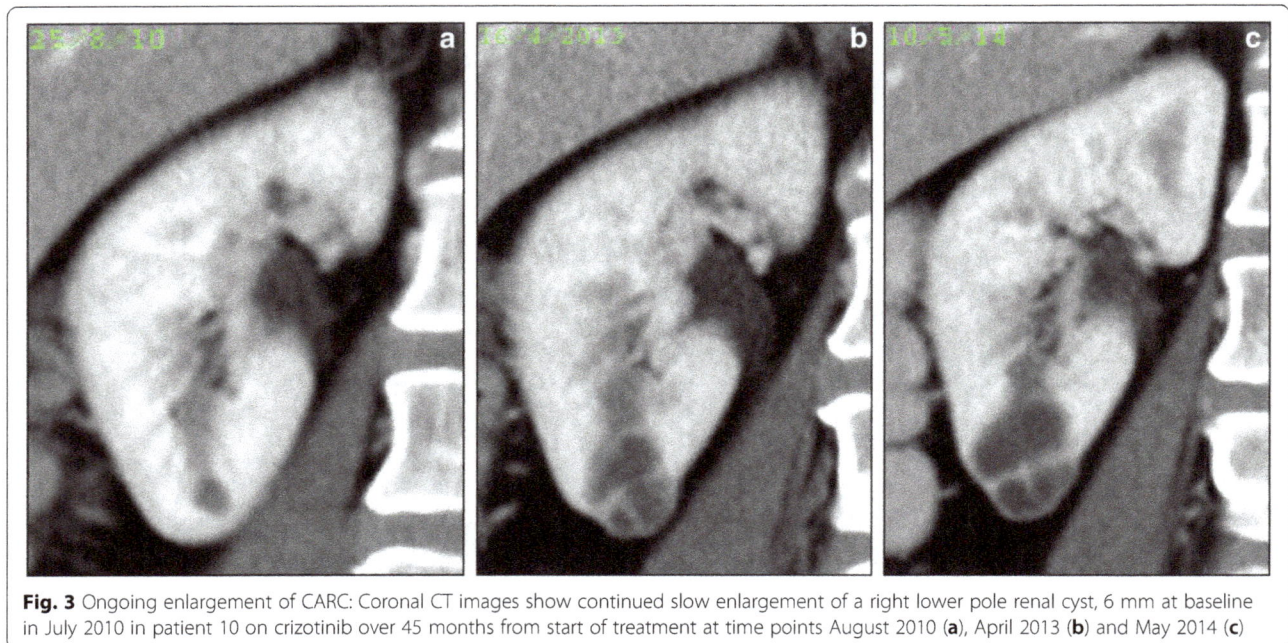

Fig. 3 Ongoing enlargement of CARC: Coronal CT images show continued slow enlargement of a right lower pole renal cyst, 6 mm at baseline in July 2010 in patient 10 on crizotinib over 45 months from start of treatment at time points August 2010 (**a**), April 2013 (**b**) and May 2014 (**c**)

respectively [14]. Thus, the prevalence of renal cysts (58%) in our patient cohort (median age 52 years) at baseline was higher than expected.

Within the limits of our small sample size, the rate of growth of renal cysts in our patients on crizotinib was noted to exceed that expected in the natural history of simple cyst evolution. A potential limitation of our study is the lack of comparison in evolution of renal cysts in *ALK*-rearranged NSCLC. There was not an apparent development of renal cysts in *ALK*-rearranged NSCLC patients who received chemotherapy on trial [10] but larger population studies would be difficult to undertake given the efficacy and availability of crizotinib in this population moving forward.

Using predefined criteria for significant change in size and complexity of renal cysts, our study confirms the previously reported increase in size and complexity of

renal cysts after commencing crizotinib. In this report we describe the highest incidence of radiologically significant renal cyst change (42%) and new complex features (27%) to date. Our definitions of significant renal cystic change differ only slightly from previous reports. Lin et al. [9] reported a 22% incidence of significant renal cystic change as defined by new renal cysts more than 4 mm in size, enlargement or regression of previous cysts by more than 4 mm or development of complicated renal cysts (Bosniak IIF or higher). Schnell et al. [10] report 2% of cysts to significantly enlarge defined as an increase by more than 50%, however this rate was determined based on cyst detection at the 6 month scan. Our cohort demographics were similar to previous reports in terms of smoking status, adenocarcinoma and median age, reflecting the expected characteristics of patients with NSCLC harbouring *ALK* gene rearrangement.

Table 3 Analysis of complex changes@ demonstrated by CARCs

No:	Patient (Ref Table 2)	No: of cysts	Number of cysts demonstrating:						
			Enlargement	New hyper-density	Septation	Mixed cystic and solid appearance	Uniform solid appearance	Poor definition of margins	Psoas/abdominal wall extension
1	#1	1	1	1	-	-	-	-	-
2	#4	5	5	-	4	5	-	2	2
3	#5	1	1	1	-	-	1	-	-
4	#8	1	1	1	1	-	-	1	-
5	#9	1	1	1		1	-	-	-
6	#10	1	1	-	1	1	-	-	-
7	#11	2	2	-	1	1	-	1	-
Total	7	12	12	4	7	8	1	4	2

Complex change@: does not include lesions with change only in size

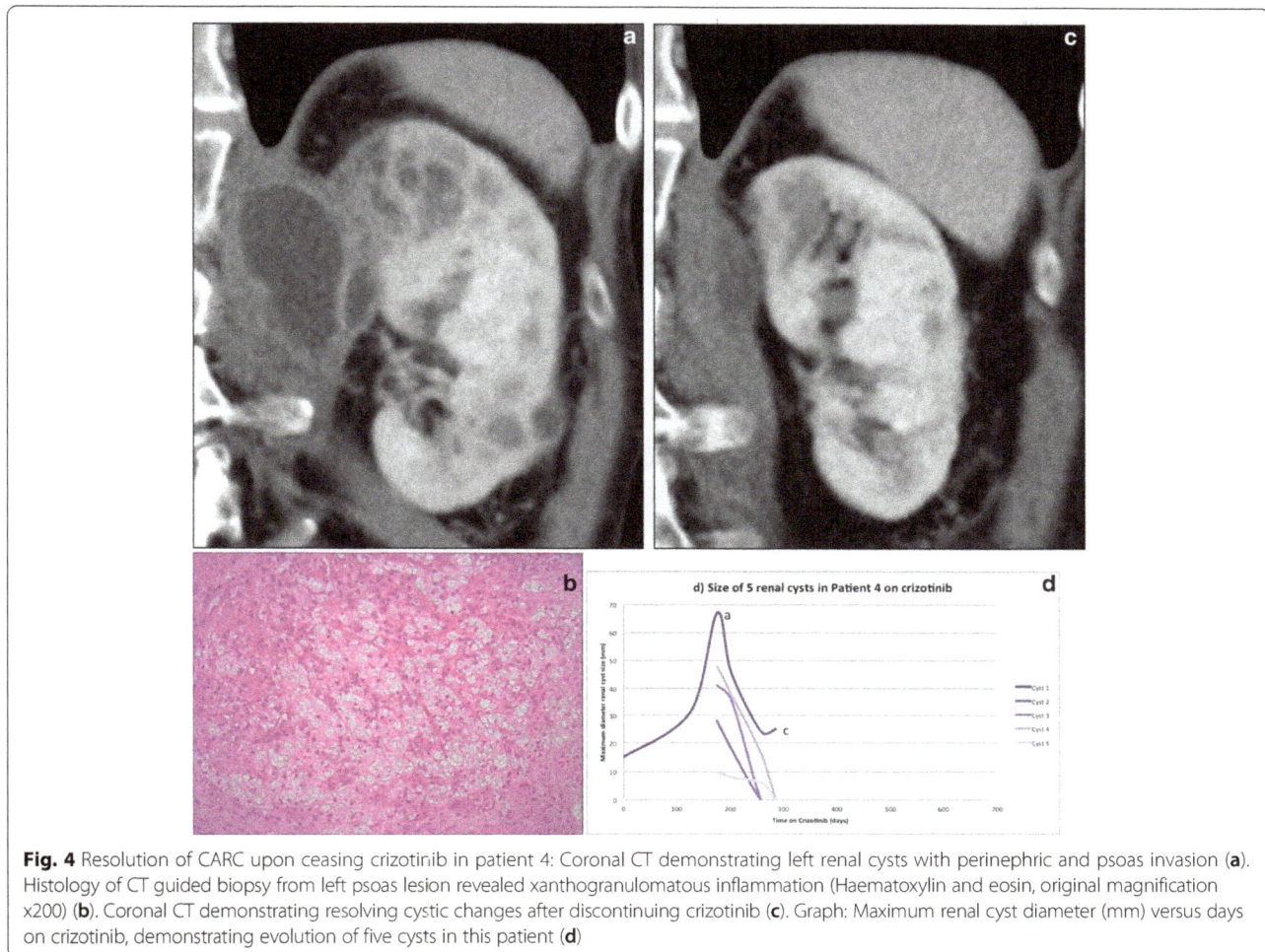

Fig. 4 Resolution of CARC upon ceasing crizotinib in patient 4: Coronal CT demonstrating left renal cysts with perinephric and psoas invasion (**a**). Histology of CT guided biopsy from left psoas lesion revealed xanthogranulomatous inflammation (Haematoxylin and eosin, original magnification x200) (**b**). Coronal CT demonstrating resolving cystic changes after discontinuing crizotinib (**c**). Graph: Maximum renal cyst diameter (mm) versus days on crizotinib, demonstrating evolution of five cysts in this patient (**d**)

We have demonstrated a variety in the pattern of cyst evolution, even within the same kidney. The clearly dominant pattern of evolution of CARCs in our study was, as reported in literature, asymptomatic cysts that enlarged and spontaneously regressed without discontinuation of crizotinib or need for intervention. It did appear that cysts regressed slightly faster in our single case in whom crizotinib was discontinued (Fig. 4) than in those who continued on treatment (Fig. 5). In addition to this dominant pattern of evolution of renal cysts, we also noted three other previously unreported patterns, namely stability of cysts detected at baseline, regression of lesions from baseline and progressive enlargement of lesions from baseline. The pattern of ongoing cyst enlargement we noted, however, likely represents only a rarer pattern of very slow spontaneous regression, as one of the 2 patients in whom this pattern was observed started showing spontaneous regression of his CARC 16 months after the end of our study period and the other patient died due to disease progression after 5 months of crizotinib therapy.

Renal cysts can be graded using the Bosniak classification system that scores the cyst complexity from I-IV [15]. Higher grades have a higher likelihood of malignancy and current recommendations for Bosniak class III/IV renal cysts include surgical resection [16]. Accurate assessment of cyst morphology and enhancement characteristics requires both non-enhanced and IV contrast enhanced scans to be performed [17]. CT scans in our study were routinely performed only in the portal venous phase. This limitation of our study was addressed by applying commonly accepted features of complexity in renal cysts to the portal venous phase scans. The two commonest complex features we noted in CARCs were the development of multiple septations and a mixed cystic and solid appearance.

The differential of renal cysts demonstrating complex features in a patient with NSCLC includes infection, renal metastases and primary renal malignancy. In two of our patients with CARCs, the imaging and clinical features were concerning enough to warrant a biopsy. In both, CT guided aspiration and biopsy revealed benign histology of xanthogranulomatous inflammation with

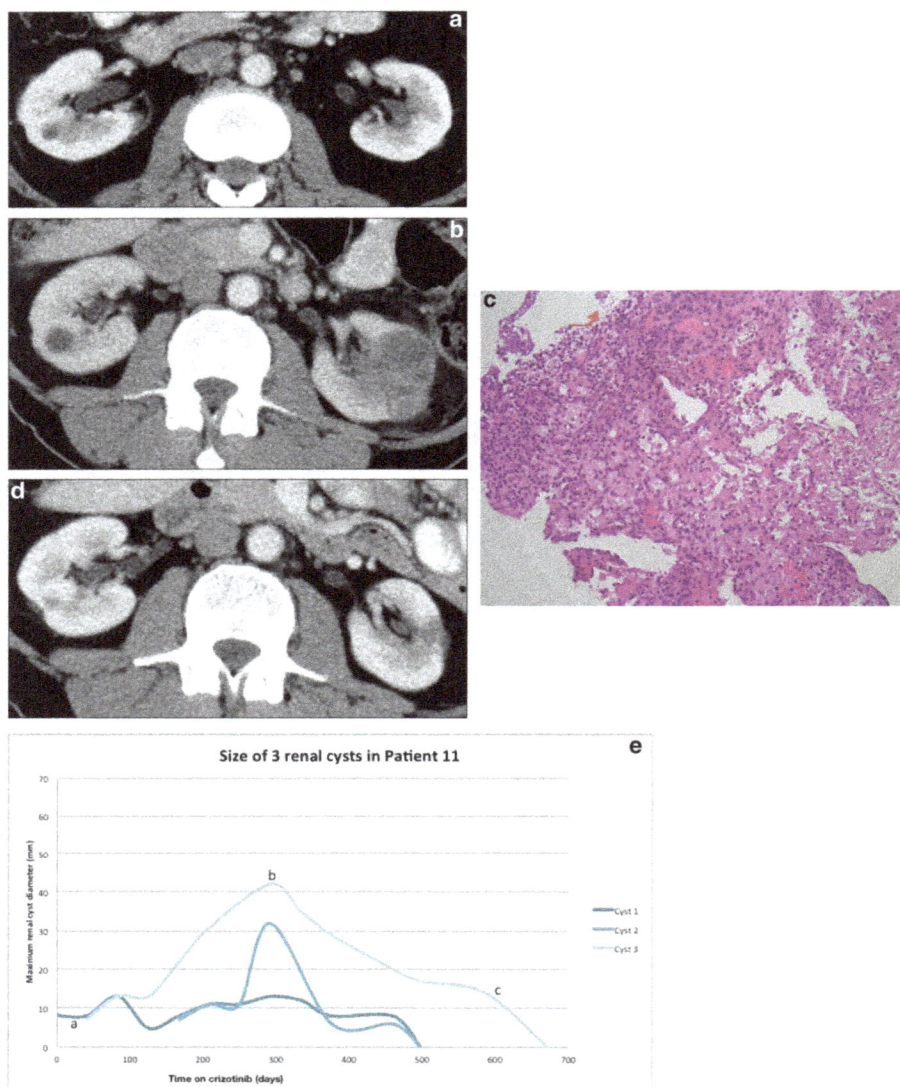

Fig. 5 Resolution of CARCs without ceasing crizotinib in patient 11: Baseline scan demonstrated an 8 mm cyst in the right kidney (**a**). Enlarging right renal cyst with no complex features and the new left renal cyst with mixed solid and cystic areas and poorly defined margins (**b**). A new right upper pole cyst with septations is not shown. CT guided aspiration/ biopsy of the left renal lesion revealed xanthogranulomatous inflammation (Haematoxylin and eosin, original magnification x200) (**c**). All three cysts spontaneously resolved with ongoing Crizotinib therapy (**d**). Graph: Maximum renal cyst diameter (mm) versus days on crizotinib, demonstrating evolution of the three cysts in this patient (**e**)

negative bacterial culture and no malignant cells evident. Several recent case reports have also documented benign pathology upon aspiration of complex cysts in patients with NSCLC treated with Crizotinib [18–20]. Prior knowledge and prompt recognition of CARCs may help avoid unnecessary biopsy/drainage and suboptimal treatment of lung cancer.

While reported regression of the CARCs may have been hastened by drainage [18–20], our experience suggests that these lesions spontaneously resolve.

Percutaneous drainage may be warranted to relieve symptoms of enlarging cysts or to investigate for infection if concerning clinical features such as fever are apparent. We propose that, when found incidentally on imaging, CARCs could simply be observed without intervention or cessation of crizotinib.

The pathogenesis of renal cyst development due to crizotinib is unknown. In response to acquired resistance to crizotinib, several more potent next generation ALK inhibitors have been developed and are now used in the clinical setting [21] Renal cysts have not been reported as a complication of these more specific ALK directed therapies indicating that cystogenesis may be driven by inhibition of other molecules targeted by crizotinib.

Crizotinib was initially developed as a c-MET inhibitor. The ligand to c-MET, hepatocyte growth factor (HGF) is thought to mediate human renal cyst formation [22]. Thus it would be paradoxical that inhibition of c-MET by crizotinib would drive cyst formation unless an unidentified feedback mechanism increased levels of HGF to drive cyst formation via another target.

Pre-clinical studies investigating an apparent link between testosterone and polycystic kidney disease have conflicting results [23, 24] and although crizotinib has been shown to reduce testosterone levels [25] we were not able to investigate testosterone levels in our retrospective analysis. Although small numbers don't allow statistical certainty, it did appear that renal cysts developed in a higher proportion of Asian patients as previously reported [9].

Conclusions

In summary, development of complex renal cysts is not an uncommon side effect of treatment with crizotinib. Cysts are typically benign, asymptomatic and resolve spontaneously on continued crizotinib therapy. As the use of crizotinib becomes more common, it is imperative that radiologists and treating physicians are aware of CARCs and their temporal evolution.

Abbreviations

ALK: Anaplastic Lymphoma Kinase; ALK-I: Anaplastic Lymphoma Kinase inhibitors; CARC: Crizotinib Associated Renal Cyst; CT: Computerised tomography; IVCECT: Intravenous contrast enhanced Computed Tomography; NSCLC: Non small cell lung cancer; PFS: Progression free survival

Acknowledgements
Not applicable.

Funding
Nil.

Authors' contributions

LBC- study design; acquisition, analysis and interpretation of data, especially patient profile, laboratory investigations and treatment response; drafting and revising the manuscript. DHSJ- study design; analysis and interpretation of data, including reading analysis of CT scans; drafting and revising the manuscript. KM- interpretation of data; including analysis of CT scans; drafting and revising the manuscript. CM - interpretation of histology data; drafting and revising the manuscript. BS -conception and design analysis and interpretation of data, especially patient profile, laboratory investigations and treatment response; drafting and revising the manuscript. BKP- conception and design; analysis and interpretation of data, including analysis of CT scans; drafting and revising the manuscript. All authors read and approved the final manuscript

Authors' information
Nil.

Competing interests
All authors declare that they have no competing interests.

Author details
[1]Department of Medical Oncology, Peter MacCallum Cancer Centre, Grattan Street, Melbourne, Australia. [2]Department of Cancer Imaging, Peter MacCallum Cancer Centre, Grattan Street, Melbourne, Australia. [3]Department of Pathology, Peter MacCallum Cancer Centre, Grattan Street, Melbourne, Australia. [4]Department of Medical Oncology, Peter MacCallum Cancer Centre; Sir Peter MacCallum Department of Oncology, University of Melbourne, Melbourne, Australia.

References

1. Soda M, Choi YL, Enomoto M, Takada S, Yamashita Y, Ishikawa S, et al. Identification of the transforming EML4-ALK fusion gene in non-small-cell lung cancer. Nature. 2007;448(7153):561–6.
2. Solomon B, Varella-Garcia M, Camidge DR. ALK gene rearrangements: a new therapeutic target in a molecularly defined subset of non-small cell lung cancer. J Thorac Oncol. 2009;4(12):1450–4.
3. Camidge DR, Bang YJ, Kwak EL, Iafrate AJ, Varella-Garcia M, Fox SB, et al. Activity and safety of crizotinib in patients with ALK-positive non-small-cell lung cancer: updated results from a phase 1 study. Lancet Oncol. 2012;13(10):1011–9.
4. Camidge D, Ou S, Shapiro G, Otterson G, Villaruz L, Villalona-Calero M, et al. Efficacy and safety of crizotinib in patients with advanced c-MET-amplified non-small cell lung cancer (NSCLC). J Clin Oncol. 2014;32:15.
5. Shaw AT, Ou S-HI, Bang Y-J, Camidge DR, Solomon BJ, Salgia R, et al. Crizotinib in ROS1-Rearranged Non–Small-Cell Lung Cancer. N Engl J Med. 2014;371:1963–71.
6. Solomon BJ, Mok T, Kim D-W, Wu Y-L, Nakagawa K, Mekhail T, et al. First-Line Crizotinib versus Chemotherapy in ALK-Positive Lung Cancer. N Engl J Med. 2014;371(23):2167–77.
7. Ou SH, Janne PA, Bartlett CH, Tang Y, Kim DW, Otterson GA, et al. Clinical benefit of continuing ALK inhibition with crizotinib beyond initial disease progression in patients with advanced ALK-positive NSCLC. Ann Oncol. 2014;25(2):415–22.
8. FDA. Crizotinib Label. http://www.accessdata.fda.gov/drugsatfda_docs/label/2013/202570s006lbl.pdf.
9. Lin Y-T, Wang Y-F, Yang JC-H, Yu C-J, Wu S-G, Shih J-Y, et al. Development of renal cysts after crizotinib treatment in advanced ALK-positive non–small-cell lung cancer. J Thoracic Oncol. 2014;9(11):1720–5.
10. Schnell P, Bartlett CH, Solomon BJ, Tassell V, Shaw AT, Pas T et al. Complex renal cysts associated with crizotinib treatment. Cancer Med. 2015;4(6):887–96.
11. Klempner SJ, Aubin G, Dash A, Ou S. Spontaneous regression of crizotinib-associated complex renal cysts during continuous crizotinib treatment. Oncologist. 2014;19(9):1008–10.
12. Baert L, Steg A. On the pathogenesis of simple renal cysts in the adult. A microdissection study. Urol Res. 1977;5(3):103–8.
13. Carrim ZI, Murchison JT. The prevalence of simple renal and hepatic cysts detected by spiral computed tomography. Clin Radiol. 2003;58:626–29.
14. Terada N, Arai Y, Kinukawa N, Terai A. The 10-year natural history of simple renal cysts. Urology. 2008;71(1):7–11.
15. Warren KS, McFarlane J. The Bosniak classification of renal cystic masses. BJU Int. 2005;95(7):939–42.
16. Whelan TF. Guidelines on the management of renal cyst disease. Can Urol Assoc J. 2010;4(2):98–9.
17. Curry NS, Cochran ST, Bissada NK. Cystic renal masses: accurate Bosniak classification requires adequate renal CT. AJR Am J Roentgenol. 2000;175(2):339–42.
18. de Carvalho L, Shimada A, da Cruz Neto M, da Silva Rocha L, Viana P, Kallas E, Katz A. Development of aseptic renal abscess in a patient with non-small-cell lung cancer with ALK translocation during Crizotinib treatment. Adv Lung Cancer. 2015;4:53–7.
19. Chan WY, Ang MK, Tan DS, Koh WL, Kwek JW. Imaging features of renal complications after crizotinib treatment for non-small-cell lung cancer: a case report. Radiol Case Rep. 2016;11(3):245–7.
20. Yoneshima Y, Okamoto I, Arimura-Omori M, Kimura S, Hidaka-Fujimoto N, Iwama E. Infected complex renal cysts during crizotinib therapy in a patient with non-small cell lung cancer positive for ALK rearrangement. Invest New Drugs. 2015;33:510–2.
21. Wu J, Savooji J, Liu D. Second- and third-generation ALK inhibitors for non-small cell lung cancer. J Hematol Oncol. 2016;9:19.

22. Horie S, Higashihara E, Nutahara K, Mikami Y, Okubo A, Kano M, et al. Mediation of renal cyst formation by hepatocyte growth factor. Lancet. 1994;344(8925):789–91.

23. Jayapalan S, Saboorian MH, Edmunds JW, Aukema HM. High dietary fat intake increases renal cyst disease progression in Han: SPRD-cy rats. J Nutr. 2000;130(9):2356–60.

24. Cowley Jr BD, Rupp JC, Muessel MJ, Gattone 2nd VH. Gender and the effect of gonadal hormones on the progression of inherited polycystic kidney disease in rats. Am J Kidney Dis. 1997;29(2):265–72.

25. Weickhardt AJ, Rothman MS, Salian-Mehta S, Kiseljak-Vassiliades K, Oton AB, Doebele RC, et al. Rapid-onset hypogonadism secondary to crizotinib use in men with metastatic nonsmall cell lung cancer. Cancer. 2012;118(21):5302–9.

17

Cement pulmonary embolism as a complication of percutaneous vertebroplasty in cancer patients

Asem Mansour[1][*] ⓘ, Nayef Abdel-Razeq[2], Hussein Abuali[1], Mohammad Makoseh[3], Nouran Shaikh-Salem[3], Kamelah Abushalha[3] and Samer Salah[3]

Abstract

Background: Vertebroplasty is a minimally invasive procedure commonly performed for vertebral compression fractures secondary to osteoporosis or malignancy. Leakage of bone cement into the paravertebral venous system and cement pulmonary embolism (cPE) are well described, mostly in patients with osteoporosis. Little is known about the clinical sequelae and outcomes in cancer patients. In this study, we report our experience with cPE following vertebroplasty performed in cancer patients.

Methods: Records of all consecutive cancer patients who underwent vertebroplasty at our institution were retrospectively reviewed. The procedure was performed via percutaneous injection of barium-opacified polymethyl-methacrylate cement.

Results: A total of 102 cancer patients with a median age of 53 (19–83) years were included. Seventy-eight (76.5%) patients had malignant vertebral fractures, and 24 (23.5%) patients had osteoporotic fractures. Cement PE was detected in 13 (12.7%) patients; 10 (76.9%) patients had malignant fractures, and the remaining three had osteoporotic fractures. Cement PE was mostly asymptomatic; however, 5 (38.5%) patients had respiratory symptoms that led to the diagnosis. Only the five symptomatic patients were anticoagulated.
Cement PE was more common with multiple myeloma (MM); it occurred in 7 (18.9%) of the 37 patients with MM compared with only three (7.3%) of the 41 patients with other malignancies. No difference in incidence was observed between patients with osteoporotic or malignant vertebral fractures.

Conclusions: Cement PE is a relatively common complication following vertebroplasty and is mostly asymptomatic. Multiple myeloma is associated with the highest risk. Large-scale prospective studies can help identify risk factors and clinical outcomes and could lead to better prevention and therapeutic strategies.

Keywords: Vertebroplasty, Cement, Pulmonary embolism, Cancer, Osteoporosis

Background

Vertebral body compression fractures are common, especially among elderly patients. The high prevalence of osteoporosis and cancer in this age group is a major contributing factor [1–3].

In addition to severe pain requiring hospital admission and parenteral opioids, these fractures can cause neurological deficits, height loss and kyphosis with associated restrictive pulmonary disease [4, 5].

Vertebroplasty is a minimally invasive procedure that is commonly performed for vertebral compression fractures secondary to both osteoporosis and malignancy [6]. The procedure is performed under image guidance and involves the injection of a cement polymer, commonly polymethylmethacrylate (PMMA), into the vertebral body to confer improved stability and pain relief [7, 8]. Vertebroplasty was first introduced at the University Hospital of Amiens, France, in 1984, when it was used to augment the post-resection defect of a benign spinal tumor [9]. Since then, it has become an

* Correspondence: amansour@khcc.jo
[1]Department of Radiology, King Hussein Cancer Center, Amman, Jordan
Full list of author information is available at the end of the article

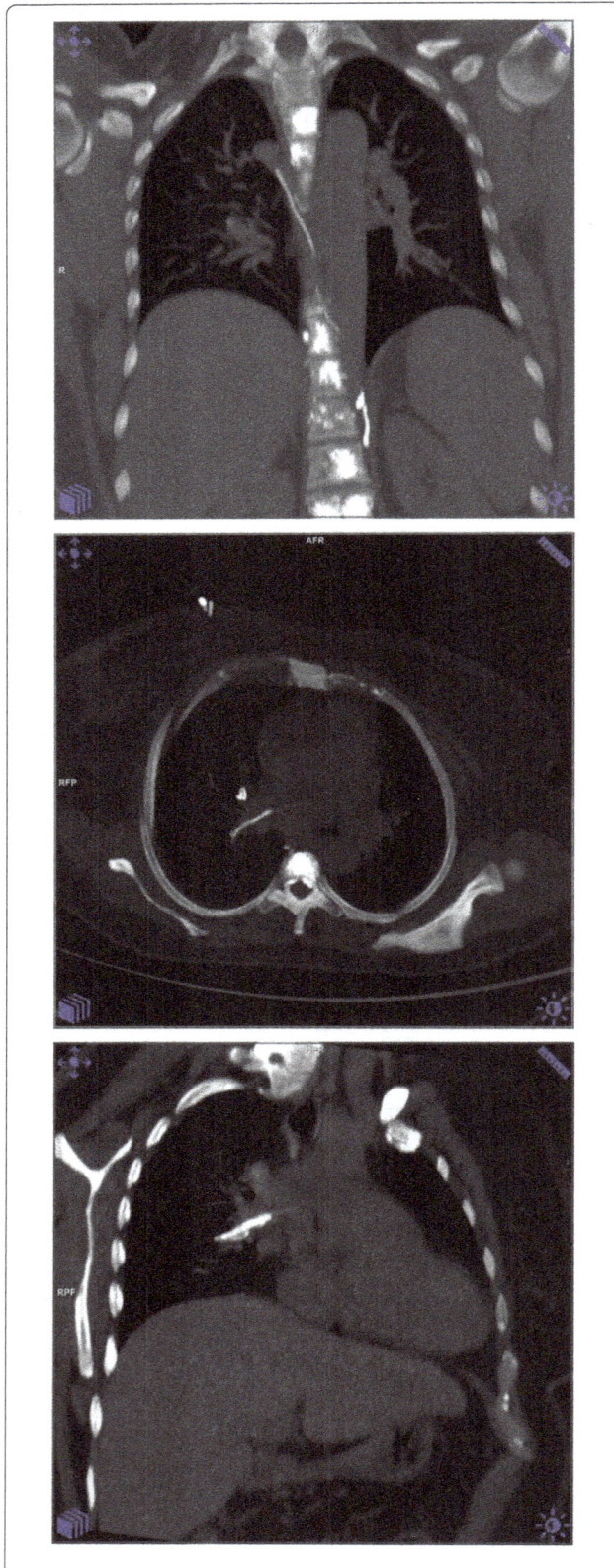

Fig. 1 Selected coronal image with maximum intensity projection of unenhanced chest CT showing multilevel vertebral augmentation by cement. There is a branching linear density along the course of the lumber veins and the azygus/hemiazygus system representing cement leak/ intravasation. Axial and coronal oblique MIP images are showing a similar linear density in the right main pulmonary artery extending to the right superior segmental branch of the right lower lobe representing cement pulmonary emboli

increasingly recommended therapeutic intervention due to its high efficacy and safety [10].

Vertebral bodies are highly vascularized and form a valveless network with the paravertebral and extradural venous plexuses. Vertebral compression fractures enhance venous drainage and facilitate migration of cement fragments into the systemic venous circulation. Leakage of bone cement into the paravertebral venous system is well described (Fig. 1) [11]. Cement pulmonary embolism (cPE) is a well-recognized complication of vertebroplasty in patients with traumatic, osteoporotic, and metastasis-induced compression fractures [12–14]. The clinical implications and complications associated with such embolisms, especially in cancer patients, are poorly characterized.

In this study, we report our experience with vertebroplasty performed for vertebral fractures in cancer patients. We also provide a literature review of published data regarding cPE in cancer and non-cancer patients.

Methods

This is a retrospective study in which the hospital's and the radiology department's databases were searched for both "vertebroplasty" and "cPE". The records of all patients who underwent vertebroplasty at our institution over the past ten years were reviewed. All imaging studies including computed tomography (CT) scans or plain chest radiographs that were performed following vertebroplasty for any indication were reviewed again by an experienced radiologist to assess for features of cPE.

The following data were extracted from patients' charts and electronic medical records: gender, age at time of vertebroplasty, type and stage of cancer, number and location of vertebral metastases, status of the patient before vertebroplasty (ambulatory or hospitalized), and history of cardiac or pulmonary diseases diagnosed before the vertebroplasty. Moreover, we gathered data pertaining to imaging tools that were utilized for diagnosis of cPE, clinical manifestations, details of treatment, hemodynamic sequelae associated with cPE, and dates of last follow-up and death.

The procedure was performed under image guidance via a percutaneous injection of barium-opacified polymethylmethacrylate cement.

Given its retrospective nature, our research was exempted from review by our Institutional Review Board (IRB).

Results

A total of 102 patients underwent vertebroplasty during the study period and were included in this report. All had a pathology-confirmed diagnosis of cancer. The median age was 53 years (range: 19–83), and 57 (55.9%) patients were female.

Pathological evaluation of the fractured vertebrae confirmed metastatic disease involvement in 78 (76.5%) patients. The fractures in the other 24 (23.5%) patients, many with active cancer, were due to osteoporosis. Vertebroplasty was performed in the lumbar spine in 57 (55.9%) patients and in the thoracic spine in 16 (15.7%) patients; 29 (28.4%) patients had the procedure performed in both lumbar and thoracic vertebrae.

Multiple myeloma was the commonest primary cancer and was identified in 37 (36.3%) patients, followed by breast cancer in 25 (24.5%) patients and lymphoma in 13 (12.7%) patients. Most patients (95.1%) were ambulatory at time of vertebroplasty; only 5 were wheelchair-bound. In addition to cancer, many patients had other comorbidities, including significant cardiac illness in 19 (18.6%) patients and significant pulmonary disease in 9 (8.8%) patients had (Table 1).

Cement PE was identified in 13 (12.7%) cases; the median age of patients with cPE was 50 years (range: 31–81). Eleven (84.6%) patients were diagnosed by CT scan (Fig. 2), while the other two patients had an initial suspicious finding on chest X-ray that was confirmed by a follow-up CT. All patients with confirmed cPE except one were ambulatory at the time of vertebroplasty.

The total number of levels injected was 252 (mean per patient: 2.47, median: 2). As such, the incidence of cPE is 5.2 episodes per 100 injections. Among the 13 patients with cPE, a total of 39 levels were injected (mean: 3.0, median: 3).

Cement PE was mostly asymptomatic, but 5 (38.5%) patients had symptoms (dyspnea, chest pain, cough, tachycardia, hypoxia) that led to the diagnosis. Only the five symptomatic patients were anticoagulated; all were treated with low molecular weight heparin (LMWH) and none had any minor or major bleeding or any other complication related to anticoagulation. Ten (76.9%) of the 13 patients had malignant vertebral fractures, while the other three (23.1%) patients had osteoporotic fractures with no known vertebral metastasis. Details of the 13 patients are listed in Table 2.

Cement PE was more common among patients with MM compared to other malignancies; it occurred in seven of 37 (18.9%) MM patients and 3 of 41 patients (7.3%) with other malignancies (HR = 0.338; 95% CI, 0.081–1.42; P = 0.18).

Table 1 Patients' characteristics

Age	
Median (years)	53
Range (years)	19–83
Sex	
Male	45 (44.1%)
Female	57 (55.9%)
Smoking history:	
Smoker	17 (16.7%)
Ex-smoker	18 (17.6%)
Never smoked	67 (65.7%)
Underlying cancer:	
Multiple Myeloma	37 (36.3%)
Breast	25 (24.5%)
Lymphoma	13 (12.7%)
Lung	5 (4.9%)
Sarcoma	4 (3.9%)
Prostate	4 (3.9%)
Others	14 (13.7%)
Timing of vertebral fracture:	
Initial presentation	57 (55.9%)
Disease recurrence	45 (44.1%)
Comorbidities:	
Hypertension	32 (31.4%)
Diabetes mellitus	26 (25.5%)
Cardiac disease	19 (18.6%)
Pulmonary disease	9 (8.8%)
Mobility:	
Ambulatory	97 (95.1%)
Wheel-chair bound	5 (4.9%)
Underlying etiology and site:	
No metastasis (Osteoporosis)	24 (23.5%)
Vertebral metastasis[a]:	78 (76.5%)
Cervical spines	61 (78.2%)
Dorsal spines	73 (93.6%)
Lumbar spines	75 (96.2%)

[a]Total > 102, reflecting multiple sites

The nature and etiology of vertebral fractures are also worth addressing. In all seven myeloma patients with cPE, the fracture was related to malignant tumor infiltration but the two lymphoma cases were related to osteoporosis and not malignancy; both lymphoma cases were in elderly women (78 and 81 years old) who had received a significant amount of steroids as part of their lymphoma treatment.

The incidence of cPE was not different in patients with osteoporotic (3/24, 12.5%) or malignant (10/78, 12.8%)

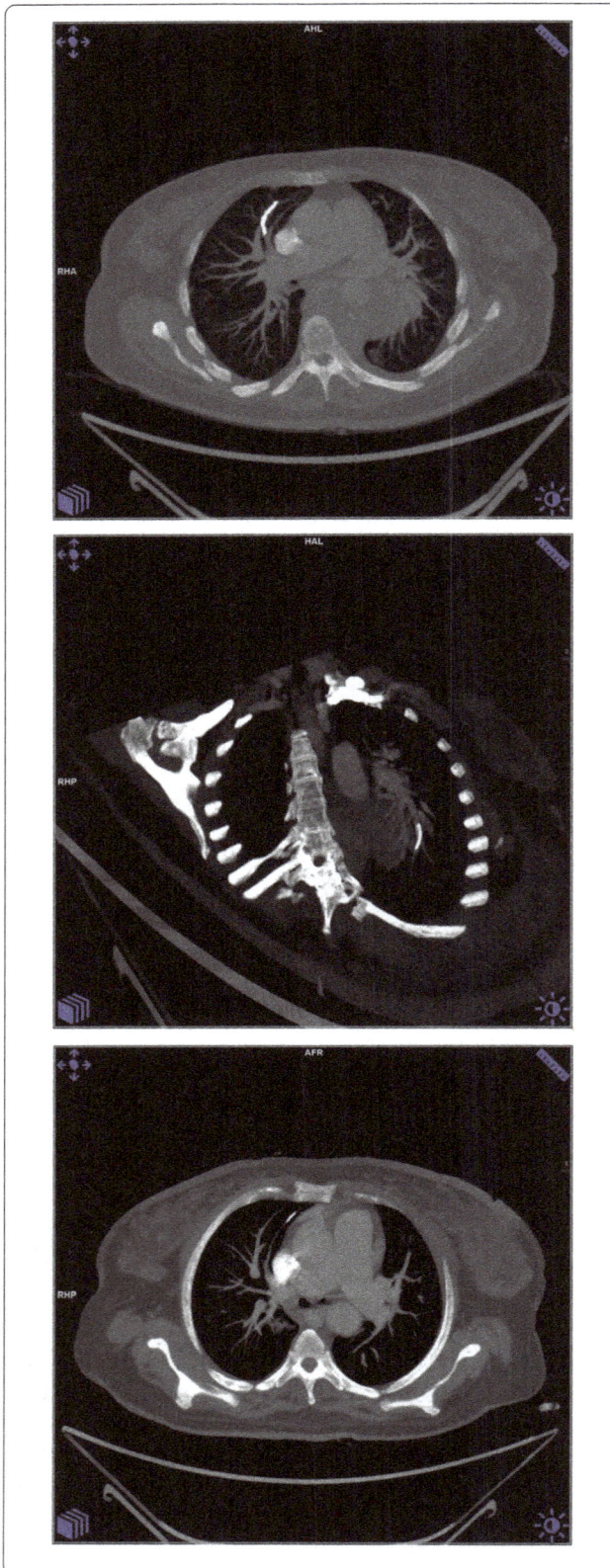

Fig. 2 Chest CT with MIP showing a curvilinear density in the anterior subsegmental branch of Right Upper lobe indicating cement PE. Oblique coronal MIP image of the same patient showing cement PE in basal subsegmental branch of LLL

vertebral fractures (HR = 0.972; 95% CI, 0.244–3.86; P = 0.99). However, patients with osteoporotic vertebral fractures were older, with a median age of 66 years compared to 51 years for patients with malignant fractures (P = 0.0076).

Survival following the vertebroplasty and associated cPE was variable; one patient survived only 6 weeks, while 3 others are alive at 48 months or more. Death was not attributed to PE in any of the patients.

Discussion

Several studies and case reports have addressed the issue of cement leakage and cPE in patients undergoing vertebroplasty, with conflicting conclusions.

Our literature search retrieved many papers addressing this topic; the majority consisted of case reports, mostly in non-cancer patients. However, some papers include a few cancer cases in series with a majority of non-cancer patients [12–14].

The reported frequency of cPE was variable. Variation in imaging modalities, screening strategies and patient populations studied contributed to this marked variation [15, 16]. In our study, the small number of patients with cPE makes it difficult to correlate the risk of cPE to the number of injections performed. Other variables including site, severity of resulting deformity, body mass index (BMI), primary tumor and additional comorbidities may contribute.

In one study, chest radiographs were available in 64 of 69 percutaneous vertebroplasty procedures and, upon retrospective review, cPE was noted in only three (4.6%) cases [17]. In another study, CT scans of the chest were obtained routinely and cPE was identified in 18 (23%) of 78 procedures performed in patients with osteoporotic, non-malignant fractures [18].

In a more recent study, VERTOS II, chest CT was obtained for all patients post-vertebroplasty regardless of symptoms; 14 (26%) of 54 patients had cPE and all were asymptomatic [19].

Data addressing the clinical manifestations and risk factors for cement pulmonary emboli in cancer patients are very limited, as much of the published literature involves patients with osteoporotic fractures. A few studies include small numbers of cancer patients among larger series of patients with vertebral fractures related to osteoporosis and not cancer [18–20].

Although data from the literature suggest that most patients with cPE as a complication of osteoporotic

Table 2 Characteristics and outcome of patients with cement pulmonary embolism

Number	Age	Gender	Underlying Etiology[b]	Primary Cancer	Location	Type of PE	Symptoms	Anticoagulation	Status	Survival (Months)
1	31	F	Malignant	Breast	T12-L2	Main	Dyspnea, Tachycardia, Hypoxia	No	Dead	8.5
2	41	F	Malignant	Breast	L1-L5	segmental	Dyspnea, Tachycardia, Hypoxia	LMWH	Dead	1.5
3	78	F	Osteoporosis	Lymphoma	L1	segmental	No	No	Alive	53
4	55	M	Osteoporosis	Lung	L2- L5	Lobar	No	No	Dead	12
5	81	F	Osteoporosis	Lymphoma	L5	subsegmental	No	LMWH	Alive	48
6	37	M	Malignant	MM	T9–12,L1	subsegmental	No	No	Dead	NA[a]
7	50	F	Malignant	MM	T5-T8	subsegmental	No	No	Dead	24
8	63	M	Malignant	MM	L1-L3	Lobar	No	No	Dead	20
9	50	M	Malignant	MM	L2-L4	subsegmental	No	No	Alive	48
10	68	M	Malignant	MM	T12,L1,L2	subsegmental	Dyspnea, Chest pain, Cough, Tachycardia, Hypoxia	No	Dead	4.5
11	60	F	Malignant	Breast	L4	subsegmental	No	Already on LMWH	Dead	11
12	45	F	Malignant	MM	L3-L5	Main	Dyspnea	LMWH	Dead	8
13	45	F	Malignant	MM	T12,L1,L2	Lobar	Dyspnea	LMWH	Dead	8

LMWH Low molecular weight heparin, *MM* Multiple Myeloma
[a]NA: Data not available, [b]all in cancer patients

compression fractures were diagnosed through screening radiographic studies and remained free of symptoms or long-term adverse pulmonary sequelae [16], five (38.5%) of our 13 patients had symptoms (dyspnea, cough, chest pain, tachycardia, hypoxia) that led to the diagnosis. While it is true that such respiratory symptoms in patients with cancer can be attributed to a variety of pulmonary disorders (lung metastasis, pleural effusions, smoking-related chronic obstructive pulmonary airway disease (COPD) or even thrombotic PE), none of the five symptomatic patients in our study had any other pathology that could explain their symptoms.

While there is no standard of care for the treatment and management of cPE, asymptomatic individuals may be effectively managed conservatively with close clinical monitoring [21]. This conclusion is supported by the fact that none of the asymptomatic patients in our series had any clinical sequelae. However, all five symptomatic patients were fully anticoagulated. Anticoagulation can help prevent progressive pulmonary artery occlusion [22].

The increasing use of vertebroplasty and the incidence of associated symptomatic and asymptomatic cPE highlight the importance of a better understanding of this commonly encountered complication. Adequate efforts should be made to identify cancer patients who are at risk of this complication and to identify appropriate screening and therapeutic strategies.

Many questions remain unanswered. Should we recommend that routine imaging studies be performed after vertebroplasty [23]? Should we anticoagulate all asymptomatic patients diagnosed by routine imaging studies performed after the procedure? Is a location (cervical, thoracic, or lumbar vertebrae) associated with higher risk? What is the natural history of cPE? Further research is needed to address these knowledge gaps regarding cPE in cancer patients.

Conclusions

Cement PE, while mostly asymptomatic, is a relatively common complication following vertebroplasty. Multiple myeloma is the commonest malignancy associated with this complication. Large-scale prospective studies can help identify risk factors and clinical outcomes, and help develop better prevention and therapeutic strategies.

Acknowledgments
Not applicable.

Funding
This research received no specific grant from any funding agency in the public, commercial, or not-for-profit sectors.

Authors' contributions

AM: reviewed all imaging studies, drafted the manuscript and coordinated the study. NA: participated in data collection and analysis. HA: reviewed all imaging studies. SS: reviewed the literature and helped draft the manuscript. MM: participated in data analysis and drafting of the manuscript. NS and KA: Both participated in data collection and analysis. All authors read and approved the final manuscript.

Competing interests

The authors declare that they have no competing interests.

Author details

[1]Department of Radiology, King Hussein Cancer Center, Amman, Jordan. [2]Istishari Hospital, Amman, Jordan. [3]Department of Internal Medicine, King Hussein Cancer Center, Amman, Jordan.

References

1. Melton LJ 3rd, Kan SH, Frye MA, Wahner JW, O'Fallon WM, Riggs BL. Epidemiology of vertebral fractures in women. Am J Epidmiol. 1989;129:1000–11.

2. Vogt TM, Ross PD, Palermo L, et al. Vertebral fracture prevalence among women screened for the fracture intervention trial and a simple clinical tool to screen for undiagnosed vertebral fractures. Fracture intervention trial research group. Mayo Clin Proc. 2000;75:888–96.

3. Papaioannou A, Watts NB, Kendler DL, Yuen CK, Adachi JD, Ferko N. Diagnosis and management of vertebral fractures in elderly adults. Am J Med. 2002;113:220–8.

4. Siminoski K, Warshawski RS, Jen H, Lee K. The accuracy of historical height loss for the detection of vertebral fractures in postmenopausal women. Osteoporos Int. 2006;17:290–6.

5. Schlaich C, Minne HW, Bruckner T, et al. Reduced pulmonary function in patients with spinal osteoporotic fractures. Osteoporos Int. 1998;8:261–7.

6. Longo UG, Loppini M, Denaro L, Brandi ML, Maffulli N, Denaro V. The effectiveness and safety of vertebroplasty for osteoporotic vertebral compression fractures. A double blind, prospective, randomized, controlled study. Clin Cases Miner Bone Metab. 2010;7:109–13.

7. Tarsuslugil S, O'Hara R, Dunne N, et al. Development of calcium phosphate cement for the augmentation of traumatically fractured porcine specimens using vertebroplasty. J Biomech. 2013;46:711–5.

8. Brodano GB, Amendola L, Martikos K, et al. Vertebroplasty: benefits are more than risks in selected and evidence-based informed patients. A retrospective study of 59 cases. Eur. Spine J. 2011;20:1265–71.

9. Mathis J, Deramond H, Belkoff S. Percutaneous Vertebroplasty and Kyphoplasty (Second Edition) Springer 2006; pp 3-5. ISBN 0-387-29078-8.

10. Katsumi K, Hirano T, Watanabe K, et al. Surgical treatment for osteoporotic thoracolumbar vertebral collapse using vertebroplasty with posterior spinal fusion: a prospective multicenter study. Int Orthop. 2016;40:2309–15.

11. Yeom JS, Kim WJ, Choy WS, Lee CK, Chang BS, Kang JW. Leakage of cement in percutaneous vertebroplasty for painful osteoporotic compression fractures. J Bone joint Surg Br. 2016;85:83–9.

12. Baumann A, Tauss J, Baumann G, Tomka M, Hessinger M, Tiesenhausen K. Cement embolization into the vena cave and pulmonal arteries after vertebroplasty: interdisciplinary management. Eur J Vasc Surg. 2006;31:558–61.

13. Duran C, Sirvanci M, Aydoğan M, Ozturk E, Ozturk C, Akman C. Pulmonary cement embolism: a complication of percutaneous vertebroplasty. Acta Radiol. 2007;48:854–9.

14. Habib N, Maniatis T, Ahmed S, et al. Cement pulmonary embolism after percutaneous vertebroplasty and kyphoplasty: an overview. Heart Lung. 2012;41:509–11.

15. Potet J, Weber-Donat G, Curis E, et al. Incidence of pulmonary cement embolism after real-time CT fluoroscopy-guided vertebroplasty. J Vasc Interv Radiol. 2013;24:1853–60.

16. Venmans A, Lohle PN, van Rooij WJ, Verhaar HJ, Mali WP. Frequency and outcome of pulmonary polymethylmethacrylate embolism during percutaneous vertebroplasty. AJNR Am J Neuroradiol. 2008;29:1983–5.

17. Choe DH, Marom EM, Ahar K, Truong MT, Madewell JE. Pulmonary embolism of polymethyl methacrylate during percutaneous vertebroplasty and kyphoplasty. AJR Am J Roentgenol. 2004;183:1097–102.

18. Kim YJ, Lee JW, Park KW, et al. Pulmonary cement embolism after percutaneous vertebroplasty in osteoporotic vertebral compression fractures: incidence, characteristics, and risk factors. Radiology. 2009;251:250–9.

19. Venmans A, Klazen CA, Lohle PN, et al. Percutaneous vertebroplasty and pulmonary cement embolism: results from VERTOS II. Am J Neuroradiol. 2010;31:1451–3.

20. Luetmer MT, Bartholmai BJ, Rad AE, Kallmes DF. Asymptomatic and unrecognized cement pulmonary embolism commonly occurs with vertebroplasty. Am J Neuroradiol. 2011;32:654–7.

21. Krueger A, Biliemel C, Zettl R, Ruchholtz S. Management of pulmonary cement embolism after percutaneous vertebroplasty and kyphoplasty: a systematic review of the literature. Eur Spine J. 2009;18:1257–65.

22. Tozzi P, Abdelmoumene Y, Corno AF, Gersbach PA, Hoogewoud HM, von Segesser LK. Management of pulmonary embolism during acrylic vertebroplasty. Ann Thorac Surg. 2002;74:1706–8.

23. Bliemel C, Buecking B, Struewer J, Piechowiak EI, Ruchholtz S, Krueger A. Detection of pulmonary cement embolism after balloon kyphoplasty: should conventional radiographs become routine? Acta Orthop Belg. 2013; 79:444–50.

18

Gastric heterotopic pancreas and stromal tumors smaller than 3 cm in diameter: clinical and computed tomography findings

Li-ming Li[1], Lei-yu Feng[2], Xiao-hua Chen[1], Pan Liang[1], Jing Li[1] and Jian-bo Gao[1*]

Abstract

Background: Identifying gastric heterotopic pancreas and stromal tumors is difficult. Few studies have reported computed tomography (CT) findings for differentiating lesions less than 3 cm in diameter. In this study, we aimed to identify clinical characteristics and CT findings that can differentiate gastric heterotopic pancreatic lesions from stromal tumors less than 3 cm in diameter.

Methods: A total of 132 patients with pathologically confirmed gastric heterotopic pancreas ($n = 66$) and stromal tumors ($n = 66$) were included. Each group was divided into primary ($n = 50$) and validation cohort ($n = 16$). Clinical characteristics and CT findings were retrospectively reviewed. CT findings included location, border, contour, growth pattern, enhancement pattern and grade, the enhancement value of tumor, enhancement ratio of tumor, and enhancement ratio of tumor to pancreas in venous phase. The findings in the two groups were compared using the Pearson χ^2 test or Student t-test. Receiver operating characteristic curves were used to determine areas under the curve and optimal cut-offs.

Results: Significant differences were observed between heterotopic pancreas and stromal tumors in the distribution of tumor location, border, contour (all $P < 0.001$), enhancement values ($P < 0.001$), enhancement ratios of tumors ($P < 0.001$), and enhancement ratios of tumors to pancreas ($P < 0.001$). No significant differences existed in growth pattern ($P = 0.203$). The area under the curve differed significantly between enhancement ratio of tumor to pancreas and enhancement ratio ($P = 0.030$). There were significant differences in above characteristics between two groups in validation cohort.

Conclusions: Heterotopic pancreas has characteristic CT features differentiating it from stromal tumors.

Keywords: Gastric, Heterotopic pancreas, Stromal tumor, Computed tomography

Background

Heterotopic pancreatic (HP) masses and stromal tumors (STs) are common gastric submucosa tumors. HP masses are typically found in autopsy or surgery, during which the frequency is approximately 0.2 to 0.25% [1, 2]. Approximately 10–15 per million people worldwide are diagnosed with gastrointestinal STs each year, with most of these tumors located in the stomach [3]. Both the management and prognosis of these two tumors are different [4–6]. STs are aggressive tumors with a potential

tendency for malignancy, and the risk increases as the tumor increases in size. They require resection once detected, and occasionally, chemotherapy is required in cases of metastasis [7]. HP is a congenital anomaly, similar to hamartoma. Most patients are recommended to undergo surveillance because HP is generally asymptomatic, and only a few patients need to be treated because of complications [8]. In view of the above, an accurate preoperative diagnosis of submucosal tumors is critical.

Identifying HP masses and STs only by clinical features is difficult because both can manifest as abdominal pain, abdominal distension, and other symptoms. Although gastroscopic biopsy is regarded as the gold standard for the diagnosis of tumors, limitations include its invasive

* Correspondence: gaojianbo_cancer@163.com
[1]Department of Radiology, The First Affiliated Hospital of Zhengzhou University, Zhengzhou 450052, Henan Province, China
Full list of author information is available at the end of the article

nature, sampling errors, diagnostic errors, long waiting times for immunohistochemistry results [9], and powerless assessing situations outside the tumor. Computed tomography (CT), as a common imaging examination method, has been used in the preoperative evaluation of submucosal tumors, and can be used as a supplemental tool in differentiating HP masses from STs [10].

Although many studies have been conducted on the imaging features of HP masses and gastric stromal tumors (STs), most have employed endoscopic ultrasonography [11, 12], with few adopting CT characteristics, and most have been case reports [10, 13]. To our knowledge, no studies have reported CT findings for differentiating gastric submucosal tumors less than 3 cm in diameter. Kim [14] reviewed CT findings of HP masses and other gastric submucosal tumors smaller than 4 cm, but size differences between the two groups inevitably led to errors in the results. Therefore, the purpose of this study was to analyze the clinical characteristics and CT findings of HP masses and STs less than 3 cm in diameter, identified in our hospital within a 5-year period, and to identify the features that differentiate one from the other.

Methods

This retrospective study was approved by the Institutional Review Board of the First Affiliated Hospital of Zhengzhou University, and the requirement for informed consent was waived.

Patients

A total of 137 patients with HP masses and 409 patients with STs in primary cohort, pathologically confirmed between June 2011 and June 2016, were selected from our hospital database. Among them, patients who fulfilled the following criteria were included: (1) available dual-phase contrast–enhanced CT images; (2) available thin-layer images; (3) lesions less than 3 cm in diameter; (4) lesions detectable on CT images; (5) lesions with a mainly solid composition. Lesions mainly with cystic components were excluded because of their particular CT findings and easy to distinguish with gastric stromal tumors [15–17]. A total of 189 patients met the inclusion criteria; however, numbers differed between the two groups, and therefore, the same numbers of STs were selected according to stratified random sampling method, based on the yearly distribution of HP masses. Finally, 100 patients (HP masses = 50, GISTs = 50) comprised our study population. A total of 32 patients (HP = 16, ST = 16) in validation cohort, pathologically confirmed between July 2016 and January 2018, were included from our hospital database using the same criterion to primary cohort. A flowchart is presented in Fig. 1.

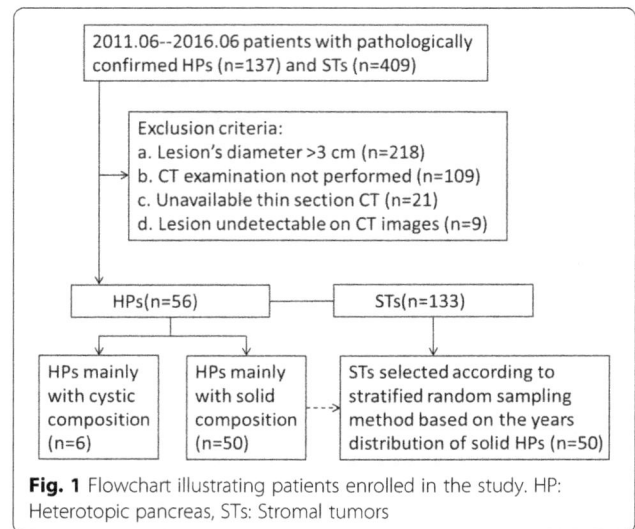

Fig. 1 Flowchart illustrating patients enrolled in the study. HP: Heterotopic pancreas, STs: Stromal tumors

CT image acquisition

CT images were obtained using a 16-channel multi-detector CT scanner (Brilliance 16, Philips Medical Systems, Cleveland, OH, USA) or a 64-channel multi-detector CT scanner (Discovery CT750 HD CT Scanner, GE Healthcare Milwaukee, WI, USA). The parameters of the Brilliance 16 scanner were as follows: detector collimation, 1.5 mm; pitch, 1.25:1; tube voltage, 120 kVp; tube current, 80–270 mAs; rotation time, 0.6 s. The parameters of the Discovery CT750 scanner were as follows: detector collimation, 0.625 mm; pitch, 1.375:1; tube voltage, 120 kVp; tube current, 80–270 mAs; rotation time, 0.5 s. For the contrast-enhanced CT study, 80–90 mL of 350 or 370 mg I/mL iodinated contrast agent was injected via a peripheral vein at a flow rate of 3.0–3.5 mL/s, using a dual high-pressure syringe. Dual-phase contrast–enhanced CT images were obtained by scanning the images 10 s and 50–65 s after attenuation of the descending thoracic aorta reached 100 Hounsfield units, using the bolus-tracking technique, for the arterial and venous phases, respectively. Axial, coronal, and sagittal CT images were reconstructed with a 3-mm section thickness and a 3-mm reconstruction interval at an Application Development Workstation (Advantage Windows 4.4; GE Medical Systems, Chicago, IL, USA).

Clinical and image analysis

A clinical attending physician (L.F.) with 5 years of experience retrospectively reviewed the clinical data, including age, sex, chief complaint, and duration of symptoms. Chief complaints were classified as gastric pain gastric pain, abdominal distension, and other symptoms, including lesions found through physical examination [18]. Duration time of symptoms was divided into ≤6 months and > 6 months.

Qualitative analysis

Two radiologists (J.G. and P.L., with 25 and 6 years of experience, respectively), who were blinded to the pathological results, analyzed the CT images by consensus. We analyzed the following CT findings: location, lesion border, contour, growth pattern, enhancement pattern, peak enhancement phase and enhancement grade, presence of prominent thickness and enhancement of overlying mucosa, presence of central umbilication, and presence of calcification, ulceration, and multiple lesions. The stomach location is anatomically divided into three portions, the upper (U), middle (M), and lower (L) parts, by the lines connecting the trisected points on the lesser and greater curvatures according to Japanese classification of gastric carcinoma: 3rd English edition [19]. Tumorous contours were classified as flat, hill-like, ovoid, round, or irregular in shape [14] (Fig. 2). Growth patterns were classified as exo-luminal, endo-luminal, or mixed. Enhancement pattern was classified as homogeneous or heterogeneous. Enhancement grade was classified as mild, moderate, or marked.

Objective analysis

Two radiologists (J.L. and X.C., both with 5 years of experience), who were aware of the gastric lesions but were blinded to the pathological results, measured the lesion diameter and CT attenuation. The CT attenuation values of the pancreas and tumors in the venous phase and plain phase were measured in Hounsfield units by two radiologists. The averages were then used to calculate the enhancement value of tumor (HU venous - HU plain), the enhancement ratio of tumor (HU venous- HU plain / HU plain) and the enhancement ratio of tumor to pancreas in venous phase (HU tumor / HU pancreas). The region of interest (ROI) ranging from 9 mm^2 to 30 mm^2 was placed to encompass the strongest enhancing portion and to avoid necrosis and calcification. The long diameter (LD) and short diameter (SD) were measured by the two radiologists. The averages were then used to calculate the LD/SD ratio.

Statistical analysis

All statistical calculations were performed using the Statistical Package for the Social Sciences (SPSS 21.0, Chicago, IL, USA), and a P-value of less than 0.05 was considered to be statistically significant. Categorical

variables including clinical characteristics (sex, chief complaint, duration of symptoms) and qualitative CT features (e.g., location, lesion border, contour, growth pattern, enhancement pattern, and enhancement grade) were described as frequencies or percentages. The Pearson χ^2 tests (including continuity correction) or Fisher's exact test were used to evaluate the differences between the two groups. Continuous variables subjected to a normality test were reported as means and standard deviation and were compared using Student's t-tests (including the correct t-test).

Receiver operating characteristic (ROC) curves of the LD/SD ratio, the enhancement value, the enhancement ratio of tumor, the enhancement ratio of tumor to pancreas were obtained to generate the area under the curve (AUC) and an optimal cut-off, where the sum of the sensitivity and the specificity was the maximum. In general, an AUC between 0.5 and 0.7 suggests low diagnostic value, an AUC between 0.7 and 0.9 suggests medium diagnostic value, and an AUC between 0.9 and 1 suggests high diagnostic value. Sensitivity, specificity, and odds ratio (ORs) with 95% confidence intervals (CIs) were analyzed for variables that differed significantly between the two groups. Variables with significant differences in primary cohort were compared in validation cohort.

Results
Clinical analysis

Table 1 summarizes the clinical characteristics between the two groups. No significant differences were observed in sex, chief complaint, and duration of symptoms. However, age distribution differed significantly between the two groups (HP masses = 41.22 ± 11.76 y; STs = 59.18 ± 11.15 y, $P < 0.001$).

Table 1 Comparison of clinical characteristics between two lesions n (%)

Clinical characteristics	HP masses ($n = 50$)	STs ($n = 50$)	P Value
Age(year)	41.22 ± 11.76	59.18 ± 11.15	< 0.001[a]
Gender			0.684
Male	21 (42)	19 (38)	
Female	29 (58)	31 (62)	
Chief complaint			0.191
Gastric pain	27 (54)	18 (36)	
Distension	7 (14)	9 (18)	
Other	16 (32)	23 (46)	
Duration of symptoms			0.680
≤ 6 months	32 (64)	30 (60)	
> 6 months	18 (36)	20 (40)	

[a]$P < 0.05$. Calculated with Student's t-test. *HP* Heterotopic pancreas, *STs* Stromal tumors

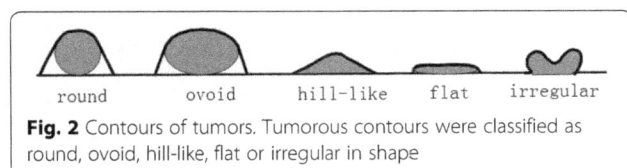

Fig. 2 Contours of tumors. Tumorous contours were classified as round, ovoid, hill-like, flat or irregular in shape

round   ovoid   hill-like   flat   irregular

Qualitative analysis

Table 2 summarizes the morphologic qualitative CT findings. A significant difference was observed in the distribution of tumor location ($P < 0.001$); most HP masses (66%, 33/50) were located in the lower part, whereas most (76%, 38/50) STs were located in the upper part. With regard to lesion border, 28 (56%) of the 50 HP masses were ill defined and 45 (90%) of the 50 STs were well defined. HP masses showed diverse shapes, and were mainly (86%, 43/50) flat, hill-like, or ovoid; few (14%, 7/50) were round or irregular in shape.

Most (88%, 44/50) STs were round or ovoid. Homogeneous enhancement in the venous phase was observed in most of the HP masses and STs, whereas marked enhancement was observed in most (62%, 31/50) HP masses and moderate enhancement were observed in most (58%, 29/50) STs. No statistical differences existed in growth pattern between the two groups ($P = 0.203$). The presence of prominent thickness and enhancement of the overlying mucosa, central umbilication, and multiple lesions was detected in only a few (10, 6, 2%) of the patients with HP masses, whereas the presence of

Table 2 Comparison of subjective CT findings between two lesions n (%)

CT findings	HP masses ($n = 50$)	STs ($n = 50$)	P Value
Location			$< 0.001^a$
The upper part	2 (4)	38 (76)	
The middle part	15 (30)	8 (16)	
The lower part	33 (66)	4 (8)	
Border			$< 0.001^a$
Well defined	22 (44)	45 (90)	
Ill defined	28 (56)	5 (10)	
Contour			$< 0.001^a$
Round	4 (8)	21 (42)	
Ovoid	24 (48)	23 (46)	
Hill-like	10 (20)	4 (8)	
Flat	10 (20)	1 (2)	
Irregular shape	3 (6)	1 (2)	
Growth pattern			0.203
Endo-luminal	38 (76)	35 (70)	
Exo-luminal	7 (14)	4 (8)	
Mixed	5 (10)	11 (22)	
Enhancement pattern			0.084
Homogeneous	46 (92)	40 (80)	
Heterogeneous	4 (8)	10 (20)	
Peak enhancement phase			0.236
Venous phase	43 (86)	48 (96)	
Arterial phase	2 (4)	0	
Both	5 (10)	2 (4)	
Enhancement grade			0.003^a
Marked	31 (62)	14 (28)	
Moderate	15 (30)	29 (58)	
Mild	4 (8)	7 (14)	
Central umbilication	3 (6)	0	0.241
Prominent enhancement of overlying mucosa	5 (10)	0	0.066
Multiple lesions	1 (2)	0	0.500
Ulceration	0	4 (8)	0.126
Calcification	0	5 (10)	0.066

$^aP < 0.05$. Calculated with χ^2 test

calcification and ulceration was detected in only a few (10, 8%) of the patients with STs. Notably, two ectopic pancreatic lesions in one patient were found, and only the bigger lesion was included in our study because the other was too small to analyze. Representative images are presented in Figs. 3, 4, and 5.

Quantitative analysis

Significant differences were observed in the variables relating to the lesion enhancement grade, including the enhancement value, the enhancement ratio, the enhancement ratio to pancreas between the two groups. HP masses had significantly higher enhancement value (HP masses = 43.54 HU ± 11.78, STs = 29.16 HU ± 13.69, $P < 0.001$), enhancement ratio (HP masses = 1.08 ± 0.45, STs = 0.77 ± 0.37, $P < 0.001$), and enhancement ratio to pancreas (HP masses = 0.93 ± 0.15, STs = 0.74 ± 0.16, $P < 0.001$) than STs.

No significant differences were found in LDs (HP masses = 15.08 mm ± 5.96, STs = 16.79 mm ± 5.96, $P > 0.05$), but significant differences were observed in SDs (HP masses = 10.29 mm ± 4.64, STs = 13.69 mm ± 5.27, $P < 0.001$) between the two groups. The mean LD/SD ratio for HP masses was significantly higher than that for STs (HP masses = 1.61 ± 0.61, STs = 1.26 ± 0.25, $P < 0.001$).

Sensitivity and specificity analysis

Using ROC analysis, cut-off values for the LD/SD ratio, the enhancement value, the enhancement ratio and the

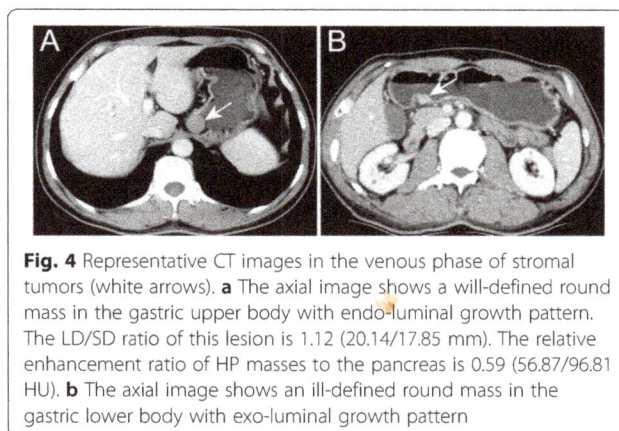

Fig. 4 Representative CT images in the venous phase of stromal tumors (white arrows). **a** The axial image shows a will-defined round mass in the gastric upper body with endo-luminal growth pattern. The LD/SD ratio of this lesion is 1.12 (20.14/17.85 mm). The relative enhancement ratio of HP masses to the pancreas is 0.59 (56.87/96.81 HU). **b** The axial image shows an ill-defined round mass in the gastric lower body with exo-luminal growth pattern

enhancement ratio to pancreas were set at 1.29, 27.50 HU, 0.66, and 0.72, respectively. The AUCs were 0.71, 0.786, 0.70, and 0.81, respectively (Fig. 6). The above continuous variables were transformed into categorical variables according to the cut-off values.

Table 3 summarizes the sensitivity, specificity, and OR of each significant variable, including location in the lower part, marked enhancement, flat and irregular shapes, ill-defined border, LD/SD > 1.29, the enhancement value > 27.50 HU, the enhancement ratio > 0.66, and the enhancement ratio to pancreas > 0.72.

Variables in the validation cohort.

Clinical characteristics and CT findings in validation cohort are summarized in the Table 4. There were significant differences in all variables between two groups in the validation cohort.

Discussion

This retrospective study included gastric lesions less than 3 cm in diameter; therefore, thin-layer images were required to analyze the CT features. Variables with significant differences in primary cohort were compared in validation cohort and there were significant differences in all above variables between two groups in validation cohort.

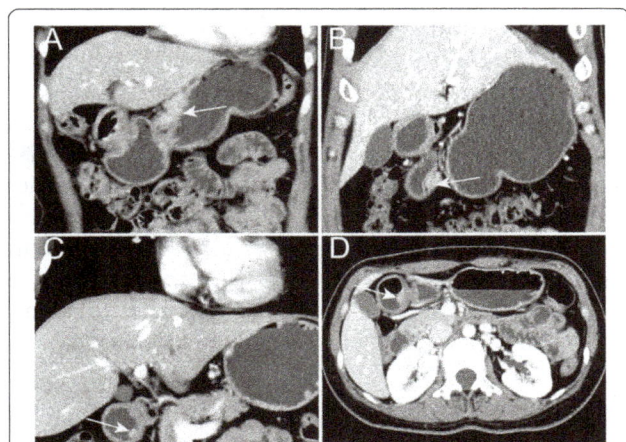

Fig. 3 Representative CT images in the venous phase of heterotopic pancreatic masses (white arrows). **a** The coronal image shows an ill-defined irregular mass in the gastric middle body with exo-luminal growth pattern. **b** The coronal image shows an ill-defined ovoid mass in the gastric lower body with mixed growth pattern. **c** The coronal image shows a will-defined flat mass in the gastric lower body with endo-luminal growth pattern. **d** The axial image shows an ill-defined hill-like mass in the gastric lower body with endo-luminal growth pattern. The LD/SD ratio of this lesion is 1.85 (15.83/8.54 mm). The relative enhancement ratio of HP masses to the pancreas is 0.94 (101.25/107.58 HU)

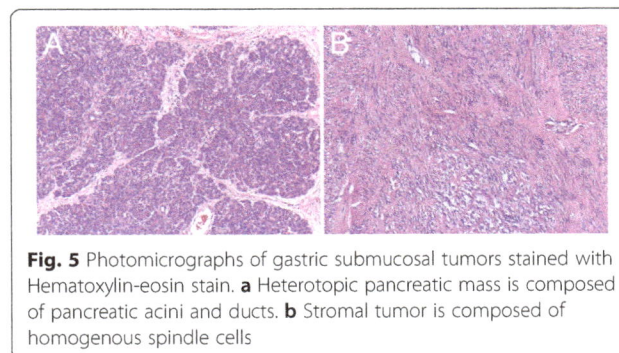

Fig. 5 Photomicrographs of gastric submucosal tumors stained with Hematoxylin-eosin stain. **a** Heterotopic pancreatic mass is composed of pancreatic acini and ducts. **b** Stromal tumor is composed of homogenous spindle cells

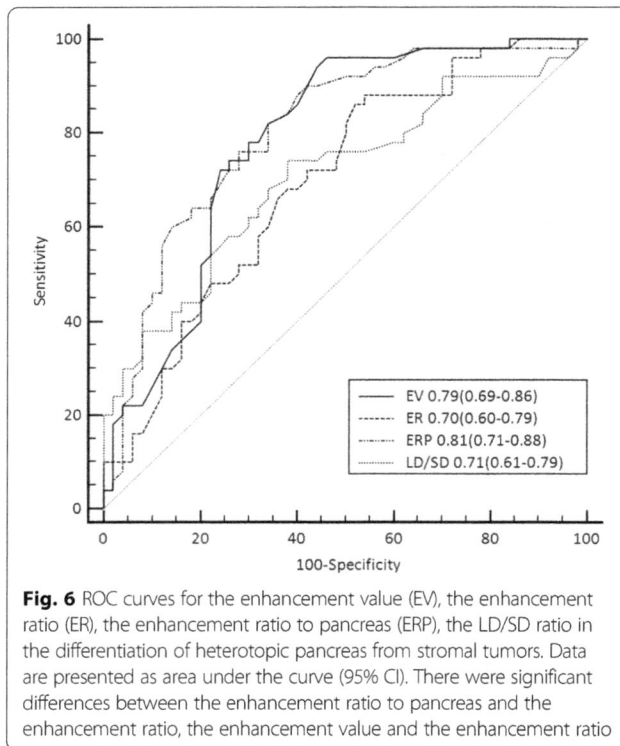

Fig. 6 ROC curves for the enhancement value (EV), the enhancement ratio (ER), the enhancement ratio to pancreas (ERP), the LD/SD ratio in the differentiation of heterotopic pancreas from stromal tumors. Data are presented as area under the curve (95% CI). There were significant differences between the enhancement ratio to pancreas and the enhancement ratio, the enhancement value and the enhancement ratio

different proportions. Approximately 27 to 76.6% of the HP masses exhibited prominent acinar features [14, 21] with lobular architecture. When this component was located in the peripheral part, the margin of the tumor was ill-defined [25]. However, the ill-defined margin was considered to be an adverse factor for the risk grading of STs in a previous study [26].

Significant differences were found in tumor contour and LD/SD ratio. In our study, 42% (21/50) of STs were round, but only 8% of (4/50) HP masses were round. Jang [27] also reported that other submucosal tumors are more likely to be round than HP masses (46.2% vs 6.7%). An HP mass is defined as ectopic flat glandular tissue with pancreatic acinar formation, and therefore commonly resembles the slender appearance of a normal pancreas and often exhibits a broad base on endoscopy [28]. HP masses of the mesentery are more elongated in shape than gastric HP masses, according to Seo [29]. In contrast, STs are real neoplasms, composed of spindle cells, epithelioid cells, or a mixture, with an obvious vertical growth trend. Our results showed that the mean SD for HP masses was significantly smaller than that for STs, but the LD did not differ significantly between the two groups. The greater LD/SD ratio also indicated a wall growth pattern for HP masses. In our study, the diagnostic value of the LD/SD ratio was medium, with an AUC of 0.707. An LD/SD ratio greater than 1.29 was found to be one of the critical imaging features of HP masses for differentiating it from STs. The LD/SD ratio trend was consistent with that mentioned in a previous study [14], but with a lower cut-off value. We concluded that the greater the diameter of an ectopic pancreatic mass, the more obvious the LD/SD ratio trend will be.

Highly significant differences were observed between the two groups in both qualitative and objective analyses. Qualitative analysis results indicated that both lesions presented homogeneous enhancement and had a greater enhancement grade in the venous phase than in the arterial phase. Hence, the CT attenuation values in the venous phase were used in subsequent calculations. In objective analysis, we assessed the enhancement grade

This study revealed significant differences in tumor location and border between the two groups, which were consistent with a previous report [20]. STs were more often located in the upper part (78%, 39/50), followed by the middle part (16%, 8/50), whereas most HP masses were located in the lower part (66%, 33/50), followed by the middle part (30%, 15/50). This trend of HP masses has been confirmed by many experts [21–23] and the hypothesis that HP masses are fragments separated from the main pancreas during the embryonic rotation process may explain this distribution [8, 24]. Most STs (90%, 45/50) exhibited well-defined margins, whereas most HP masses (56%, 28/50) exhibited ill-defined margins. These ill-defined margins were related to the histological structure of the HP masses. HP masses consisted of pancreatic acini, ductal components, and islets at

Table 3 Sensitivity and specificity of CT findings in diagnosis of HP masses

CT findings	Sensitivity (%)	Specificity (%)	OR (95% CI)
Enhancement value > 27.50 HU	96 (48/50)	54 (27/50)	28.17 (8.59, 92.39)
Lower part	66 (33/50)	92 (46/50)	22.32 (8.06,61.48)
Enhancement ratio to pancreas > 0.72	92 (46/50)	56 (28/50)	14.64 (5.27, 40.68)
Ill-defined border	56 (28/50)	90 (45/50)	11.45 (3.89, 33.72)
Flat or hill-like	26 (32/50)	96 (48/50)	8.43 (0.64, 32.74)
Enhancement ratio > 0.66	88 (44/50)	46 (23/50)	6.25 (2.40, 16.29)
LD/SD ≥1.29	68 (34/50)	68 (34/50)	4.52 (1.98, 10.26)
Marked enhancement	62 (31/50)	72 (36/50)	4.20 (1.83, 9.58)

OR odds ratio, *CI* confidence interval, *LD* long diameter, *SD* short diameter

Table 4 Clinical characteristics and CT findings for validation cohort

Features	HP masses ($n = 16$)	STs($n = 16$)	P Value
Age(year)	43.56 ± 12.49	57.51 ± 7.49	0.001[a]
Location (the lower part/other)	12/4	1/15	< 0.001
Border (ill defined/ well defined)	10/6	4/12	0.033
Contour (flat or hill-like/other)	6/10	1/15	0.026
Enhancement grade (marked/ other)	13/3	2/14	0.001
CT enhancement value (> 27.50 HU/< 27.50 HU)	13/3	5/11	0.004
Relative enhancement ratio (> 0.66/< 0.66)	13/3	4/12	0.001
Relative enhancement ratio to pancreas (> 0.72/< 0.72)	13/3	6/10	0.012
LD/SD(> 1.29/< 1.29)	12/4	6/10	0.033

[a]$P < 0.05$. Calculated with Student's t-test. Other calculated with χ2 test. *LD* long diameter, *SD* short diameter

by using the CT enhancement value and the enhancement ratio, rather than the values in the venous phase. The application of the enhancement value and ratio may reduce the influence of differences in machine and individual variations, which have been a factor in many previous studies [30, 31]. The presence of marked enhancement is a crucial finding with regard to avoiding misdiagnosis of HP masses and distinguishing them from STs. The study by Kim [14] indicated that the enhancement grade of HP masses has a close relationship with histological components. HP masses with predominant acini present greater enhancement than those with predominant ducts [22, 32]. Additionally, the enhancement ratio of tumor to pancreas is also crucial for distinguishing HP masses from STs. The average ratio of HP masses was significantly greater than that of STs and closer to 1, which is consistent with previous magnetic resonance imaging findings [27]. The AUC of the enhancement ratio to pancreas was greater than that of the enhancement value and the enhancement ratio, which indicated the ratio of the CT value of an HP mass to that of the pancreas is more valuable for identification than the variables (the enhancement value, the enhancement ratio) of the lesion itself.

In our study, both tumors predominantly exhibited an endo-luminal growth pattern; 30% of STs exhibited a predominantly exo-luminal or mixed growth pattern, which was lower than the proportion reported in a previous study on tumors less than 4 cm in diameter [14]. In addition, STs with a mean diameter of 10 cm also exhibit an obvious exo-luminal growth pattern [33]. We concluded that the larger a tumor is, the more obvious the exo-luminal growth pattern will be. The smaller a tumor is, the more difficult identification will be.

In our study, some findings, such as the presence of prominent thickness of the overlying mucosa, central umbilication, and multiple lesions, were detected in only a few (10, 6, 2%, respectively) patients with HP masses, and other findings, such as calcification and ulceration were detected in only a few (10, 8%, respectively) patients with STs. We assessed whether these findings constitute specific characteristics. First, central umbilication suggesting a rudimentary duct is present radiographically in only 16 to 25% of HP masses [14, 34], but present endoscopically in 35 to 60% of HP masses [12, 35]. Endoscopic ultrasonography is superior to CT in the assessment of mucosal surfaces. To our knowledge, no studies have reported STs with central umbilication, but ulceration may be confused with central umbilication, which was observed in 8% of STs in our study. Second, recurrent inflammatory changes caused by HP masses may explain the prominent thickness and enhancement of the overlying mucosa indicating microscopic gastritis in HP masses in a previous study [14]. Third, only one patient with HP exhibited multiple lesions; however, a previous study reported the presence of multiple lesions as a typical characteristic of succinate dehydrogenase deficient STs [36]. Therefore, the presence of multiple lesions is a rare and non-specific feature. Finally, HP with calcification has been reported [37], indicating that calcification is also not a specific feature.

Our study had several limitations. First, two CT scanners were used in our retrospective study, resulting in nonconformity of the scanned parameters and volumes of contrast media. However, we believe that morphological features may be unaffected by nonconformity, and the application of the enhancement values, enhancement ratios, and the enhancement ratios to pancreas may greatly reduce the influence of nonconformity. Second, histological analysis was not performed and radiologic-pathologic correlation was not assessed in our study because a complete pathological specimen was not available for all the included patients, and we could not guarantee that the sample and the ROI were at the same level. Third, HPs of mainly cystic composition were excluded. This induces a bias, but considering their particular CT findings the diagnosis of mainly cystic HP does not constitute a significant radiological problem. Finally, logistic regression analysis, texture analysis, and nomography [38] were not performed in this study. Larger prospective investigations are needed to confirm the present findings.

Conclusions

In conclusion, HP has characteristic CT features for differentiating it from STs in the stomach. No significant differences were observed in growth patterns between the two lesions less than 3 cm in diameter. An LD/SD ratio greater than 1.29, an enhancement value greater than 27.50 HU, an enhancement ratio greater than 0.66, and an enhancement ratio to pancreas greater than 0.72 were critical CT features for differentiating HP masses from stromal tumors in our study.

Abbreviations

AUC: The area under the curve; CI: 95% confidence intervals; CT: Computed tomography; HP: Heterotopic pancreatic; LD: Long diameter; ORs: Odds ratio; ROC: Receiver operating characteristic; SD: Short diameter; STs: Stromal tumors

Acknowledgements

The study was supported by the Department of Radiology of the First Affiliated Hospital of Zhengzhou University.

Funding

This work was supported in part by the National Natural Science Foundation of China, No.81701687.

Authors' contributions

Study concept and design: LML and PL; Imaging data collection: LML and LYF; Imaging preliminary valuation: XHC and JL; Imaging final valuation: PL and JBG; Statistical analysis: LML and LYF; Manuscript preparation: LML; All authors have read and approved the final manuscript.

Competing interests

The authors declare that they have no competing interest.

Author details

[1]Department of Radiology, The First Affiliated Hospital of Zhengzhou University, Zhengzhou 450052, Henan Province, China. [2]Department of Internal Medicine, The First Affiliated Hospital of Zhengzhou University, Zhengzhou 450052, Henan Province, China.

References

1. Agale SV, Agale VG, Zode RR, Grover S, Joshi S. Heterotopic pancreas involving stomach and duodenum. J Assoc Physicians India. 2009;57:653–4.
2. Tanaka K, Tsunoda T, Eto T, Yamada M, Tajima Y, Shimogama H, et al. Diagnosis and management of heterotopic pancreas. Int Surg. 1993;78:32–5.
3. Søreide K, Sandvik OM, Søreide JA, Giljaca V, Jureckova A, Bulusu VR. Global epidemiology of gastrointestinal stromal tumours (GIST): a systematic review of population-based cohort studies. Cancer Epidemiol. 2016;40:39–46. https://doi.org/10.1016/j.canep.2015.10.031
4. Seo SW, Hong SJ, Han JP, Choi MH, Song JY, Kim HK, et al. Accuracy of a scoring system for the differential diagnosis of common gastric subepithelial tumors based on endoscopic ultrasonography. J Dig Dis. 2013; 14:647–53. https://doi.org/10.1111/1751-2980.12099
5. Min YW, Park HN, Min BH, Choi D, Kim KM, Kim S. Preoperative predictive factors for gastrointestinal stromal tumors: analysis of 375 surgically resected gastric subepithelial tumors. J Gastrointest Surg. 2015;19:631–8. https://doi.org/10.1007/s11605-014-2708-9
6. He G, Wang J, Chen B, Xing X, Wang J, Chen J, et al. Feasibility of endoscopic submucosal dissection for upper gastrointestinal submucosal tumors treatment and value of endoscopic ultrasonography in pre-operation assess and post-operation follow-up: a prospective study of 224 cases in a single medical center. Surg Endosc. 2016;30:4206–13. https://doi.org/10.1007/s00464-015-4729-1
7. von Mehren M, Randall RL, Benjamin RS, Boles S, Bui MM, Casper ES, et al. Gastrointestinal stromal tumors, version 2.2014. J Natl Compr Cancer Netw. 2014;12:853–62.
8. Trifan A, Târcoveanu E, Danciu M, Huţanaşu C, Cojocariu C, Stanciu C. Gastric heterotopic pancreas: an unusual case and review of the literature. J Gastrointestin Liver Dis. 2012;21:209–12.
9. Zhang XC, Li QL, Yu YF, Yao LQ, Xu MD, Zhang YQ, et al. Diagnostic efficacy of endoscopic ultrasound-guided needle sampling for upper gastrointestinal subepithelial lesions: a meta-analysis. Surg Endosc. 2016;30: 2431–41. https://doi.org/10.1007/s00464-015-4494-1
10. Subasinghe D, Sivaganesh S, Perera N, Samarasekera DN. Gastric fundal heterotopic pancreas mimicking a gastrointestinal stromal tumour (GIST): a case report and brief review. BMC Res Notes. 2016;9:185. https://doi.org/10.1186/s13104-016-1995-5
11. Rawat KS, Buxi TB, Yadav A, Ghuman SS, Bhalla S, Dhawan S. Ectopic pancreas in the Duodenojejunal flexure-computed tomographic and endoscopic Ultrasonographic images. Indian J Surg. 2015;77:332–4. https://doi.org/10.1007/s12262-015-1284-x
12. Park SH, Kim GH, Park DY, Shin NR, Cheong JH, Moon JY, et al. Endosonographic findings of gastric ectopic pancreas: a single center experience. J Gastroenterol Hepatol. 2011;26:1441–6. https://doi.org/10.1111/j.1440-1746.2011.06764.x
13. Christodoulidis G, Zacharoulis D, Barbanis S, Katsogridakis E, Hatzitheofilou K. Heterotopic pancreas in the stomach: a case report and literature review. World J Gastroenterol. 2007;13:6098–100.
14. Kim JY, Lee JM, Kim KW, Park HS, Choi JY, Kim SH, et al. Ectopic pancreas: CT findings with emphasis on differentiation from small gastrointestinal stromal tumor and leiomyoma. Radiology. 2009;252:92–100. https://doi.org/10.1148/radiol.2521081441
15. Jin HB, Lu L, Yang JF, Lou QF, Yang J, Shen HZ, et al. Interventional endoscopic ultrasound for a symptomatic pseudocyst secondary to gastric heterotopic pancreas. World J Gastroenterol. 2017;23:6365–70. https://doi.org/10.3748/wjg.v23.i34.6365
16. Fléjou JF, Potet F, Molas G, Bernades P, Amouyal P, Fékété F. Cystic dystrophy of the gastric and duodenal wall developing in heterotopic pancreas: an unrecognised entity. Gut. 1993;34:343–7.
17. Rodriguez AA, Berquist W, Bingham D. Gastric outlet obstruction caused by heterotopic pancreas in an adolescent. Dig Dis Sci. 2015;60:835–7. https://doi.org/10.1007/s10620-014-3314-0
18. Lee NJ, Hruban RH, Fishman EK. Gastric heterotopic pancreas: computed tomography with Clinicopathologic correlation. J Comput Assist Tomogr. 2017;41:675–8. https://doi.org/10.1097/RCT.0000000000000606
19. Japanese Gastric Cancer Association. Japanese classification of gastric carcinoma: 3rd English edition. Gastric Cancer. 2011;14:101–12. https://doi.org/10.1007/s10120-011-0041-5
20. Rezvani M, Menias C, Sandrasegaran K, Olpin JD, Elsayes KM, Shaaban AM. Heterotopic pancreas: histopathologic features, imaging findings, and complications. Radiographics. 2017;37:484–99. https://doi.org/10.1148/rg.2017160091

21. Zhang Y, Sun X, Gold JS, Sun Q, Lv Y, Li Q, et al. Heterotopic pancreas: a clinicopathological study of 184 cases from a single high-volume medical center in China. Hum Pathol. 2016;55:135–42. https://doi.org/10.1016/j.humpath.2016.05.004

22. Lin YM, Chiu NC, Li AF, Liu CA, Chou YH, Chiou YY. Unusual gastric tumors and tumor-like lesions: radiological with pathological correlation and literature review. World J Gastroenterol. 2017;23:2493–504. https://doi.org/10.3748/wjg.v23.i14.2493

23. Wei R, Wang QB, Chen QH, Liu JS, Zhang B. Upper gastrointestinal tract heterotopic pancreas: findings from CT and endoscopic imaging with histopathologic correlation. Clin Imaging. 2011;35:353–9. https://doi.org/10.1016/j.clinimag.2010.10.001

24. Ulrych J, Fryba V, Skalova H, Krska Z, Krechler T, Zogala D. Premalignant and malignant lesions of the heterotopic pancreas in the esophagus: a case report and review of the literature. J Gastrointestin Liver Dis. 2015;24:235–9. https://doi.org/10.15403/jgld.2014.1121.242.uly

25. Kim JH, Lim JS, Lee YC, Hyung WJ, Lee JH, Kim MJ, et al. Endosonographic features of gastric ectopic pancreases distinguishable from mesenchymal tumors. J Gastroenterol Hepatol. 2008;23:e301–7. https://doi.org/10.1111/j.1440-1746.2008.05351.x

26. Brand B, Oesterhelweg L, Binmoeller KF, Sriram PV, Bohnacker S, Seewald S, et al. Impact of endoscopic ultrasound for evaluation of submucosal lesions in gastrointestinal tract. Dig Liver Dis. 2002;34:290–7.

27. Jang KM, Kim SH, Park HJ, Lim S, Kang TW, Lee SJ, et al. Ectopic pancreas in upper gastrointestinal tract: MRI findings with emphasis on differentiation from submucosal tumor. Acta Radiol. 2013;54:1107–16. https://doi.org/10.1177/0284185113491251

28. Matsumoto T, Tanaka N, Nagai M, Koike D, Sakuraoka Y, Kubota K. A case of gastric heterotopic pancreatitis resected by laparoscopic surgery. Int Surg. 2015;100:678–82. https://doi.org/10.9738/INTSURG-D-14-00182.1

29. Seo N, Kim JH. Characteristic CT features of heterotopic pancreas of the mesentery: "another pancreas" in the mesentery. Clin Imaging. 2014;38:27–30. https://doi.org/10.1016/j.clinimag.2013.09.008

30. Ma Z, Liang C, Huang Y, He L, Liang C, Chen X, et al. Can lymphovascular invasion be predicted by preoperative multiphasic dynamic CT in patients with advanced gastric cancer? Eur Radiol. 2017;27:3383–91. https://doi.org/10.1007/s00330-016-4695-6

31. Chen XH, Ren K, Liang P, Chai YR, Chen KS, Gao JB. Spectral computed tomography in advanced gastric cancer: can iodine concentration non-invasively assess angiogenesis? World J Gastroenterol. 2017;23:1666–75. https://doi.org/10.3748/wjg.v23.i9.1666

32. Park SH, Han JK, Choi BI, Kim M, Kim YI, Yeon KM, et al. Heterotopic pancreas of the stomach: CT findings correlated with pathologic findings in six patients. Abdom Imaging. 2000;25:119–23.

33. Pinaikul S, Woodtichartpreecha P, Kanngurn S, Leelakiatpaiboon S. 1189 gastrointestinal stromal tumor (GIST): computed tomographic features and correlation of CT findings with histologic grade. J Med Assoc Thail. 2014;97:1189–98.

34. Cho JS, Shin KS, Kwon ST, Kim JW, Song CJ, Noh SM, et al. Heterotopic pancreas in the stomach: CT findings. Radiology. 2000;217:139–44.

35. Attwell A, Sams S, Fukami N. Diagnosis of ectopic pancreas by endoscopic ultrasound with fine-needle aspiration. World J Gastroenterol. 2015;21:2367–73. https://doi.org/10.3748/wjg.v21.i8.2367

36. Miettinen M, Lasota J. Succinate dehydrogenase deficient gastrointestinal stromal tumors (GISTs) - a review. Int J Biochem Cell Biol. 2014;53:514–9. https://doi.org/10.1016/j.biocel.2014.05.033

37. Oka R, Okai T, Kitakata H, Ohta T. Heterotopic pancreas with calcification: a lesion mimicking leiomyosarcoma of the stomach. Gastrointest Endosc. 2002;56:939–42.

38. Hayano K, Tian F, Kambadakone AR, Yoon SS, Duda DG, et al. Texture analysis of non-contrast-enhanced computed tomography for assessing angiogenesis and survival of soft tissue sarcoma. J Comput Assist Tomogr. 2015;39:607–12. https://doi.org/10.1097/RCT.0000000000000239

Image quality of arterial phase and parenchymal blood volume (PBV) maps derived from C-arm computed tomography in the evaluation of transarterial chemoembolization

Tanja Zitzelsberger[1], Roland Syha[1*], Gerd Grözinger[1], Sasan Partovi[2], Konstantin Nikolaou[1] and Ulrich Grosse[1]

Abstract

Background: To evaluate the benefits of arterial phase imaging and parenchymal blood volume (PBV) maps acquired by C-arm computed tomography during TACE procedure in comparison to cross-sectional imaging (CSI) using CT or MRI.

Methods: From January 2014 to December 2016, a total of 29 patients with HCC stage A or B (mean age 65 years; range 47 to 81 years, 86% male) were included in this study. These patients were referred to our department for TACE treatment and received peri-interventional C-arm CT. Dual phase findings of each lesion in terms of overall image quality, conspicuity, tumor size and feeding arteries were compared between arterial phase imaging and PBV using 5-point semi-quantitative Likert-scale, whereby pre-interventional CSI served as reference standard.

Results: A significantly higher overall image quality of the PBV maps compared to arterial phase C-arm CT acquisitions (4.34 (±0.55) vs. 3.93 (±0.59), $p = 0.0032$) as well as a higher conspicuity of HCC lesions (4.27 ± 0.74 vs. 3.83 ± 1.08, $p < 0.0001$) was observed. Arterial phase imaging led to an overestimation of tumor size (mean size, 26.5 ± 15.9 mm) compared to PBV (24.9 ± 15.2 mm, $p = 0.0004$) as well as CSI (25.2 ± 15.1 mm), $p = 0.021$). Regarding detectability of tumor feeding arterial vessels, significantly more feeding vessels were detected in arterial phase C-arm CT ($n = 1.67 ± 0.92$ vessels) compared to PBV maps ($n = 1.27 ± 0.63$ vessels) ($p = 0.0001$). One lesion was missed in pre-interventional CT imaging, but detected by C-arm CT.

Conclusion: The combination of PBV maps and arterial phase images acquired by C-arm CT during TACE procedure enables precise detection of the majority of HCC lesions and tumor feeding arteries and has therefore the potential to improve patient outcome.

Keywords: Hepatocellular carcinoma, Transarterial chemoembolization, C-arm computed tomography, Parenchymal blood volume, Image quality

---

* Correspondence: roland.syha@gmx.net
[1]Department of Diagnostic and Interventional Radiology, University of Tuebingen, Hoppe-Seyler-Straße 3, 72076 Tuebingen, Germany
Full list of author information is available at the end of the article

Background

Hepatocellular Carcinoma (HCC) is one of the leading cancer entities in the industrialized countries with rising incidence [1]. Within the standard of care, transarterial chemoembolization (TACE) is recommended as first-line therapy in certain patients with compensated liver function in intermediate stage HCC (stage B in the Barcelona Clinic Liver Cancer (BCLC) staging system). TACE may contribute to downstaging or bridging to orthotopic liver transplantation in early stage HCC (BCLC stage A) according to the Barcelona Clinic Liver Cancer (BCLC) staging system [2] and the EASL-EORTC guidelines [3]. The goal of TACE treatment is to embolize the tumor's arterial blood supply and to deliver high chemotherapeutic drug concentrations to the viable tumor tissue, with the goal to achieve a high rate of tumor necrosis while preserving the surrounding heathy liver parenchyma and diminish systemic toxicity [4]. Therefore, during TACE treatment, several digital subtraction angiography series (DSA) are typically necessary to precisely identify the tumor and its feeding vasculature. In patients with complex hepatic arterial branching patterns, an increased number of DSA acquisitions at different angles are usually required to identify the tumor feeding arteries, which in turn leads to an increased radiation and contrast medium exposure.

In this context, cone beam computed tomography (CBCT) is an evolving and attractive tool, due to its capability of peri-interventional 3D imaging in combination with high vascular contrast and high spatial resolution [5]. In recent studies, CBCT has demonstrated a high diagnostic accuracy for detecting hepatic tumor lesions and small feeding arteries to hepatic neoplasms for the guidance of trans-arterial chemoembolization (TACE) [6–8]. Previous studies have also shown that peri-interventional CBCT during a TACE procedure influences diagnosis as well as treatment in up to 81%, due to improved tumor feeder detection, catheter navigation and treatment effect assessment [9, 10]. An advanced development of these techniques is represented by dual-phase cone-beam computed tomography (CBCTHA), which allows an assessment of post-processed maximum intensity projections and parenchymal blood volume (PBV) maps, in addition to acquiring native and contrast-enhanced images [11]. Promising experiences with these techniques in the initial evaluation and treatment of HCC have been published lately [12–14]. However, it remains unclear which of the images acquired with C-arm CT are suited best to delineate tumor size and tumor feeding arteries.

Therefore, the aim of this retrospective study was to compare the image quality of arterial phase and PBV maps acquired with CBCT during TACE treatment, whereby pre-interventional acquired cross-sectional images (CT or MRI) served as reference standard.

Methods

Patients

From January 2014 to December 2016 a total of 29 patients with HCC (mean age at examination: 65 years (range 47 to 81 years), 86% male), which were referred to our department for TACE treatment, received peri-interventional C-arm CT and were included in this retrospective study. Patients with early stage HCC (BCLC A) as well as intermediate stage HCC (BCLC B) were included. Exclusion criteria of this study were in accordance with the CIRSE guidelines [15]:

- Decompensated cirrhosis (Child C).
- Extrahepatic spread.
- Severely reduced portal vein flow.
- Renal insufficiency (creatinine ≥ 2 mg/dl or creatinine clearance ≤ 30 ml/min).
- Bilirubin level > 2 mg/dl.
- Advanced hepatic encephalopathy.

Underlying cause for liver cirrhosis and HCC development were Hepatitis-C-virus infection ($n = 11$), alcohol abuse ($n = 9$), NASH ($n = 2$) and hemochromatosis ($n = 1$). In six patients, the underlying cause for developing HCC was cryptogenic. Seventeen patients of this collective had received previous TACE treatment. Detailed patient information is listed in Table 1. The study was approved by the institutional review committee and was in compliance with HIPAA regulations. Due to the retrospective nature of the study, informed consent for retrospective data analysis was waved by the institutional review board.

Pre-interventional imaging

All patients underwent cross-sectional imaging (multiphase CT, $n = 25$ or MRI, $n = 4$) before TACE following the national guidelines for the assessment of HCC [16]. Median interval between baseline imaging and TACE was 8 days with a range of 4–22 days. Multiphase CT included a non-enhanced, arterial phase (30s after injection of contrast media) as well as portal venous phase (70s after injection of contrast media). The CT exam was performed on a 128 row detector CT with one or two x-ray tubes (SOMATOM Definition AS+ or Definition Flash, Siemens Healthcare, Forchheim, Germany). MRI consisted of a T2 weighted turbo-spin-echo sequence, an unenhanced and dynamic contrast enhanced T1 weighted gradient-echo sequences (VIBE) as well as diffusion-weighted sequences acquired at a field strength of 1.5 T (Magnetom Avanto fit/ Magnetom Aera, Siemens Germany).

All HCC lesions were classified based on morphology in diffuse ($n = 9$, 17%) or encapsulated ($n = 43$, 83%) lesions. According to LIRADS criteria, encapsulated HCC was defined as a predominantly round lesion with the presence of a capsule and clear wash-out in cross-

Table 1 Baseline characteristics 1

Characteristics	No. of Patients
Sex	
Male	25
Female	4
Age at examination (median)	
< 65	15
≥ 65	14
Number of tumors	
1	11
2	6
> = 3	6
Tumor size	
< 3 cm	38
3-5 cm	9
> 5 cm	5
BCLC[a]	
A	16
B	13
Cause of liver cirrhosis	
Hepatitis C	11
Alcohol related	9
Hemochromatosis	1
Non-alcoholic steatohepatitis	2
Cryptogenic	6
MELD[b] score	8.2
Previous TACE[c]	17

[a]Barcelona clinic liver cancer
[b]Model of End Stage Liver Disease
[c]transarterial chemoembolization

sectional imaging. Diffuse HCC lesions were defined as predominantly irregular or lobular lesions without a capsule [17]. The number and extent of HCC lesion was noted.

Transarterial chemoembolization (TACE)
In all patients, endovascular intervention was performed using the same robotic digital subtraction angiography system (Artis Zeego Q, VE 40 A, Siemens, Forchheim, Germany). Percutaneous arterial access was achieved through the common femoral artery (19 G needle) under local anesthesia with placement of a 4F sheath (Terumo, Leuven, Belgium). A 4F straight catheter (Terumo, Leuven, Belgium) was utilized for aortography, while a 4F Cobra (C2) or sidewinder (SIM1) catheter was used for entering the coeliac trunk. A 2.7F coaxial microcatheter (Progreat; Terumo, Leuven, Belgium) was used for selective and super-selective access of the hepatic arteries. In case of extrahepatic tumor supply (two patients

with a right inferior phrenic artery and one patient with a lumbar artery supply), an embolization of these additional feeders using pushable microcoils was performed. In all cases, a superselective TACE with DEB (100-300 μm DC-Beads (BTG, Langweid/Augsburg, Germany) loaded with 50 mg Epirubicin was conducted.

C-arm computed tomography
C-Arm CT consisted of an unenhanced rotation (mask run) and contrast enhanced rotations (return and fill run) with contrast medium injection from the proper hepatic artery for acquisition of parenchymal blood volume (PBV) maps. The following C-Arm CT image acquisition parameters were used: time per rotation 4 s, total examination time 16 s, 200° total angle, per frame 0.8°, 248 frames, matrix 616 × 480, pixel size 616 μm, projection on 30x40cm flat panel. The actual tube current and tube voltage were automatically adjusted to the individual patient by the system. For contrast enhancement, 30 ml diluted contrast medium (7.5 ml Ultravist 370, Bayer Schering, Leverkusen, Germany and 22.5 saline solution) was administered by an automated power injector (Accutron-HP-D, Medtron, Saarbrücken, Germany), using a flow rate of 3 ml/s. Contrast injection was performed immediately after the mask run. Contrast enhanced acquisition was performed in a steady state of liver perfusion [13, 14]. Image reconstruction was conducted on a multimodality workstation (MMWP VD 10, Siemens Healthcare, Forchheim, Germany). Fill run and mask run were subtracted. A non-rigid registration algorithm was performed to mitigate the motion between the two runs. The arterial input function value is calculated from an automated histogram analysis of the vessel tree. This arterial input function value is then applied as a scaling factor to obtain the PBV map [12].

All arterial phases and processed PBV maps were analyzed concerning number and extent of HCC lesions as well as the number of tumor feeding vessels.

Image analysis
A retrospective analysis of image quality and diagnostic value of arterial phase and PBV maps was performed by two experienced board certified readers (4 and 6 years of experience in dedicated interventional radiology and angiography). For this purpose, standardized reconstructions in the axial plane were acquired and clinical data of the patients were recorded.

The overall image quality of arterial phase C-arm CT and PBV maps as well as the conspicuity of HCC lesion was evaluated on a 5-point semi-quantitative Likert-scale: (1) non diagnostic image quality; (2) poor image quality; (3) moderate image quality; (4) good image quality; (5) excellent image quality.

Moreover, a 5-point Likert-Scale was used to assess the presence of artifacts (1 = compromising diagnostic image quality, 2 = present, but not compromising diagnostic image quality, 3 = no artifacts presents) and noise (1 = severe, 2 = moderate, 3 = mild, 4 = minimal, 5 = none). In addition, the delineation of central hepatic arteries as well as the visualization of the gallbladder wall was evaluated: (1) marked blurring of organ contours, (2) subtle blurring of organ contours, (3) moderate delineation of organ contours, (4) very good delineation of organ contours and (5) excellent delineation of organ contours. Complete covering of the entire liver on C-arm CT was assessed by: (1) non diagnostic, (2) incomplete but diagnostically irrelevant, (3) entire liver covered, diagnostic standard.

Tumor size was determined based on maximum diameter on axial images and was measured in arterial phase, PBV map and cross sectional images (CSI). As a quantitative measure, the contrast-to-noise ratio (CNR) was computed using the following formula (μ_R and μ_L represent the mean values of the ROI and normal liver parenchyma):

$$CNR = | \mu_R - \mu_L | / \text{noise liver}$$

Statistics

All statistical analyses were performed using the software package JMP 11 (SAS Institute Inc., Vary, NC Arithmetic means (mean) and standard deviations (SD) were calculated and mean values were tested for statistical significant differences using a non-parametric Wilcoxon signed rank test. A p-value of less than 0.05 was considered significant.

Correlation analysis was performed using Spearman rank correlation coefficients. Spearman correlations are interpreted as follows in this study: $|r| > 0.90$ = very strong correlation; $0.6 < |r| < 0.9$ = strong correlation; $0.4 < |r| < 0.6$ = moderate correlation; $|r| < 0.4$ = weak correlation.

A Bland-Altman-analysis was performed for comparison of different measurement methods (arterial phase C-arm CT, PBV, CSI) of maximum tumor diameter. Mean difference (MD) and 95% confidence interval (CI) were determined.

Results

Subjective image quality analysis

According to a 5-point Likert scale, overall image quality of arterial phase C-arm CT acquisition and reconstructed PBV maps ($n = 29$) was good (4) or excellent (5) in 80% and in 97% of the cases, respectively. A significant better image quality of the PBV maps compared to arterial phase C-arm CT acquisition ($p = 0.0032$) was

observed. None of the C-arm CT acquired arterial phase or PBV maps showed a poor (2) or non-diagnostic (1) image quality.

As displayed in Table 2, arterial phase acquisitions showed a significantly higher amount of noise and artifacts compared to PBV maps ($p = 0.195$ and $p = 0.0001$). None of the acquisitions and/or reconstructions showed major artifacts affecting diagnostic image quality. Central hepatic arteries showed significantly sharper delineation in PBV maps compared to arterial phase C-arm CT acquisitions ($p = 0.0213$), whereas the wall of the gallbladder tended to be more clearly delineated in arterial phase C-arm CT images, however this finding was not significant ($p = 0.1353$). Mean values, standard deviations and p-values of the investigated parameters are listed in Table 2.

Complete acquisition of the liver was achieved in 59% ($n = 17$) of all cases. However, the diagnostic quality (1) was not restricted by missing parts of the liver in any of the affected cases due to exact patient positioning in knowledge of the localization of the lesions from the pre-interventional imaging. Missing parts of the liver consisted of partly not covered segments 2 and 3 ($n = 5$), segments 5 and 6 ($n = 2$), segment 2 ($n = 1$), segment 4 ($n = 1$), segment 6 ($n = 1$), segment 7 ($n = 1$), and segment 2, 3, 5, and 6 ($n = 1$).

Lesion characterization and detection of tumor feeding vessels

A total of 52 hypervascularised HCC lesions were detected in arterial phase C-arm CT and reconstructed PBV maps. Mean diameter of HCC lesions was 26.6 mm (±15.8 mm) in arterial phase C-arm CT and 24.9 mm (±15.1) in PBV maps resulting in a significantly higher diameter in arterial phase C-arm CT images ($p = 0.0004$). An excellent correlation was seen between both methods (rho = 0.93). The lesions showed similar, but significantly higher conspicuity in PBV maps. Mean conspicuity was 4.27 (±0.74) in PBV maps as opposed to 3.83 (± 1.08) ($p < 0.0001$) in arterial phase images. Both methods showed a strong correlation (rho = 0.74). Calculated CNR was significantly higher in PBV maps compared to arterial phase C-arm CT with a mean CNR of 22.84 (±39.75) compared to 3.39 (± 2.51) ($p < 0.0001$). Regarding

Table 2 Image quality analysis using 5-point Likert Scale

Parameter	C-arm CT arterial phase	PBV map	p-value
Overall quality ($n = 29$)	3.93 (±0.59)	4.34 (±0.55)	0,0032*
Artifacts ($n = 29$)	2.79 (±0.56)	2.21 (±0.56)	0,0001*
Gallbladder wall ($n = 27$)	4 (±0.73)	3.7 (±0.61)	0,1353
Large vessels ($n = 29$)	4.14 (±0.52)	4.48 (±0.51)	0,0213*
Noise ($n = 29$)	3.48 (±0.57)	3.79 (±0.41)	0,195

* statistically significant

detectability of tumor feeders, significantly more feeding vessels were detected in arterial phase C-arm CT (1.67 ± 0.92) compared to PBV maps (1.27 ± 0.63) ($p = 0.0001$).

Comparison to cross-sectional imaging

Of 52 HCC lesions detected on CBCT imaging, a corresponding lesion in pre-interventional cross-sectional imaging was found in 51 cases (98%). One lesion was not seen in pre-interventional CT imaging. An example of arterial phase imaging, PBV map and CSI imaging is given at Fig. 1.

The maximum diameter of HCC lesions in pre-interventional CSI was 25.2 mm (± 15.1) compared to 24.9 mm (± 15.2) in PBV ($p = 0.20$, MD = $- 0.25$ mm, CI = $- 0.73$ to 0.22 mm). Maximum tumor diameter in arterial phase C-arm CT (26.5 ± 15.9) was significantly higher compared to CSI ($p = 0.0212$, MD = 1.27 mm CI = 0.11 to 2.44 mm).

Results of the Bland-Altman plot are shown in Fig. 2. Spearman's correlation coefficient rho revealed an excellent correlation between maximum tumor diameter in CSI and arterial phase C-arm CT (rho = 0.9168) as well as in CSI and PBV maps (rho = 0.9814).

Discussion

Due to the opportunities of peri-interventional 3D imaging in combination with high contrast resolution and high spatial resolution of the arterial vasculature, the use of C-arm computed tomography during TACE treatments of HCC has steadily increased in recent years. Numerous studies have evaluated its clinical usefulness [9, 18] and hence the Cardiovascular and Interventional Radiological Society of Europe (CIRSE) as well as the Society of Interventional Radiology (SIR) recommend its use in TACE procedures [19].The exact localization of tumor is crucial to increase the selectivity of drug delivery into the targeted tumor tissue, thereby limiting non-target embolization and preserving healthy liver tissue. Eventually, such an approach will optimize tumor response to liver directed therapy [20]. However, detection of small or less vascularized tumors is reported to be limited using conventional angiography, especially in

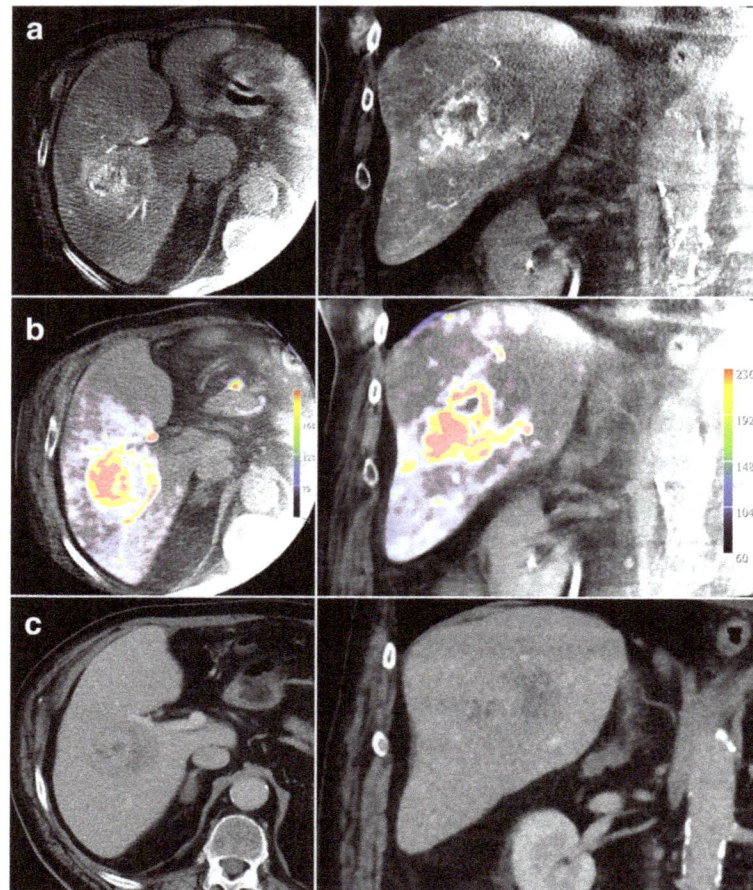

Fig. 1 Images of HCC lesion at liver segment V of a 82-year old male patient in arterial phase (**a**), PBV map (**b**) as well as pre-interventional CT at portal venous phase (**c**)

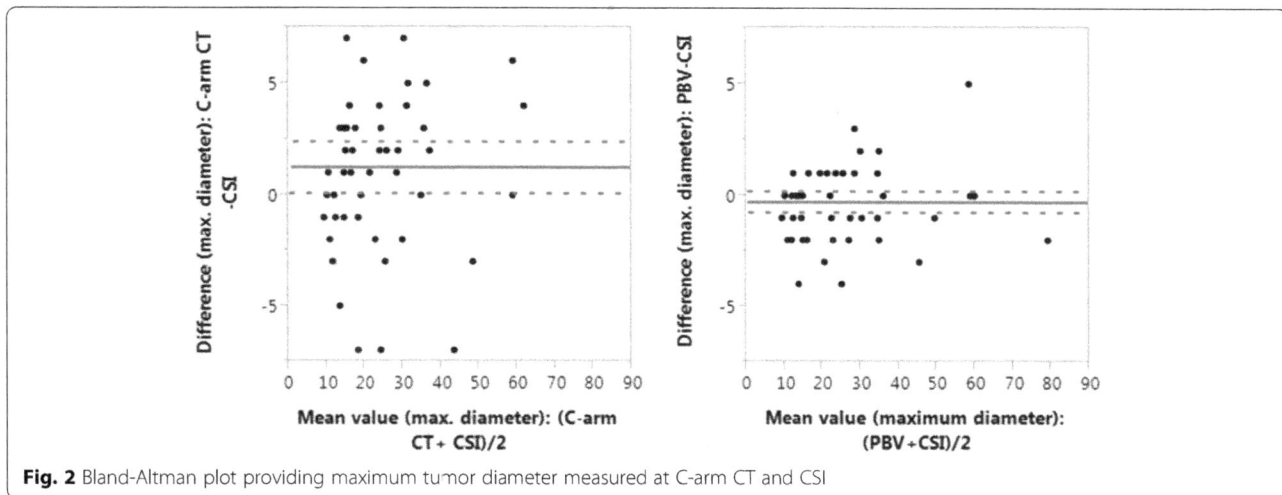

Fig. 2 Bland-Altman plot providing maximum tumor diameter measured at C-arm CT and CSI

advanced cirrhosis with heterogeneous perfused liver parenchyma [21]. C-arm CT allows intra-procedural acquisition of arterial phase images in a volume of interest, whereas dual phase C-arm CT enables acquisition of the liver parenchyma during different parenchymal phases and the acquisition of parenchymal blood volume (PBV) information as well as perfusion data [11, 22].

As compared to conventional CT acquisition, C-arm CT is associated with limitations concerning image quality, mostly due to the increased photon scatter and increased image noise generated by the small acquired FOV [22]. This disadvantage might result in an incomplete visualization of the entire liver, as it was seen in 12 (41%) of our patients. However, due to correct patient positioning, all HCC lesions could be detected in this study. The assessment of overall image quality revealed a significantly superior image quality of PBV maps compared to arterial phase C-arm CT acquisition as well as lower amount of noise and artifacts, which is most likely related to advanced post-processing techniques involved in the generation of PBV maps compared to the arterial phase images.

The high spatial resolution of C-arm CT due to the flat detector technology in conjunction with improved depiction of soft tissue details has already demonstrated an improved visibility of small HCCs [23] and direct contrast agent administration to hepatic arteries results in markedly higher tumor-to-liver contrast ratio compared to CSI [22]. Loffroy et al. [7] investigated detectability of HCC lesions by C-arm dual-phase CT compared to contrast enhanced MRI and showed that dual-phase C-arm CT is more useful and reliable than single-phasic imaging to depict HCC lesions. Lucatelli et al. [8] found that C-arm CT has a significantly higher diagnostic performance detecting smaller or less vascularized lesions than multidetector CT. In contrast to this data, our retrospective study investigates the value of

arterial phase images and PBV maps acquired with CBCT during TACE treatment as compared to pre-interventional cross-sectional imaging modalities.

In this study, we found a higher conspicuity of tumor lesions in PBV maps compared to arterial phase images, which is most likely explained by the above mentioned improved image quality of PBV maps compared to arterial phase images. Furthermore, lesion size was slightly overestimated in arterial phase images compared to PBV maps and CSI. This finding was in line of the study published by Tacher et al. [24] using a semiautomatic tumor segmentation software in measuring tumor volume on CE-MRI and dual phase CBCT images. For patient outcomes, the exact detection and treatment of tumor lesions and its feeders is of utmost importance [25]. Using C-arm CT during TACE, one lesion was detected (size 32x22mm) which had been missed by pre-interventional multiphasic CT. This is likely related to the higher tumor-to-liver contrast ratio using CBCT. This observation is concordant with the literature. Several studies showed an equal or even better sensitivity of tumor detection of HCC in C-arm CT compared to MDCT [26], especially in smaller tumors.

Virmani et al. investigated the utility of C-arm CT to optimize the catheter position during TACE and correction of catheter position was necessary in almost 39% based on C-arm CT assessment [27]. Traditionally, the detection of tumor feeders has been performed using conventional fluoroscopy and DSA. However, due to the two-dimensional character of this technique, the detection is limited by the potential misidentification or poor visualization of tumor feeders, mainly due to superimposed vessels. This could result in unnecessary or insufficient treatment, thereby potentially negatively impacting the individual patient outcome. Moreover, it has been demonstrated that in a significant percentage of cases, MDCT and MRI cannot correctly define the intra- and/or extrahepatic arterial feeders [28]. C-arm CT offers a 3-dimensional visualization of the liver vessel with high vessel-to-liver contrast resolution and high spatial resolution. Therefore, sensitivity for detecting tumor feeders has been found to range between 73 and 100% [6, 29]. These results are supported by this study which showed significantly more feeding vessels in the C-Arm CT arterial phase compared to PBV maps and CSI, probably due to the higher contrast concentration caused by direct intra-arterial injection of contrast material. This leads to markedly improved visualization of smaller vessels compared to CTA acquired in MDCT during intravenous application of the contrast agent. Furthermore, volume rendering and planar reformats that complement digital subtraction angiography allow for clarification of three-dimensional vascular relationships and provide a road map that simplifies the complex vascular anatomy in cirrhotic patients [30].

In summary, whereas overall image quality, conspicuity of HCC lesions and determination of tumor size was better in PBV maps, arterial phase images are necessary in order to accurately detect tumor feeders.

The study has several limitations. First, the study has a retrospective design and the size of the patient cohort is limited. Therefore, these results have to be interpreted with care and cannot be transferred to other C-arm CT vendors and protocols. Another possible limitation is the use of two different modalities in pre-interventional imaging, which is due the retrospective study design. However we only used 1.5 T scanners for MRI imaging and 128 slices scanners for CT. Subgroup analysis of the two different imaging techniques didn't show any significant difference in lesion diameters between CT vs CBCT and MRI vs CBCT.

Conclusion

The combination of PBV maps and arterial phase images acquired by C-arm CT during the TACE procedure enables for precise detection of the majority of HCC lesions and tumor feeding arteries and may therefore potentially increase patient outcomes.

Abbreviations
BCLC: Barcelona Clinic Liver Cancer; CBCT: Cone beam computed tomography; CBCTHA: Dual-phase cone-beam computed tomography; CIRSE: Cardiovascular and Interventional Radiological Society of Europe; CNR: Contrast to noise ratio; CSI: Cross sectional imaging; CT: Computed tomography; CTA: Computed tomography angiography; DSA: Digital subtraction angiography; HCC: Hepatocellular carcinoma; HIPAA: Health Insurance Portability and Accountability Act; MDCT: Multidetector computed tomography; MRI: Magnetic resonance imaging; NASH: Nonalcoholic steatohepatitis; PBV: Parenchymal blood volume; SD: Standard deviation; TACE: Transarterial chemoembolization

Funding
This research did not receive any specific grant from funding agencies in the public, commercial, or not-for-profit sectors.

Authors' contributions
TZ searched the data base for patients with HCC and c-arm CT, collected clinical data and drafted the manuscript. GG, SP and NK contributed to conception and design of the study and revised the manuscript for important intellectual content. RS, UG designed the study, interpreted data, and revised the manuscript for important intellectual content. All authors read and approved the final manuscript.

Competing interests
There are no conflicts of interest. The authors disclose any financial competing interests but also any non-financial competing interests.

Author details
[1]Department of Diagnostic and Interventional Radiology, University of Tuebingen, Hoppe-Seyler-Straße 3, 72076 Tuebingen, Germany. [2]Department of Radiology, Section of Interventional Radiology, University Hospitals Cleveland Medical Center, Case Western Reserve University, Cleveland, OH, USA.

References
1. Maillard E. Epidemiology, natural history and pathogenesis of hepatocellular carcinoma. Cancer Radiother. 2011;15(1):3–6.
2. Llovet JM, Bru C, Bruix J. Prognosis of hepatocellular carcinoma: the BCLC staging classification. Semin Liver Dis. 1999;19(3):329–38.
3. European Association For The Study Of The L, European Organisation For R, Treatment Of C: EASL-EORTC clinical practice guidelines: management of hepatocellular carcinoma. J Hepatol. 2012;56:908–43.
4. Bouvier A, Ozenne V, Aube C, Boursier J, Vullierme MP, Thouveny F, Farges O, Vilgrain V. Transarterial chemoembolisation: effect of selectivity on tolerance, tumour response and survival. Eur Radiol. 2011;21(8):1719–26.
5. van den Hoven AF, Prince JF, de Keizer B, Vonken EJ, Bruijnen RC, Verkooijen HM, Lam MG, van den Bosch MA. Use of C-arm cone beam CT during hepatic Radioembolization: protocol optimization for extrahepatic shunting and parenchymal enhancement. Cardiovasc Intervent Radiol. 2016;39(1):64–73.
6. Iwazawa J, Ohue S, Mitani T, Abe H, Hashimoto N, Hamuro M, Nakamura K. Identifying feeding arteries during TACE of hepatic tumors: comparison of C-arm CT and digital subtraction angiography. AJR Am J Roentgenol. 2009; 192(4):1057–63.
7. Loffroy R, Lin M, Rao P, Bhagat N, Noordhoek N, Radaelli A, Blijd J, Geschwind JF. Comparing the detectability of hepatocellular carcinoma by C-arm dual-phase cone-beam computed tomography during hepatic arteriography with conventional contrast-enhanced magnetic resonance imaging. Cardiovasc Intervent Radiol. 2012;35(1):97–104.
8. Lucatelli P, Argiro R, Ginanni Corradini S, Saba L, Cirelli C, Fanelli F, Ricci C, Levi Sandri GB, Catalano C, Bezzi M. Comparison of image quality and diagnostic performance of cone-beam CT during drug-eluting embolic Transarterial chemoembolization and multidetector CT in the detection of hepatocellular carcinoma. J Vasc Interv Radiol. 2017;
9. Tacher V, Radaelli A, Lin M, Geschwind JF. How I do it: cone-beam CT during transarterial chemoembolization for liver cancer. Radiology. 2015; 274(2):320–34.
10. Kakeda S, Korogi Y, Ohnari N, Moriya J, Oda N, Nishino K, Miyamoto W. Usefulness of cone-beam volume CT with flat panel detectors in conjunction with catheter angiography for transcatheter arterial embolization. J Vasc Interv Radiol. 2007;18(12):1508–16.
11. Chu WF, Lin CJ, Chen WS, Hung SC, Chiu CF, Wu TH, Guo WY. Radiation doses of cerebral blood volume measurements using C-arm CT: a phantom study. AJNR Am J Neuroradiol. 2014;35(6):1073–7.
12. Vogl TJ, Schaefer P, Lehnert T, Nour-Eldin NE, Ackermann H, Mbalisike E, Hammerstingl R, Eichler K, Zangos S, Naguib NN. Intraprocedural blood volume measurement using C-arm CT as a predictor for treatment response of malignant liver tumours undergoing repetitive transarterial chemoembolization (TACE). Eur Radiol. 2016;26(3):755–63.
13. Peynircioglu B, Hizal M, Cil B, Deuerling-Zheng Y, Von Roden M, Hazirolan T, Akata D, Ozmen M, Balkanci F. Quantitative liver tumor blood volume measurements by a C-arm CT post-processing software before and after

Image quality of arterial phase and parenchymal blood volume (PBV) maps derived from C-arm...

169

hepatic arterial embolization therapy: comparison with MDCT perfusion. Diagnostic and interventional radiology (Ankara, Turkey). 2015;21(1):71–7.

14. Zhuang ZG, Zhang XB, Han JF, Beilner J, Deuerling-Zheng Y, Chi JC, Wang J, Qian LJ, Zhou Y, Xu JR. Hepatic blood volume imaging with the use of flat-detector CT perfusion in the angiography suite: comparison with results of conventional multislice CT perfusion. J Vasc Interv Radiol. 2014;25(5):739–46.

15. Basile A, Carrafiello G, Ierardi AM, Tsetis D, Brountzos E. Quality-improvement guidelines for hepatic transarterial chemoembolization. Cardiovasc Intervent Radiol. 2012;35(4):765–74.

16. Sommer CM, Stampfl U, Kauczor HU, Pereira PL. National S3 guidelines on hepatocellular carcinoma. Radiologe. 2014;54(7):642–53.

17. Witjes CD, Willemssen FE, Verheij J, van der Veer SJ, Hansen BE, Verhoef C, de Man RA, Ijzermans JN. Histological differentiation grade and microvascular invasion of hepatocellular carcinoma predicted by dynamic contrast-enhanced MRI. J Magn Reson Imaging. 2012;36(3):641–7.

18. Pellerin O, Lin M, Bhagat N, Shao W, Geschwind JF. Can C-arm cone-beam CT detect a micro-embolic effect after TheraSphere radioembolization of neuroendocrine and carcinoid liver metastasis? Cancer Biother Radiopharm. 2013;28(6):459–65.

19. Wallace MJ, Kuo MD, Glaiberman C, Binkert CA, Orth RC, Soulez G. Three-dimensional C-arm cone-beam CT: applications in the interventional suite. J Vasc Interv Radiol. 2009;20(7 Suppl):S523–37.

20. Mahnken AH, Spreafico C, Maleux G, Helmberger T, Jakobs TF. Standards of practice in transarterial radioembolization. Cardiovasc Intervent Radiol. 2013; 36(3):613–22.

21. Sumida M, Ohto M, Ebara M, Kimura K, Okuda K, Hirooka N. Accuracy of angiography in the diagnosis of small hepatocellular carcinoma. AJR Am J Roentgenol. 1986;147(3):531–6.

22. Bapst B, Lagadec M, Breguet R, Vilgrain V, Ronot M. Cone beam computed tomography (CBCT) in the field of interventional oncology of the liver. Cardiovasc Intervent Radiol. 2016;39(1):8–20.

23. Tognolini A, Louie JD, Hwang GL, Hofmann LV, Sze DY, Kothary N. Utility of C-arm CT in patients with hepatocellular carcinoma undergoing transhepatic arterial chemoembolization. J Vasc Interv Radiol. 2010;21(3): 339–47.

24. Tacher V, Lin M, Chao M, Gjesteby L, Bhagat N, Mahammedi A, Ardon R, Mory B, Geschwind JF. Semiautomatic volumetric tumor segmentation for hepatocellular carcinoma: comparison between C-arm cone beam computed tomography and MRI. Acad Radiol. 2013;20(4):446–52.

25. Lencioni R. Chemoembolization in patients with hepatocellular carcinoma. Liver cancer. 2012;1(1):41–50.

26. Zheng J, Li J, Cui X, Ye H, Ye L. Comparison of diagnostic sensitivity of C-arm CT, DSA and CT in detecting small HCC. Hepato-Gastroenterology. 2013;60(126):1509–12.

27. Virmani S, Ryu RK, Sato KT, Lewandowski RJ, Kulik L, Mulcahy MF, Larson AC, Salem R, Omary RA. Effect of C-arm angiographic CT on transcatheter arterial chemoembolization of liver tumors. J Vasc Interv Radiol. 2007;18(10): 1305–9.

28. Matoba M, Tonami H, Kuginuki M, Yokota H, Takashima S, Yamamoto I. Comparison of high-resolution contrast-enhanced 3D MRA with digital subtraction angiography in the evaluation of hepatic arterial anatomy. Clin Radiol. 2003;58(6):463–8.

29. Minami Y, Yagyu Y, Murakami T, Kudo M. Tracking navigation imaging of Transcatheter arterial chemoembolization for hepatocellular carcinoma using three-dimensional cone-beam CT angiography. Liver cancer. 2014;3(1): 53–61.

30. Pung L, Ahmad M, Mueller K, Rosenberg J, Stave C, Hwang GL, Shah R, Kothary N. The role of cone-beam CT in Transcatheter arterial chemoembolization for hepatocellular carcinoma: a systematic review and meta-analysis. J Vasc Interv Radiol. 2017;28(3):334–41.

20

CT during celiac artery angiography for localization of clinically suspected small insulinomas

Feng Duan[*†], Yan-hua Bai[†], Li Cui[†], Jie-yu Yan, Xiao-hui Li and Xiu-qi Wang

Abstract

Background: To identify location and number of insulinomas before operation is very important for improving the cure rate. The objective of the study was to assess performance of CT during celiac artery angiography for preoperative localization of clinically suspected small insulinomas (< 2 cm in diameter).

Methods: From January 2013 to November 2016, 42 patients with hypoglycemic symptoms underwent celiac artery angiography, superior mesenteric artery angiography and CT during celiac artery angiography by a combined CT/digital subtraction angiography system, MIYABI Angio CT plus an Artiszeeceiling (SIEMENS, Germany). Patient group consisted of 13 males and 29 females, age 17–69 years (average, 45.4 ± 13.5 y). After diagnosis, all 42 patients were operated. Obtained images were retrospectively analyzed and compared with findings from post-operation pathology.

Results: All interventional radiology procedures were performed successfully with no complications. Sensitivity of angiography alone for insulinoma was 76.1% (32/42), at combined CT/digital subtraction angiography, 4 more nodules were found (sensitivity, 85.7%, 36/42), while 6 false-negatives were observed (all false negative lesions were less than 2 cm). A total of 64 ml to 80 ml contrast media was used per patient.

Conclusion: CT during celiac artery angiography is a sensitive diagnostic procedure for localizing insulinomas. Combined with angiography, it can prioritize the pancreatic region for exploration and guide a pancreatic resection.

Keywords: Computed tomography· digital subtraction angiography · celiac artery ·insulinoma· interventional radiology

Background

Insulinoma is a rare tumor of the pancreas, with an estimated incidence of 0.4 per 100, 000 person/year [1]. To date, resection is the best treatment option. Therefore, preoperative localization of the tumor is very important. This information can help surgeons to make decisions on type and extent of the surgical resection [2]. However, small insulinomas (< 2 cm in diameter), in patients with clinical and biochemical evidence of endogenous hyper-insulinemia, are often difficult to localize in the pancreas. This is because there are still some false-positive and falls-negative diagnoses using non-invasive imaging modalities. CT during celiac artery angiography is a novel imaging modality and may enhance sensitivity for detection of small insulinomas. Therefore, we evaluated the benefit of CT during celiac artery angiography for localization of primary tumors in patients with clinically and biochemically suspected small insulinomas.

* Correspondence: duanfeng@vip.sina.com

[†]Feng Duan, Yan-hua Bai and Li Cui contributed equally to this work.
Department of Interventional Radiology, the General Hospital of Chinese People's Liberation Army, Beijing 100853, China

Methods

This retrospective study was approved by the Hospital Ethics Committee. Informed consent was obtained from all patients included in the study.

General information

From January 2013 to November 2016, 42 patients with hypoglycemic symptoms underwent CT during celiac artery angiography examinations. Patient group consisted of 13 males and 29 females, age between 17 and 69 (average of 45.4 ± 13.5), and blood sugar level varied between 0.81 and 3.05 mmol/L (average of 2.08 ± 0.67 mmol/L).

All examinations were performed using a MIYABI Angio-CT plus an Artiszee ceiling (SIEMENS, Germany), a combined CT/digital subtraction angiography (DSA) system. The two modalities were combined into a single system to provide both morphological and functional data from the same tumor in a single imaging session.

Firstly, celiac and superior mesenteric arteriography was performed via selective catheterization using a 4-F hepatic artery catheter (Terumo, Tokyo, Japan). Selective gastro-duodenal arteriography and splenic arteriography (if necessary) were performed using 4-F hepatic artery catheter as well. The total contrast media volume (Ultravist 370, Bayer, Germany) and injection rate were 20 ml and 4 ml/s for celiac and superior mesenteric arteriography, 12 ml and 3 ml/s for selective gastro-duodenal arteriography, and 16 ml and 4 ml/s for selective splenic arteriography. A total of 64 to 80 ml contrast media was used per patient.

Secondly, CT during celiac artery angiography was performed using the following scanning parameters: 16 detector rows, 5 mm section, pitch factor of 0.75, reconstruction interval of 1.5 mm, gantry rotation time of 0.6 s, tube voltage of 130 kV, and automatically determined tube mA. After infusion of 24 ml Ultravist-saline mixture (1:1) at 4 ml/s for 4 s, arterial-phase scanning was started. Venous-phase scanning started 12 – 15 s after perfusion of contrast medium began, and late-phase scanning was started 18 – 23 s after initiating contrast material infusion. The scanning time (approximately 4 – 6 s) varied depending on pancreas size. The total volume of non-diluted contrast medium for enhanced CT scan was 12 ml.

Angiographic procedures were performed by radiologists who had at least 10 years of experience with abdominal angiography. CT images were evaluated by two experienced radiologists. Statistical analyses were performed by the author (D.F.). A commercial statistical software package (SPSS for Windows, version 16.0; SPSS, Chicago, Ill) was used for data analysis. The t test was used to test differences between preoperative and postoperative blood glucose levels. P values< 0.05 were considered to indicate statistically significant difference.

Results

All interventional radiology procedures were performed successfully with no complications. Subsequently, all 42 patients were operated, and in total 47 tumor nodules were collected. Most of the tumor nodules were grayish white, and only a few were grayish red or cherry red. All tumors ranged between a diameter of 0.5–3.5 cm (mean, 1.56 ± 0.8 cm), there were 3 lesions larger than 2 cm (2.5 cm, 2.5 cm and 3.5 cm, respectively), and the rest were less than 2 cm. All 3 patients with lesions larger than 2 cm were with multiple lesions. Excised lesions were of medium hardness, and of which 6 were from the head (Fig. 1), 10 from the body, 14 from the tail (Fig. 2a, b), 9 from the neck, and 8 from the uncinate process of the pancreas, with a multiple tumor rate of 9.5% (4/42 cases). Based on pathology results, all were benign insulinomas. Angiography imaging was consistent with surgery in 76.1% (32/42) of the cases (Fig. 3a), combined with angiography images, 4 more nodules were found in CT images, and CT imaging was consistent with surgery in 85.7% (36/42) of the cases (Fig. 3b), while 6 false-negatives were observed (all false negative lesions were less than 2 cm). A total of 64 to 80 ml contrast media was used per patient.

DSA manifestation of small insulinomas was characterized by homogeneous staining of the tumor, clear borders of majority of the tumors, enlargement of feeding arteries and increased tumor vessel density. Plain CT scans showed no significant differentiation or local

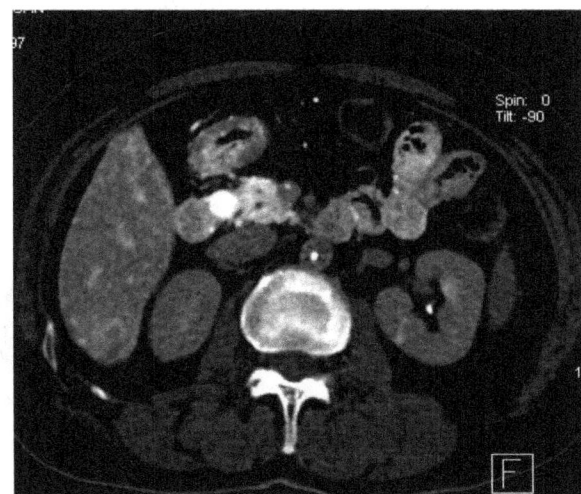

Fig. 1 CT during celiac artery angiography shows an insulinoma in the pancreas head

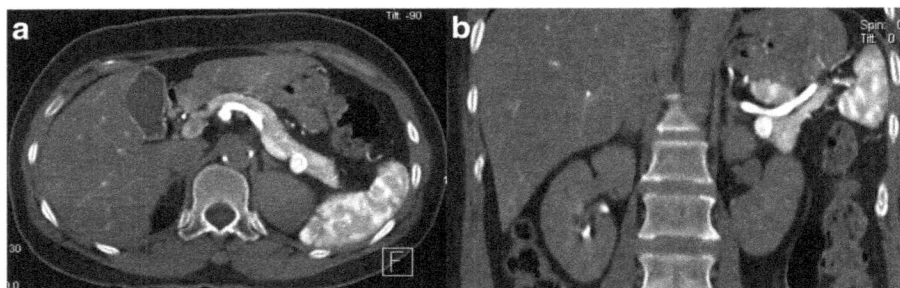

Fig. 2 CT during celiac artery angiography shows an insulinoma in the pancreas tail. **a** Transverse CT view. **b** Coronal CT view

elevated outline, and tumor density was not different from normal pancreas. Contrast enhanced scans indicated tumor nodules with clear borders, which present washout of contrast.

The hypoglycemic symptoms of all patients improved after operation. Blood glucose levels before operation were between 0.81 and 3.05 mmol/L (average of 2.08 ± 0.67 mmol/L), while blood glucose levels after operation were between 4.76 and 11.2 mmol/L (average of 7.30 ± 2.21 mmol/L), p<0.01.

Discussion

Insulinomas are classified as neuroendocrine tumors derived of beta cells in the pancreas, which secrete insulin, according to the 2010 WHO, 2007 ENETS and 2010 UICC-pTNM (NETs) classification [3]. Most insulinomas are functional, with typical symptoms according to the Whipple triad. During a typical hypoglycemia episode, blood glucose decreases to < 2.8 mmol/l, which is quickly relieved after intake of glucose. Although clinical symptoms are evident, insulinomas are often small, with more than 80% of the insulinomas smaller than 2 cm in diameter [4]. In this group of patients, 92.9% of the insulinomas are < 2 cm. Because of their small size, they are likely to be missed during conventional imaging exams.

Common detection methods for insulinomas currently include non-invasive imaging modalities, such as ultrasonography (US), computed tomography (CT), magnetic resonance imaging (MRI) and 18-Fluoro-DOPA PET/CT scanning, and invasive pre-operative diagnostic procedures, such as endoscopic ultrasound (EUS), DSA, intra-arterial calcium stimulation test (ASVS), and trans-hepatic peri-pancreatic venous blood sampling (TPVB). There are pros and cons for each method, for example, the sensitivity of non-invasive preoperative imaging, for localization of lesions, is between 73.08 and 90% [5–8]. Conventional enhanced images sometimes are not able to accurately capture the most prominent phase of enhancement of a particular lesion, which makes it possible to get an equivocal results at conventional imaging [9]. Especially for small lesions, non-invasive imaging is not sufficient for preoperative localization of insulinomas. In case of the various invasive exam methods, endoscopic ultrasound is highly sensitive for diagnosis. However, findings can be sometimes false positive. Quality of findings obtained by endoscopic ultrasound imaging depends to a large extent on the experience of the examiner. Furthermore, some insulinomas are missed by preoperative EUS, because they are completely isoechoic [10, 11]. Conventional angiography DSA has low resolution. Especially lesions, which overlay with duodenum or spleen, can hardly be distinguished. It has been reported that the diagnosis accuracy of selective DSA on pancreas is 72–83.3% [12]. ASVS can only provide information on regional location

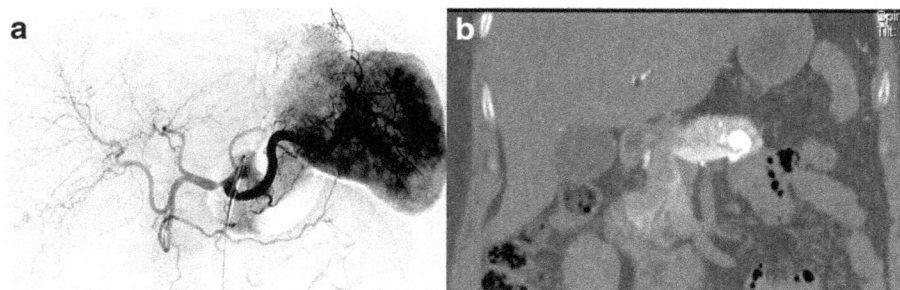

Fig. 3 A 55-year old female. **a** Celiac artery angiography does not show any lesion. **b** CT during celiac artery angiography indicates a suspected lesion in the pancreas tail. Lesion is considered to overlay with spleen

of insulinomas, but cannot confirm size or exact position (for instance on pancreas surface or not). Importantly, insufficient preoperative imaging may affect the choice of operational methods in a negative way (e. g., if a minimally invasive laparoscopic enucleation is applicable) [13].

The combination of angiography with CT during celiac artery angiography showed several advantages: 1) it can provide greater enhancement of pancreatic tumors by the administration of contrast material directly into the proper artery. 2) CT provides significantly higher spatial resolution than DSA, thus it provides more precise diagnosis for small lesions, especially lesions, which overlay with duodenum or spleen. 3) Only local injection of contrast medium is required, so the dosage of contrast medium is greatly reduced compared to conventional CT. In our study, the dose of contrast medium for CT was 12 ml, and even with the addition of contrast medium for angiography, the total dose of contrast media was still lower than applied with a conventional CT. 4) Two exams can be performed simultaneously, and through integration of the two exam findings small insulinomas can more precisely be located. In particular, for iso-attenuating insulinomas, adjuvant observation of blood flow in the suspected lesions can help with identification of tumor regions [14]. Although current DSA includes dyna-CT function, its resolution is still lower than conventional CT. Moreover, the reconstruction region of dyna-CT is relatively small [15]; in some cases not the entire pancreas can be included. Consequently small insulinomas can likely be missed.

Limitations of the modality presented here include: 1, the study did not carry out a comparison of CT during celiac artery angiography and other "conventional" imaging modalities. Because the study was retrospective, the preoperative imaging algorithm was not standardized; the number of cases for each examination is too small to carry out comparative study. As the number of cases increases, we will conduct a comparative study with the conventional imaging modality; 2, CT during celiac artery angiography is an invasive exam method, thus it has a higher increased risk than noninvasive exams; 3, this exam still relies on the difference between tumorous arterial blood supply and normal tissue blood supply to identify tumor lesions. For that reason false negatives can incur when tumors have normal arterial blood supply. In this case, ASVS can be combined to increase the sensitivity.

Conclusion

Together we conclude that CT during celiac artery angiography is a sensitive diagnostic procedure for localization of insulinomas. In combination with angiog-raphy, it can cover the pancreatic region for a prioritized exploration and guide pancreatic resections.

Abbreviations
ASVS: intra-arterial calcium stimulation test; CT: Computed Tomography; DSA: digital subtraction angiography; EUS: endoscopic ultrasound; MRI: magnetic resonance imaging; TPVB: trans-hepatic peri-pancreatic venous blood sampling; US: ultrasonography

Acknowledgements
We would like to extend our sincere gratitude to our departmental chair for all these support. Also, we would like to give many thanks to our physicians, engineers, nurses as well as other staff of the department.

Authors' contributions
DF, BYH and CL designed this study. DF, LXH and WXQ performed the angiography procedures. YJY and CL collected data. DF, BYH, CL and YJY wrote this manuscript. DF, BYH and CL revised the manuscript. All authors read and approved the final manuscript.

Competing interests
The authors declare that they have no competing interests.

References
1. Service FJ, McMahon MM, O'Brien PC, Ballard DJ. Functioning insulinoma – incidence, recurrence, and long-term survival of patients: a 60-year study. Mayo Clin Proc. 1991;66:711–9.
2. Thompson SM, Vella A, Service FJ, Grant CS, Thompson GB, Andrews JC. Impact of variant pancreatic arterial anatomy and overlap in regional perfusion on the interpretation of selective arterial calcium stimulation with hepatic venous sampling for preoperative localization of occult insulinoma. Surgery. 2015;158:162–72.
3. Ito T, Lee L, Hijioka M, Kawabe K, Kato M, Nakamura K, et al. The up-to-date review of epidemiological pancreatic neuroendocrine tumors in Japan. J Hepatobiliary Pancreat Sci. 2015;22:574–7.
4. Jyotsna VP, Rangel N, Pal S, Seith A, Sahni P, Ammini AC. Insulinoma: Diagnosis and surgical treatment. Retrospective analysis of 31 cases. Indian J Gastroenterol. 2006;25:244–7.
5. Li X, Zhang F, Chen H, Yu H, Zhou J, Li M, et al. Diagnosis of insulinoma using the ratios of serum concentrations of insulin and C-peptide to glucose during a 5-hour oral glucose tolerance test. Endocr J. 2017;64:49–57.
6. Varma V, Tariciotti L, Coldham C, Taniere P, Buckels JA, Bramhall SR. Preoperative localisation and surgical management of insulinoma: single Centre experience. Dig Surg. 2011;28:63–73.
7. Katayama A, Iseda I, Tone A, Matsushita Y, Inoue K, Tsukamoto K, et al. The usefulness of super-selective computed tomography angiography (CTA) for diagnosing and localizing a small insulinoma. Intern Med. 2010;49:1983–6.
8. McAuley G, Delaney H, Colville J, Lyburn I, Worsley D, Govender P, et al. Multimodality preoperativeimaging of pancreatic insulinomas. ClinRadiol. 2005;60:1039–50.
9. Clarke SE, Saranathan M, Rettmann DW, Hargreaves BA, Vasanawala SS. High resolution multi-arterial phase MRI improves lesion contrast in chronic liver disease. Clin Invest Med. 2015;38:E90–9.
10. Kann PH, Ivan D, Pfützner A, Forst T, Langer P, Schaefer S. Preoperative diagnosis of insulinoma: low body mass index, young age, and female gender are associated with negativeimaging by endoscopic ultrasound. Eur J Endocrinol. 2007;157:209–13.
11. Kann PH, Rothmund M, Zielke A. Endoscopic ultrasound imaging of insulinomas: limitations and clinical relevance. ExpClinEndocrinol Diabetes. 2005;113:471–4.

12. Fu W, Li J, Wen J, Lin G, Wei Z, Deng J, et al. Management of islet cell
     tumours: a single hospital experience. Hepato-Gastroenterology. 2015;62:
     723–6.
13. Tagaya N, Kasama K, Suzuki N, Taketsuka S, Horie K, Furihata M, et al.
     Laparoscopic resection of the pancreas and review of the literature.
     SurgEndosc. 2003;17:201–6.
14. Zhu L, Xue HD, Sun H, Wang X, He YL, Jin ZY, et al. Isoattenuating
     insulinomas at biphasic contrast-enhanced CT: frequency, clinicopathologic
     features and perfusion characteristics. Eur Radiol. 2016;26:3697–705.
15. Hohenforst-Schmidt W, Banckwitz R, Zarogoulidis P, Vogl T, Darwiche K,
     Goldberg E, et al. Radiation exposure of patients by cone beam CT during
     endobronchial navigation - a phantom study. J Cancer. 2014;5:192–202.

21

^{11}C-acetate PET/MRI in bladder cancer staging and treatment response evaluation to neoadjuvant chemotherapy

Antti Salminen[1,8]* (iD), Ivan Jambor[2,8], Harri Merisaari[8], Otto Ettala[1], Johanna Virtanen[2], Ilmari Koskinen[3], Erik Veskimae[4], Jukka Sairanen[3], Pekka Taimen[5], Jukka Kemppainen[6,8], Heikki Minn[7,8†] and Peter J. Boström[1†]

Abstract

Background: To evaluate the accuracy of ^{11}C-acetate Positron Emission Tomography/Magnetic Resonance Imaging (PET/MRI) in bladder cancer (BC) staging and monitoring response to neoadjuvant chemotherapy (NAC).

Methods: Eighteen patients were prospectively enrolled. Fifteen treatment naive patients underwent ^{11}C-acetate PET/MRI before transurethral resection of bladder tumor (TUR-BT) for primary tumor evaluation. Five patients with muscle invasive BC were imaged after NAC and prior to radical cystectomy (RC) with extended pelvic lymph node dissection (ePLND) for NAC treatment response evaluation. Two patients were part of both cohorts. ^{11}C-acetate PET/MRI findings were correlated with histopathology. Accuracy for lymph node detection was evaluated on patient and the ePLND template (10 regions) levels.

Results: The sensitivity, specificity and accuracy of ^{11}C-acetate PET/MRI for the detection of muscle invasive BC was 1.00, 0.69 and 0.73 while the area under the receiver operating characteristic curve (95% confidence interval) was 0.85 (0.55–1.0), respectively. All five NAC patients underwent chemotherapy as planned and ^{11}C-acetate PET/MRI correctly staged three patients, overstaged one and understaged one patient compared with RC and ePLND findings. A total of 175 lymph node were removed, median of 35 (range, 27–43) per patient in five patients who had RC and ePLND while 12 (7%) harboured metastases. Sensitivity, specificity, accuracy and AUC for N-staging were 0.20, 0.96, 0.80 and 0.58 on the ePLND template (10 regions) level.

Conclusions: ^{11}C-acetate PET/MRI is feasible for staging of BC although sensitivity for the detection of nodal metastases is low. Monitoring response to NAC shows promise and warrants evaluation in larger studies.

Keywords: Bladder cancer, ^{11}C-acetate, PET/MRI, Neoadjuvant chemotherapy

Background

Approximately 77,000 new cases of bladder cancer (BC) are diagnosed annually in USA [1]. In Europe, based on EU science hub estimates, incidence of new BC cases was 131,000 in 2015, but there is large variability between

different countries [2]. Staging is based on TNM system [3]. Ta tumors are treated with transurethral resection of bladder tumor (TUR-BT). T1 and carcinoma in situ (Tis) tumors have risk of progression and intravesical immunotherapy with Bacillus-Calmette-Guerin (BCG) instillations is used to obtain local control and organ preservation [4]. Muscle invasive bladder cancer (MIBC) is an aggressive disease and standard treatment is radical cystectomy (RC), accompanied by pelvic lymph node dissection (PLND) [5]. In addition to radical surgery, neoadjuvant chemotherapy (NAC) has been demonstrated to increase overall survival

* Correspondence: antti.salminen@tyks.fi
†Heikki Minn and Peter J. Boström contributed equally to this work.
[1]Department of Urology, University of Turku and Turku University hospital, Kiinamyllynkatu 4-8, 20520 Turku, Finland
[8]Department of Radiology, Icahn School of Medicine at Mount Sinai, New York, USA
Full list of author information is available at the end of the article

in MIBC and is recommended by consensus guidelines [5, 6].

Staging of BC remains suboptimal with standard imaging modalities such as computed tomography (CT) and anatomical (T2- and T1-weighted imaging) magnetic resonance imaging (MRI) [7, 8]. Compared to contrast enhanced CT, MRI has better soft tissue contrast which may improve local tumor evaluation [9]. Locoregional staging in particular is difficult, since normal-sized lymph nodes may harbour metastases. The use of ultra-small paramagnetic particles of iron oxide (USPIO) has shown some promise in the detection of nodal metastases with MRI [10, 11] but still remains an experimental approach with very limited availability.

Positron emission tomography-CT (PET/CT) imaging has been widely investigated in BC in an attempt to improve nodal staging but with limited success [12–15]. PET/MRI is a novel combination of two imaging modalities which could potentially offer advantages for evaluation of MIBC over PET/CT. Only a limited experience in staging of BC is available with PET/MRI and specifically studies of tracers with low excretion in urine are lacking [16]. Hence, we undertook the current study to evaluate ^{11}C-acetate PET/MRI in initial staging and estimation of response to NAC in patients with BC.

Methods

Patients

The study was approved by the ethical committee of Hospital District of Southwest Finland and registered at ClinicalTrials.gov (NCT01918592). Candidates for study were screened in cystoscopy units in three participating university hospitals. Eligible patients signed written consent after verbal and written information.

Imaging protocol

All patients were imaged with an Ingenuity TF PET/MRI scanner (Philips Medical Systems, Cleveland, OH). Details of the physical performance of the system have already been reported [17]. Before imaging, each patient had a Foley catheter inserted holding 10 ml glycine in balloon and the bladder was consequently filled with 100 ml sterile saline. The patients were placed supine on the scanner table. After completed MR-based attenuation correction (see below) the table was rotated for PET scan and a median dose of 713 (range, 654–796) MBq of ^{11}C-acetate was injected intravenously and PET acquisition (two 4-min table positions) covering the whole pelvis was immediately started.

MR-based attenuation correction (MRAC) was performed using the vendor-provided method. The anatomical MR acquisition (atMR) for MRAC was performed using Repetition Time/Echo Time (TR/TE)

4.0/2.3 ms and flip angle 10°. Subsequently, MRAC algorithm converts the atMR images by segmentation and classification to attenuation correction maps containing air (0.0 cm^{-1}), lung (0.022 cm^{-1}) and soft tissue (0.096 cm^{-1}). This MRAC map was then used in PET image reconstruction. All quantitative corrections were applied to this reconstruction taking into account detector dead time, radioactivity decay, random, scatter and photon attenuation. PET images were reconstructed in a 144×144 matrix with an isotropic voxel size of 4 mm following a fully 3-D maximum-likelihood ordered subsets expectation maximum (LM-OSEM) algorithm with 3 iterations and 33 subsets using TOF technology.

After the PET scan, bladder was emptied and radioactive urine was safely disposed. Bladder was re-filled with 100 ml sterile saline and MRI examination was performed.

T2-weighted imaging was performed using single-shot turbo spin echo sequence with TR/TE 3618/130, field of view (FOV) 300×300 mm^2, acquisition voxel size $1.25 \times 1.25 \times 3.00$ mm^3, reconstruction voxel size $0.69 \times 0.69 \times 3.00$ mm^3 in axial (acquisition time 1:30 min), sagittal (acquisition time 1:30 min) and coronal (acquisition time 1:12 min) planes. Diffusion weighted imaging (DWI) covering whole pelvis was performed using a single shot SE-EPI sequence, monopolar diffusion gradient scheme, and the following parameters: TR/TE 3148/45, FOV 300×300 cm^2, acquisition voxel size $2.5 \times 2.5 \times 4.0$ mm^3, reconstruction voxel size $1.25 \times 1.25 \times 4.00$ mm^3, b value 0 and 800 s/mm^2, diffusion gradient timing (Δ) 21.6 ms, diffusion gradient duration (δ) 8.3 ms, diffusion time (Δ-δ/3) 18.8 ms, SENSE [18] factor of 2, partial-Fourier acquisition 0.69, SPAIR fat suppression acquisition time 1:47 min per position (two positions in total). Additional T2-weighted imaging in axial plane with the same slice location as DWI covering whole pelvis was obtained using TR/TE 3148/45, FOV 300×300 cm^2, acquisition voxel size acquisition voxel size $1.25 \times 1.25 \times 4.00$ mm^3, reconstruction voxel size $0.69 \times 0.69 \times 4.00$ mm^3, acquisition time 1:05 min per position (two positions in total). Additional B0 and B1 mapping were performed. Multiple additional experimental DWI acquisitions, a spin locking method were acquired but not analyzed in the current study [19]. Detailed importable PET/MRI protocol is provided in the supporting material.

PET/MRI images were evaluated by two radiologists (IJ, JV) in conjunction with an experienced nuclear medicine physician (JK). Primary tumor size, possible muscle invasion and metastatic spread was evaluated [20]. Lymph nodes were evaluated on

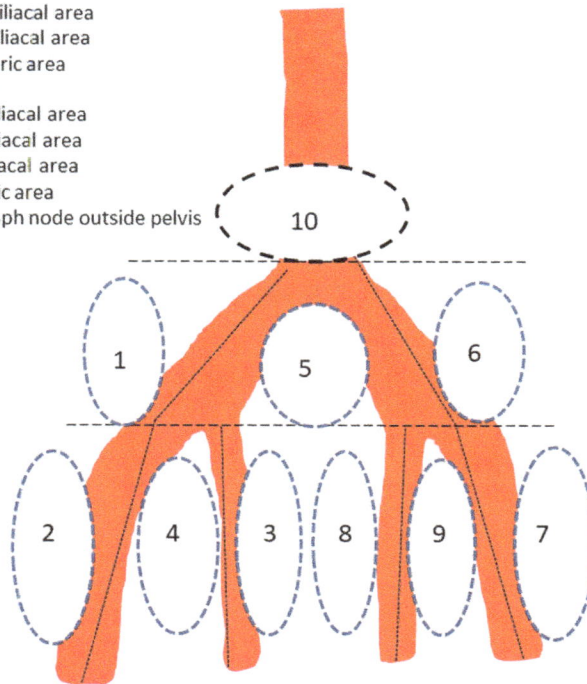

1. Right common iliacal area
2. Right external iliacal area
3. Right internal iliacal area
4. Right obturatoric area
5. Presacral area
6. Left common iliacal area
7. Left external iliacal area
8. Left internal iliacal area
9. Left obturatoric area
10. Suspicious lymph node outside pelvis

Fig. 1 Examined lymph node areas in radical cystectomy

pre-determined 10 regions (suspicion of metastasis vs. benign) as described in Fig. 1.

Treatment

A diagnostic TUR-BT followed imaging after a median of 11 (range 1–21) days (Fig. 2) in the primary tumor evaluation of 15 patients. A complete resection was performed in each case and imaging findings did not affect the extent of the procedure. Further treatment after TUR-BT was done according to standard guidelines [5, 21]. In addition to 15 patients who underwent PET/MRI *before* TUR-BT, three MIBC

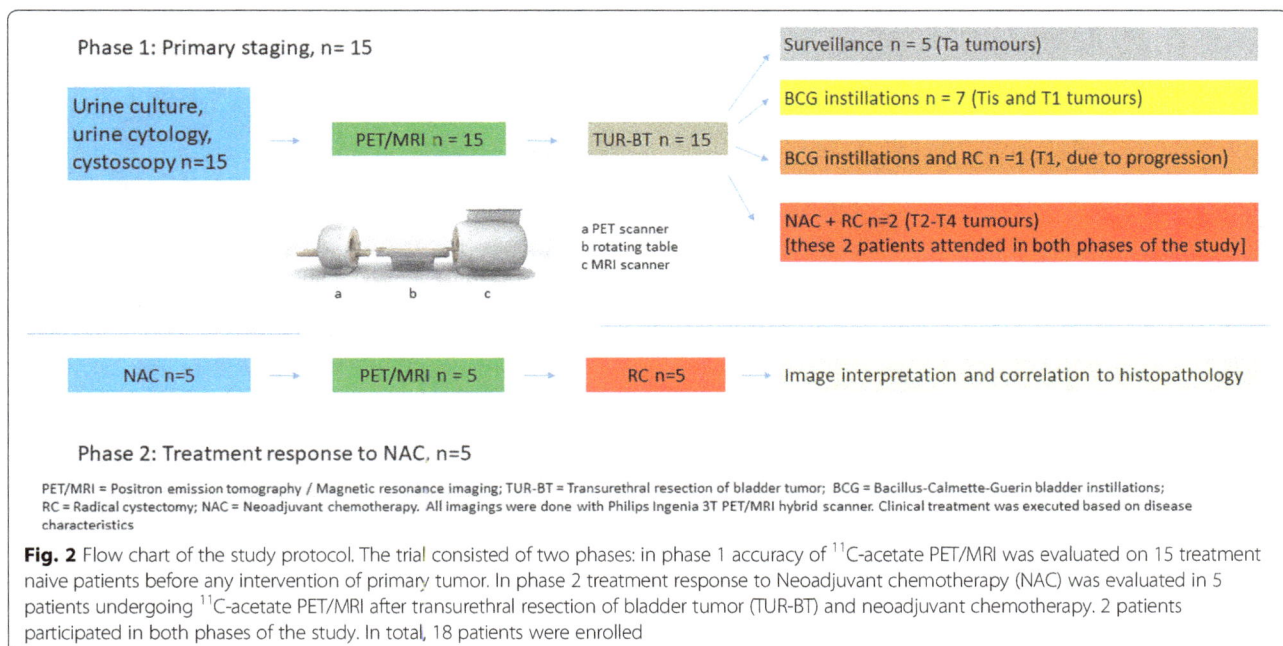

PET/MRI = Positron emission tomography / Magnetic resonance imaging; TUR-BT = Transurethral resection of bladder tumor; BCG = Bacillus-Calmette-Guerin bladder instillations; RC = Radical cystectomy; NAC = Neoadjuvant chemotherapy. All imagings were done with Philips Ingenia 3T PET/MRI hybrid scanner. Clinical treatment was executed based on disease characteristics

Fig. 2 Flow chart of the study protocol. The trial consisted of two phases: in phase 1 accuracy of ^{11}C-acetate PET/MRI was evaluated on 15 treatment naïve patients before any intervention of primary tumor. In phase 2 treatment response to Neoadjuvant chemotherapy (NAC) was evaluated in 5 patients undergoing ^{11}C-acetate PET/MRI after transurethral resection of bladder tumor (TUR-BT) and neoadjuvant chemotherapy. 2 patients participated in both phases of the study. In total, 18 patients were enrolled

patients were enrolled *after* TUR-BT for NAC treatment response evaluation.

NAC treatment response was evaluated in five patients (Table 1). Two patients in this study phase were part of both phases. Five patients received either 3 or 4 cycles of cisplatin-gemcitabine according to treating hospital policy. Second ^{11}C-acetate PET/MRI imaging was performed a median of 21 (range, 11–33) days after completion of NAC. Finally, open RC and extended (E) PLND were performed according to predetermined ten fields described in Fig. 1. Delay from NAC completion to RC was 36 days (range 28-47 days). The selected EPLND template was based on commonly known lymphatic spread pathways [22]. In addition to extent of primary tumour, each predetermined PLND area was separately analysed from the PET/MRI data sets. For the histopathological examination, the RC specimen and the ten PLND areas were sent separately and were analysed by an experienced uropathologist (PT).

Statistics

The statistical analysis was performed using Matlab (version r2013a, The MathWorks Inc., Natick, MA). Sensitivity, specificity and accuracy of ^{11}C-acetate PET/MRI for BT staging in 15 patients who underwent PET/MRI before TUR-BT was compared with TUR-BT histopathology specimens as ground truth. The classification was performed in binary class: benign + non-muscle invasive (Ta/Tis/T1) vs muscle invasive (T2-T4). In five patients presenting with MIBC who underwent RC and PLND, regional classification (10 regions of interest, in total 50 regions) between benign vs malignant LNs was performed. Additional patient level analysis was performed. Receiver operating characteristic curve analysis was used

Table 1 Patients' characteristics

	Primary tumor	NAC[a]
No of patients in phase of study	15	5
Gender (Male/Female)	13/2	5
Age (years)	67 (55–79)	65 (57–69)
ASA-score	2 (1–3)	2
BMI (kg/m²)	27 (23–31)	26 (23–30)
Treatment modality		
TUR-BT and surveillance	5	N/A
TUR-BT and BCG	7	N/A
TUR-BT, NAC, RC and EPLND	2	5
TUR-BT, BCG and RC[b]	1	N/A

Mean values and range are given, when feasible. *ASA-score* The American Society of Anesthesiologists physical status grading system; *BMI* body mass index, *TUR-BT* Transurethral resection of bladder tumor, *BCG* Bacillus-Calmette-Guerin bladder instillations, *RC* radical cystectomy, *EPLND* extended pelvic lymph node dissection, *N/A* not applicable
[a]2 patients participated in both phases of the study
[b]RC due to disease progression

to evaluate ability of ^{11}C-acetate PET/MRI for primary staging and detection of lymph node metastases. Area under the receiver operating characteristic curve (AUC) values were calculated using the trapezoid rule. Ninety-five percent confidence interval for AUC values were calculated from 100,000 bootstrap samples. SUV measurements were compared using Bonferroni multiple comparison test [23].

Results

In total, 15 patients underwent the primary tumour evaluation and five response evaluation with two patients participating in both groups giving a total of 18 participants. Patient characteristics are presented in Table 1. Despite careful and hygienic catheterization three patients (17%, 3/18) developed urinary tract infection after imaging. Two patients subsequently required hospitalization while one patient received antimicrobial treatment at home. In these three patients underlying bacteriuria could not be ruled out since bacteriuria had not been screened before or at the time of enrolment.

Primary staging

All primary tumors were urothelial cancer and demonstrated positive uptake of ^{11}C-acetate. The median maximum standardized uptake value (SUVmax) was 2.9 (range, 1.3–4.7). There was no difference between SUVmax of MIBC versus superficial (clinical stage Tis-T1) BC.

The sensitivity, specificity, accuracy and AUC (95% confidence interval) values of ^{11}C-acetate PET/MRI for the detection of MIBC (primary BT staging) were 1.00, 0.69 and 0.73, and 0.85 (0.55–1.00), respectively (Figs. 3 and 4). The individual differences for all 15 patients between ^{11}C-acetate PET/MRI and TUR-BT are presented in Table 2.

Therapy response evaluation

All five patients with MIBC underwent NAC and had RC and EPLND. NAC was generally well tolerated and all 5 patients received the planned amount of cycles but dose adjustment of anticancer drugs was necessary for 2 patients before surgery. Comparison of ^{11}C-acetate PET/MRI and histopathological evaluation on patient level are presented in Table 3. Compared to histopathology ^{11}C-acetate PET/MRI correctly staged three patients (Figs. 4 and 5), overstaged one (Fig. 6) and understaged one patient. True negative findings in BT were reported in two patients and true positive in one patient, respectively. Details are presented in the Supporting Material.

Lymph node metastases detection

The median number of evaluated nodes per patient was 35 (range 27–43). Of a total 175 LNs removed, 12 (7%)

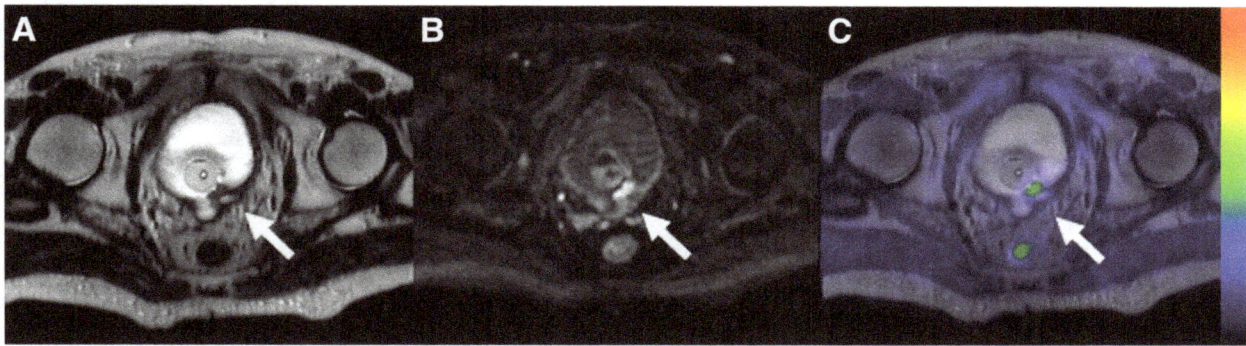

Fig. 3 Pre-transurethral resection ^{11}C-acetate PET/MRI (**a**, **b**, **c**) in a 75-year old male patient (number 3 in primary imaging) showing a heterogenous lobulated mass on the left side of mid-line **without** extension (white arrow) to perivesical fat on T2-weighted image (**a**) or an area of increased diffusion signal restriction (white arrow) extending beyond the bladder wall (**b** - b value 800 s/mm^2 trace diffusion weighted image). The lesion had increased ^{11}C-acetate uptake (**c** - PET fused with T2-weighted image, SUV is scaled from 0.0 to 3.2). The imaging findings were suggestive of T1 stage. The transurethral resection of bladder tumor specimen revealed stage T1, thus the findings of ^{11}C-acetate PET/MRI correctly staged the tumor

harboured metastases. On patient level, two of the five patients had nodal metastatic disease (Table 4, Fig. 5). All metastatic LNs were found around the iliac arteries and none were identified outside the pelvis (Fig. 6). The sensitivity, specificity and accuracy of ^{11}C-acetate PET/MRI for the detection of LN metastases on the predetermined 10 nodal areas were 0.2, 0.96, 0.88, respectively, and AUC (95% confidence interval) value was 0.58. The corresponding values on patient level were 0.5, 0.67, 0.6, and 0.58 respectively (Table 4).

Discussion

This prospective registered clinical trial is the first study to demonstrate feasibility of ^{11}C-acetate PET/MRI in BC staging and its potential to assist in monitoring response to NAC. Compared to CT, MRI as the anatomic

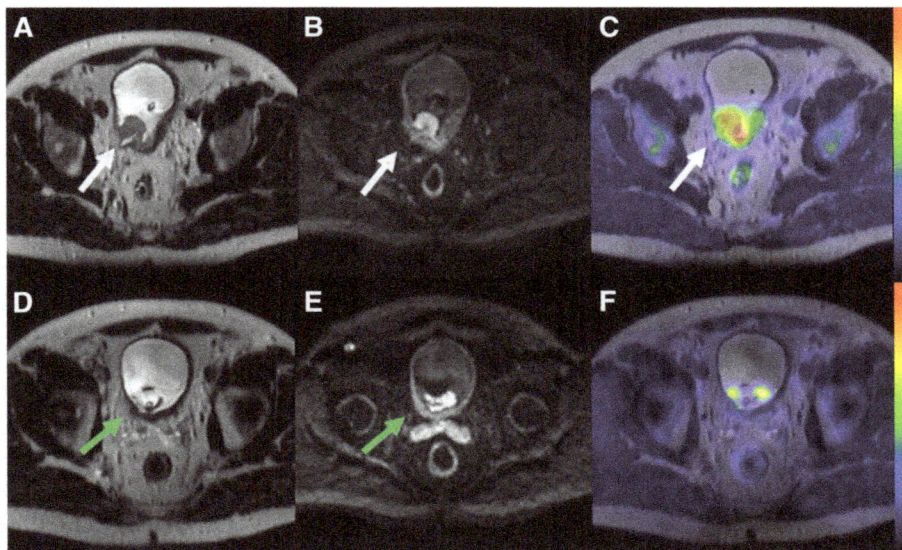

Fig. 4 Comparison of local bladder cancer staging (T-stage) on pre-transurethral resection (**a**, **b**, **c**) and post-chemotherapy ^{11}C-acetate PET/MRI (**d**, **e**, **f**) in a 63-year-old male patient (number 12 in primary imaging). A heterogenous lobulated mass on the right side of mid-line **with** extension (white arrow) to perivesical fat seen on T2-weighted image (**a**), an area of increased diffusion signal restriction (white arrow) beyond the bladder wall (**b** - b value 800 s/mm^2 trace diffusion weighted image), an associated right sided hydroureter, and increased ^{11}C-acetate uptake (**c** - PET fused with T2-weighted image, SUV is scaled from 0.0 to 3.5) suggestive of T3 stage. On post-chemotherapy ^{11}C-acetate PET/MRI, residual abnormal wall thickening (green arrow) on T2-weighted image (**d**) and diffusion signal restriction extending to perivesical fat (**e** - b value 800 s/mm^2 trace diffusion weighted image) was presented suggestive of T3 stage. The final cystectomy specimen revealed stage T2, thus the findings of ^{11}C-acetate PET/MRI were considered as true positive for muscle invasion

Table 2 ^{11}C-acetate PET/MRI primary staging

Patient no	PET-MRI	TUR-BT pathology
1	T1	Tis
2	T1	Ta
3	T1	T1
4	T2	T1
5	T2	T1
6	T3	T2
7	T1	T1
8	T1	Ta
9	T1	Ta
10	T1	Ta
11	T1	T1
12	T3	T2
13	T3	T1
14	T2	Ta
15	T1	T1

PET/MRI positron emission tomography – magnetic resonance imaging, *TUR-BT* transurethral resection of bladder tumor. T-stage according to the TNM classification

modality may be favoured since CT is poor for evaluation of muscle invasion. Similar to prostate cancer [24], ^{11}C- acetate PET/MRI does not seem to offer a satisfactory solution for the detection of metastatic LNs in pelvis due to limited accuracy.

^{11}C-acetate PET/MRI demonstrated accuracy of 0.73 in primary tumor staging, detection of MIBC. In previous studies higher accuracy of MRI alone has been reported [25]. Green et al. [25] noted, however, that differentiation between T1 high grade tumor and T2 tumor is challenging even with known histopathology

Table 3 Treatment response evaluation to neoadjuvant chemotherapy using ^{11}C-acetate PET/MRI. Patients 1 and 2 participated in both phases of the trial, underwent PET/MRI before any intervention and secondary PET/MRI was performed after completion of NAC. Patients 3–5 were enrolled after TUR-BT and underwent PET/MRI after completion of NAC. Imaging after NAC prior RC was compared to RC pathology

Patient	PET/MRI		RC	
	Primary tumour	LNM +/−	Primary tumour	LN n tot / n+
1	T0	+	T0	27 / 0
2	T4	+	T2	42 / 3
3[a]	T0	−	T3	27 / 9
4	T0	−	T0	43 / 0
5	T3	−	T2	36 / 0
				175 / 12

PET/MRI positron emission tomography – magnetic resonance imaging, *RC* radical cystectomy, *LNM* lymph node metastasis (+) = suspicion of presence; (−) = suspicion of absence
[a]Patient had bilateral hip prostheses which distorted the image quality

and TUR-BT stage. Two studies of PET/MRI after TUR-BT or with proven history of BC using 2-deoxy-2-[^{18}F]fluoro-D-glucose (^{18}F-FDG) report high activity in urinary system and in inflammatory tissue [26, 27]. This is clearly detrimental for evaluation of BT because of suboptimal target-to-background ratio. In the current trial, treatment naive patients with suspicion of muscle invasion in cystoscopy were imaged minimizing the impact of inflammatory reaction post TUR-BT. ^{11}C-acetate did not miss any MIBC cases and we hypothesise that ^{11}C- acetate could outperform ^{18}F-FDG since accuracy of ^{18}F-FDG is limited by urine extraction. Although overstaging affected accuracy in the current trial, it is less significant as clinical challenge than understaging, which is a common cause of treatment delay, meaning execution of RC and ePLND.

Only three studies, all published in 2012, reported evaluation of ^{11}C-acetate PET/CT in bladder cancer. Vargas et al. reported on 16 patients and compared MRI, CT and ^{11}C-acetate PET/CT before cystectomy and PLND. They concluded that while all three modalities had similar accuracy PET/CT carried a risk of understaging [28]. Orevi et al. found in a study of 13 patients that ^{11}C-acetate PET/CT was positive in 10 LNs, of which five were malignant giving a specificity of 50% [13]. Finally, Schröder et al. demonstrated that ^{11}C-acetate PET/CT showed specificity of 50% and sensitivity of 80% for the detection of LN metastases. They also noted that intravesical instillation therapy with BCG yielded falsely high positive findings in the resected tumor bed of bladder wall as well as in LNs. [15]. Similar problems were seen by Vargas et al. [28]. In comparison to all these three PET/CT studies [13, 15, 28] in the current trial, specificity of 50% on patient level for detection of regional metastases was found. If one patient with hip prostheses was discarded, sensitivity would have been 100%. It is tempting to assume that ^{11}C-acetate PET/MRI is comparable or better than PET/CT for primary tumor evaluation. However, there are no studies directly comparing PET/CT to PET/MRI in bladder cancer staging and, therefore, the issue remains a matter of further research.

Our registered prospective trial is the third ^{11}C -acetate study evaluating LNs in BC. However, ^{11}C -acetate and PET-MRI have not been used as a surrogate modality before [13, 28, 29]. A pilot study demonstrating the utility of ^{18}F-FDG PET/MRI in BC staging has already been conducted [26]. The results seem to favour PET/MRI in LN evaluation compared to MRI alone, but the number of study subjects was low and needs to be verified in larger studies. Orevi et al. demonstrated that ^{11}C-choline and acetate were comparable in evaluation of lymph node metastases [13], and recent meta-analytic study [29] reports for both tracers low sensitivity and

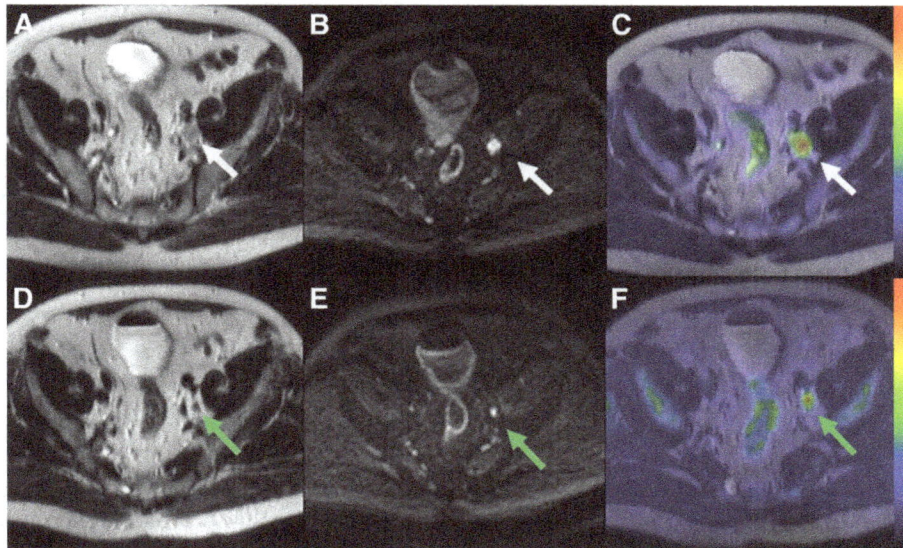

Fig. 5 Comparison of lymph node staging (N-stage) on pre-transurethral resection (**a**, **b**, **c**) and post-chemotherapy ^{11}C-acetate PET/MRI (**d**, **e**, **f**) in patient number 12, the same patient as in Fig. 4. 17 mm right obturator lymph node (**a** - white arrow on T2-weighted image) demonstrated increased diffusion signal restriction (**b** - b value 800 s/mm^2 trace diffusion weighted image) and increased ^{11}C-acetate uptake (**c** - PET fused with T2-weighted image, SUV is scaled from 0.0 to 3.5) suggestive of lymph node metastasis. On post-chemotherapy ^{11}C-acetate PET/MRI, lymph node decreased in size and measured 4 mm (**d** - green arrow on T2-weighted image) with increased diffusion signal (**e** - b value 800 s/mm^2 trace diffusion weighted image) and increased ^{11}C-acetate uptake (**f** - PET fused with T2-weighted image, SUV is scaled from 0.0 to 3.0). SUVmax values of the lymph node on the pre-transurethral resection (**c**) and post-chemotherapy ^{11}C-acetate PET/MRI (**f**) were 3.4 and 2.8, respectively. The lymph node was confirmed to be lymph node metastasis measuring 3 mm on extended pelvic lymph node dissection, thus the findings of ^{11}C-acetate PET/MRI were considered as true positive

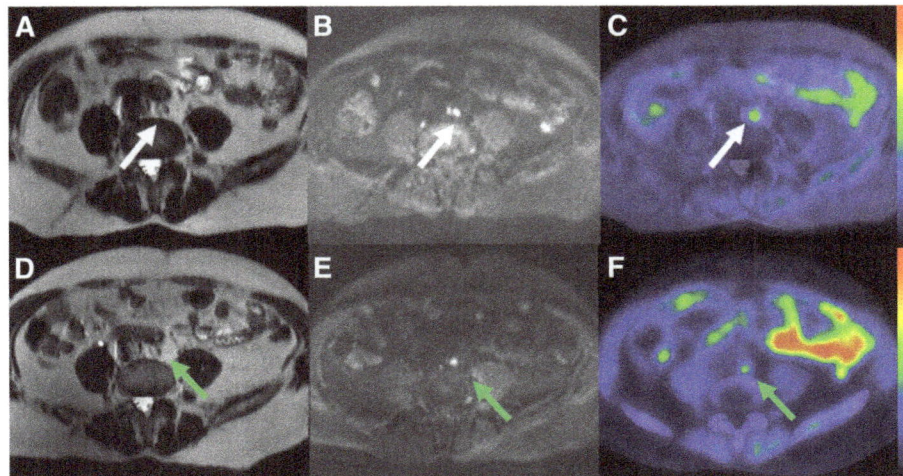

Fig. 6 Comparison of lymph node staging (N-stage) on pre-transurethral resection (**a**, **b**, **c**) and post-chemotherapy ^{11}C-acetate PET/MRI (**d**, **e**, **f**) in a 66-year-old male (patient number 6 in primary imaging). 8 mm retroaortic lymph node (**d** - white arrow on T2-weighted image) demonstrated increased diffusion signal restriction (**b** - b value 800 s/mm^2 trace diffusion weighted image), and increased ^{11}C-acetate uptake (**c** - PET fused with T2-weighted image, SUV is scaled from 0.0 to 2.8) suggestive of lymph node metastasis. On post-chemotherapy ^{11}C-acetate PET/MRI, lymph did not decrease in size and measured 7 mm (**d** - green arrow on T2-weighted image) with increased diffusion signal (**e** - b value 800 s/mm^2 trace diffusion weighted image) and increased ^{11}C-acetate uptake (**f** - PET fused with T2-weighted image, SUV is scaled from 0.0 to 2.8). SUVmax values of the lymph node on the pre-transurethral resection (**c**) and post-chemotherapy ^{11}C-acetate PET/MRI (**f**) was 1.7, 1.3, respectively. No lymph node metastases were found on extended pelvic lymph node dissection, thus the findings of ^{11}C-acetate PET/MRI were considered as false positive

Table 4 ^{11}C-acetate PET/MRI lymph node evaluation

Area of interest	Sensitivity	Specificity	Accuracy	AUC
LN areas ($n = 50$)	0.20	0.96	0.88	0.58
On patient level[a] ($n = 5$)	0.50	0.67	0.60	0.58

[a]evaluation of LN positivity. Only 2 patients had LN metastases and the other had hip prostheses

moderate specificity while heterogeneity of publications limits further conclusions. Our sensitivity of 20% in LN staging is in line with the meta-analysis and we could conclude that the optimal tracer for evaluating urinary tract and pelvic LNs remains to be found.

Studies comparing PET/CT vs. PET/MRI for the detection of lymph nodes are lacking. ^{18}F-FDG PET is widely available and has been studied in multiple studies enrolling BC patients, but prior studies were mainly performed with PET/CT and some compared to CT alone [30–32]. Overall, the results are conflicting. Swinnen et al. found no benefit from adding PET to CT alone [30]. ^{18}F-FDG is highly active in urinary system and forced urinary protocols and delayed execution of PET imaging have been shown to improve performance of ^{18}F-FDG PET/CT [33]. Using these methods, excessive hydration and use of diuretics can also be considered an extra burden for the patient. Although the published evidence does not support routine use of PET-imaging for BC staging, our results indicate that ^{11}C-acetate is a viable tracer option in BC staging.

Our study has several limitations. First, the number of patients especially evaluated for NAC response was low. Furthermore, patient no. 3 in NAC treatment response group had bilateral hip prostheses, which caused B_0 field distortions and the image quality was not optimal. We hypothesize that the patient's largest metastatic 2.0 cm LN would not have been missed if B_0 field distortions were fully compensated. Although excellent therapy responses were found (Figs. 4 and 5) the low number of patients precludes definite conclusion about the value of ^{11}C -acetate PET/MRI in setting of therapy response evaluation. In contrast, compared to previous studies a higher number of treatment ($n = 15$) naive patients underwent baseline imaging, and allowed us to evaluate performance of ^{11}C -acetate PET/MRI without contribution of inflammation to findings. To decrease heterogeneity in future studies, BCG or chemotherapy ideally should not be given before initial PET-MRI or PET-CT. In the current trial T1-weighted imaging and dynamic contrast enhanced MRI were not performed. Before conducting this trial, we have performed very careful optimization of MRI acquisition protocol, done multiple iterations of the acquisition protocol, and carefully optimized the acquisition protocol with special attention on DWI. As can be seen in Figs. 3, 4, 5 and 6, DWI was the "workhorse "for TNM staging of BC. In order to increase openness of our trial, promote #opensource research (#OpenSourceTrial), we share our optimized MRI acquisition protocol in supporting material.

Conclusion

In conclusion, we found a moderate accuracy for staging of primary BC using ^{11}C-acetate PET/MRI in this pilot prospective registered clinical trial. In contrast, only a limited sensitivity for detection of metastatic lymph nodes and response to neoadjuvant chemotherapy was found. Our findings do not advocate for routine use of ^{11}C-acetate PET/MRI in staging of BC but consideration of its potential role in future organ preservation trials with combined use of imaging and other markers, such as molecular information, is warranted.

Abbreviations

AUC: Area under curve; BC: Bladder cancer; BCG: Bacillus-Calmette-Guerin bladder instillation therapy; CT: Computed tomography; DWI: Diffusion weighted imaging; FDG: 2-deoxy-2-[^{18}F]fluoro-D-glucose; FOV: Field of view; LM-OSEM: Maximum-likelihood ordered subsets expectation maximum; MIBC: Muscle invasive bladder cancer; MRAC: MR-based attenuation correction; MRI: Magnetic resonance imaging; NAC: Neoadjuvant chemotherapy; PET/CT: Positron emission tomography – Computed tomography; PET/MRI: Positron emission tomography – Magnetic resonance imaging; PLND: Pelvic lymph node dissection; RC: Radical cystectomy; SUV: Standardized uptake value; TE: Echo Time; Tis: Tumor in situ; TNM: Tumor – node – metastases Classification for malignant tumors; TR: Repetition Time; TUR-BT: Transurethral resection of bladder tumor; USPIO: Ultra small paramagnetic particles of iron oxide

Funding

The study was funded by Finnish Governmental Special Funding grant to the department of Urology, Turku University hospital, and by a research grants by the Sigrid Juselius Foundantion, the Finnish Urology association and Finnish cultural foundation.

Authors' contributions

AS, IJ, PB designed the study; AS, IJ, OE, H.M. and PB wrote the manuscript; AS, IJ, HM performed statistical analysis; IJ, JK, JV performed imaging interpretation; PT performed pathological analysis; AS, IK, JS, EV enrolled the patients; All authors critically evaluated manuscript. All authors read and approved the final manuscript.

Competing interests

The authors declare that they have no competing interests.

Author details

[1]Department of Urology, University of Turku and Turku University hospital, Kiinamyllynkatu 4-8, 20520 Turku, Finland. [2]Department of Radiology, University of Turku and Turku University Hospital, Turku, Finland. [3]Department of Urology, University of Helsinki and Helsinki University hospital, Helsinki, Finland. [4]Department of Urology, University of Tampere and Tampere University hospital, Tampere, Finland. [5]Department of Pathology, Institute of Biomedicine, University of Turku and Turku University hospital, Turku, Finland. [6]Department of Clinical Physiology and nuclear imaging, University of Turku and Turku University hospital, Turku, Finland. [7]Department of Oncology and Radiotherapy, University of Turku and Turku University hospital, Turku, Finland. [8]Department of Radiology, Icahn School of Medicine at Mount Sinai, New York, USA.

References

1. https://seer.cancer.gov/statfacts/html/urinb.html (site visited 6.12.2017).
2. https://ec.europa.eu/jrc/en/publication/epidemiology-bladder-cancer-europe (site visited 30.5.2018).
3. Brierley JD, Gospodarowicz MK, Wittekind C. TNM Classification of Malignant Tumours, 7th Edition 2009.
4. Anastasiadis A, de Reijke TM. Best practice in the treatment of nonmuscle invasive bladder cancer. Ther Adv Urol. 2012;4(1):13–32.
5. Alfred Witjes J, Lebret T, Compérat EM, Cowan NC, De Santis M, Bruins HM, Hernández V, Espinós EL, Dunn J, Rouanne M, Neuzillet Y, Veskimäe E, van der Heijden AG, Gakis G, Ribal MJ. Updated 2016 EAU guidelines on muscle-invasive and metastatic bladder Cancer. Eur Urol. 2016;
6. Advanced Bladder Cancer Overview Collaboration. Neoadjuvant chemotherapy for invasive bladder cancer. Cochrane Database Syst Rev. 2005;2:CD005246. Review
7. Shariat S, et al. Discrepancy between Clinical and Pathologic Stage: Impact on Prognosis after Radical Cystectomy. Eur Urol. 2007;51:137–51.
8. Turker P, Bostrom PJ, Wroclawski ML, van Rhijn B, Kortekangas H, Kuk C, Mirtti T, Fleshner NE, Jewett MA, Finelli A, Kwast TV, Evans A, Sweet J, Laato M, Zlotta AR. Upstaging of urothelial cancer at the time of radical cystectomy: factors associated with upstaging and its effect on outcome. BJU Int. 2012;110(6):804–11.
9. Lin WC, Chen JH. Pitfalls and limitations of diffusion-weighted magnetic resonance imaging in the diagnosis of urinary bladder Cancer. Transl Oncol. 2015;8(3):217–30.
10. Birkhäuser FD, Studer UE, Froehlich JM, Triantafyllou M, Bains LJ, Petralia G, Vermathen P, Fleischmann A, Thoeny HC. Combined ultrasmall superparamagnetic particles of iron oxide-enhanced and diffusion-weighted magnetic resonance imaging facilitates detection of metastases in normal-sized pelvic lymph nodes of patients with bladder and prostate cancer. Eur Urol. 2013;64(6):953–60.
11. Triantafyllou M, Studer UE, Birkhäuser FD, Fleischmann A, Bains LJ, Petralia G, Christe A, Froehlich JM, Thoeny HC. Ultrasmall superparamagnetic particles of iron oxide allow for the detection of metastases in normal sized pelvic lymph nodes of patients with bladder and/or prostate cancer. J Cancer. 2013;49(3):616–24.
12. Goodfellow H, Viney Z, Hughes P, Rankin S, Rottenberg G, Hughes S, Evison F, Dasgupta P, O'Brien T, Khan MS. Role of fluorodeoxyglucose positron emission tomography (FDG PET)-computed tomography (CT) in the staging of bladder cancer. BJU Int. 2014;114(3):389–95.
13. Orevi M, Klein M, Mishani E, Chisin R, Freedman N, Gofrit ON. 11C-acetate PET/CT in bladder urothelial carcinoma: intraindividual comparison with 11C-choline. Clin Nucl Med. 2012;37(4):e67–72.
14. Maurer T, Horn T, Souvatzoglou M, Eiber M, Beer AJ, Heck MM, Haller B, Gschwend JE, Schwaiger M, Treiber U, Krause BJ. Prognostic value of 11C-choline PET/CT and CT for predicting survival of bladder cancer patients treated with radical cystectomy. Urol Int. 2014;93(2):207–13.
15. Schöder H, Ong SC, Reuter VE, Cai S, Burnazi E, Dalbagni G, Larson SM, Bochner BH. Initial results with (11)C-acetate positron emission tomography/computed tomography (PET/CT) in the staging of urinary bladder cancer. Mol Imaging Biol. 2012;14(2):245–51.
16. Rosenkrantz AB, Friedman K, Chandarana H, Meisaether A, Moy L, Ding YS, Jhaveri K, Beltran L, Jain R. Current status of hybrid PET/MRI in oncologic imaging. AJR Am J Roentgenol. 2015;22:1–11.
17. Zaidi H, Ojha N, Morich M, et al. Design and performance evaluation of a whole-body ingenuity TF PET/MRI system. Phys Med Biol. 2011;56:3091.
18. Pruessmann KP, Weiger M, Scheidegger MB, Boesiger P. SENSE: sensitivity encoding for fast MRI. Magn Reson Med. 1999;42(5):952–62.
19. Jambor I, Pesola M, Merisaari H, Taimen P, Boström PJ, Liimatainen T, Aronen HJ. Relaxation along fictitious field, diffusion-weighted imaging, and T2 mapping of prostate cancer: prediction of cancer aggressiveness. Magn Reson Med. 2016;75(5):2130–40.
20. Gandhi N, Krishna S, Booth CM, Breau RH, Flood TA, Morgan SC, Schieda N, Salameh JP, McGrath TA, McInnes M. Diagnostic accuracy of MRI for tumor staging of bladder cancer: systematic review and meta-analysis. BJU Int. 2018; https://doi.org/10.1111/bju.14366. [Epub ahead of print]
21. Babjuk M, Böhle A, Burger CO, Cohen D, Compérat EM, Hernández V, Kaasinen E, Palou J, Rouprêt M, van Rhijn BW, Shariat SF, Soukup V, Sylvester RJ, Zigeuner R. EAU Guidelines on Non-Muscle-invasive Urothelial Carcinoma of the Bladder: Update 2016, Eur Urol. 2016.
22. Roth B, Wissmeyer MP, Zehnder P, Birkhäuser FD, Thalmann GN, Krause TM, Studer UE. A new multimodality technique accurately maps the primary lymphatic landing sites of the bladder. Eur Urol. 2010;57(2):205–11.
23. DeGroot MH, Schervish MJ. Kolmogorov–Smirnov tests. In: Prob- ability and statistics. 4th ed. London: Pearson; 2011. p. 657–8.
24. Jambor I, Borra R, Kemppainen J, Lepomäki V, Parkkola R, Dean K, Alanen K, Arponen E, Nurmi M, Aronen HJ, Minn H. Improved detection of localized prostate cancer using co-registered MRI and 11C-acetate PET/CT. Eur J Radiol. 2012;81(11):2966–72.
25. Green DA, Durand M, Gumpeni N, Rink M, Cha EK, Karakiewicz PI, Scherr DS, Shariat SF. Role of magnetic resonance imaging in bladder cancer: current status and emerging techniques. BJU Int. 2012;110(10):1463–70.
26. Rosenkrantz AB, Balar AV, Huang WC, Jackson K, Friedman KP. Comparison of Coregistration accuracy of pelvic structures between sequential and simultaneous imaging during hybrid PET/MRI in patients with bladder Cancer. Clin Nucl Med. 2015;40(8):637–41.
27. Rosenkrantz AB, Friedman KP, Ponzo F, Raad RA, Jackson K, Huang WC, Balar AV. Prospective pilot study to evaluate the incremental value of PET information in patients with bladder Cancer undergoing 18F-FDG simultaneous PET/MRI. Clin Nucl Med. 2017;42(1):e8–e15.
28. Vargas HA, Akin O, Schoder H, et al. Prospective evaluation of MRI, (11)C-acetate PET/CT and contrast-enhanced CT for staging of bladder cancer. Eur J Radiol. 2012;
29. Kim SJ, Koo PJ, Pak K, Kim IJ, Kim K. Diagnostic accuracy of C-11 choline and C-11 acetate for lymph node staging in patients with bladder cancer: a systematic review and meta-analysis. World J Urol. 2018;36(3):331–40.
30. Swinnen G, Maes A, Pottel H, Vanneste A, Billiet I, Lesage K, et al. FDG-PET/CT for the preoperative lymph node staging of invasive bladder cancer. Eur Urol. 2010;57:641–7.
31. Lodde M, Lacombe L, Friede J, Morin F, Saourine A, Fradet Y. Evaluation of fluorodeoxyglucose positron-emission tomography with computed tomography for staging of urothelial carcinoma. BJU Int. 2010;106:658–63.
32. Kibel AS, Dehdashti F, Katz MD, Klim AP, Grubb RL, Humphrey PA, et al. Prospective study of 18F-fluorodeoxyglucose positron emission tomography/computed tomography for staging of muscle-invasive bladder carcinoma. J Clin Oncol. 2009;27:4314–20.
33. Harkirat S, Anand S, Jacob M. Forced diuresis and dual-phase F-fluorodeoxyglucose-PET/CT scan for restaging of urinary bladder cancers. Indian J Radiol Imaging. 2010;20(1):13–9. https://doi.org/10.4103/0971-3026. 59746.

22

Ultrasound shear wave elastography of breast lesions: correlation of anisotropy with clinical and histopathological findings

Ya-ling Chen[1,2], Yi Gao[1,2], Cai Chang[1,2*], Fen Wang[1,2], Wei Zeng[1,2] and Jia-jian Chen[3]

Abstract

Background: Ultrasound shear-wave elastography (SWE) may increase specificity of breast lesion assessment with ultrasound, but elasticity measurements may change with transducer orientation, defined as anisotropy. In this study, we aimed to observe the anisotropy of SWE of breast lesions, and its correlation with clinical and histopathological findings.

Methods: This retrospective study was approved by institutional review board. From June 2014 to June 2015, a total of 276 women (mean age, 48.75 ± 12.12 years) with 276 breast lesions (174 malignant, 102 benign) were enrolled for conventional ultrasound and SWE before surgical excision. Elasticity modulus in the longest diameter and orthogonal diameter were recorded, including maximum elasticity (Emax), mean elasticity (Emean), standard deviation (Esd) and ratio between mean elasticity of lesion and normal fatty tissue (Eratio). Anisotropy coefficients including anisotropic difference (AD) and anisotropy factors (AF) were calculated, and correlations with malignancy, tumor size, palpability, movability, lesion location and histopathology were analyzed.

Results: The average Emax, Emean, Esd and Eratio of the longest diameter were significantly higher than orthogonal diameter ($P < 0.05$). AUCs of ADs and AFs were inferior to quantitative parameters ($P < 0.001$), with AUCs of AFs superior to ADs ($P < 0.001$). ADs showed no significant correlation with malignancy, palpability, movability, distance from nipple and skin, and histopathological patterns. ADmean was significantly higher in inner half than outer half of the breast ($P = 0.034$). Higher AFs were significantly correlated with larger lesion size ($P = 0.042$), palpability ($P < 0.05$), shorter distance from nipple and skin ($P < 0.05$) and higher suspicion for malignancy ($P < 0.001$). AFs were significantly higher in IDC than DCIS ($P < 0.05$), higher in Grade II/III than Grade I IDC ($P < 0.001$), and correlated with ER/PR(+) ($P < 0.05$).

Conclusions: AF of SWE was an indicator for malignancy and more aggressive breast cancer.

Keywords: Breast lesion, Ultrasound, Elasticity, Shear wave elastography, Anisotropy, BI-RADS

Background

Ultrasound (US) is a useful routine tool in screening and differentiation of benign and malignant breast lesions [1, 2]. The Breast Imaging-Reporting and Data System (BI-RADS) lexicon of American College of Radiology (ACR) has been widely applied in clinical practice [3]. In recent years, breast ultrasonic elastography has become a new promising technique obtaining more accurate characterization of breast lesions [4, 5]. Among the currently used elastography technique, shear wave elastography (SWE) induces shear waves which propagate transversely in the tissue, and has been confirmed as a quantitative stiffness measurement technique of high reproducibility and less operator dependency, compared to external mechanical compression based strain elastography [4, 6]. Previous studies demonstrated that combination of conventional US with SWE features significantly improved specificity of breast mass assessment without loss of sensitivity [7–11], and thus could reduce unnecessary biopsies of low-suspicion BI-RADS category 4A masses.

* Correspondence: changcai1962@163.com
[1]Department of Ultrasound, Fudan University Shanghai Cancer Center, No. 270 Dong-An Road, Shanghai 200032, China
[2]Department of Oncology, Shanghai Medical College, Fudan University, No. 270 Dong-An Road, Shanghai 200032, China
Full list of author information is available at the end of the article

When performing SWE examination, the imaging planes used in reported studies of SWE have varied. In some studies, SWE images were acquired in a single transducer orientation for each mass [7, 9]. However, in other studies, two orthogonal planes were obtained routinely, either radial/antiradial planes or transverse/longitudinal planes [10, 12], and diagnostic performance was improved by combining conventional ultrasound with two-view SWE (two orthogonal planes) compared with combining with single-view SWE (single transducer orientation) [12].

Anisotropy is an orientation-dependent property that exists in fiber-rich tissues, which implies different properties in different directions. In terms of ultrasound elastograpy, anisotropy could be defined as different imaging features with the change of orientation of the transducer, resulting in different measurements of elasticity when assessing along different axes. Recently, Zhou et al. has demonstrated the anisotropy of elasticity of normal breast glandular and fatty tissue by comparing measurements of radial and antiradial planes [13]. Previous studies observed anisotropy in solid breast lesions [14], and Skerl et al. discovered anisotropy in SWE as an indicator of malignancy [15]. Nevertheless, in the aforementioned study, the anisotropy factor (AF) was calculated with Emean, which was defined as mean elasticity of the stiffest area using a region of interest size (ROI) of 2 mm, rather than the measurements of the whole lesions. Besides, anisotropy of other quantitative parameters such as Emax, Esd and Eratio has not been analyzed yet [15].

The aim of this study is to observe the anisotropy of each SWE quantitative parameter of breast lesions between two orthogonal planes, and its correlation with clinical and histopathological findings in Chinese patients.

Materials and methods

Patients

A retrospective analysis of 284 consecutive women with 284 breast lesions detected by palpation and/or imaging was performed from June 2014 to June 2015. All participants were inpatients from department of Breast Surgery of our center, and underwent conventional US and 2-dimensional (2D) SWE before surgical excision. Eight patients with large masses (over 4 cm) which couldn't be covered by SWE colour overlay were excluded. Finally, 276 women (mean age, 48.75 ± 12.12 years; age range, 21–84 years) with 276 breast lesions constituted the study cohort.

Image acquisition

Conventional US and 2D SWE were performed using the Aixplorer® US system (SuperSonic Imagine, Aix-en-Provence, France) with a SL15–4 multifrequency linear-array transducer by one of three radiologists with 5–20 years'

experience in breast imaging (Y.L.C., Y.G. and F.W.). Prior to this clinical trial, all participating investigators had performed over 4000 breast US examinations in two years, and had practiced breast SWE on over 200 cases for the last 6 months. We firstly used the default preset of breast, with center frequency at "GEN", dynamic range at 70 dB, tissue tuner 1480 m/s. We decreased the center frequency to "PEN" if lesions were deeply located, while increased to "RES" with superficial location. The clockwise location, distance from the nipple and the skin were recorded.

SWE was carried out at default scale – 180 kPa. Three acquisitions through the longest diameter of the lesion (View A) and another three acquisitions through the orthogonal diameter plane (View B) were obtained and saved for analysis.

Image evaluation

Before SWE examination, independent and blinded review of conventional US images was performed by two investigators (C.C. and W.Z.) with 20 years of experience in breast US, and classified into appropriate categories according to ACR BI-RADS US [3].

Quantitative SWE features were measured on each SWE images of View A and View B using the quantification tool built in Aixplorer® US system. By using a circular ROI covering as much as the entire lesion and any immediately adjacent stiff areas on the SWE images, we measured maximal elasticity (Emax), mean elasticity (Emean), standard deviation of elasticity (Esd) of the whole lesion. The ratio between the mean elasticity of the lesion and normal fatty tissue (Eratio) was calculated with the same circular ROI of 2 mm of diameter placed on the stiffest portion of the lesion (or its immediately adjacent tissue) and normal fatty tissue respectively. Average values for each parameter of three acquisitions in both View A and View B were calculated.

Anisotropy

To evaluate the anisotropic properties of SWE of breast lesions, anisotropy coefficients were calculated to quantify the differences in elasticity between View A and View B through the equations below [15]. The anisotropic difference (AD) for Emax, Emean, Esd and Eratio was calculated as

$$\mathrm{ADmax} = \mathrm{Emax_{View\ A}} - \mathrm{Emax_{View\ B}},\ \mathrm{ADmean} = \mathrm{Emean_{View\ A}} - \mathrm{Emean_{View\ B}}$$

$$\mathrm{ADsd} = \mathrm{Esd_{View\ A}} - \mathrm{Esd_{View\ B}},\ \mathrm{ADratio} = \mathrm{Eratio_{View\ A}} - \mathrm{Eratio_{View\ B}}$$

The anisotropy factor (AF) was calculated as the square of AD to evaluate the general anisotropy of the lesion independent on the stiffer plane:

$$AF = AD^2$$

Clinical findings

Clinical data of each patient was recorded, such as palpability, movability and location of the lesions. When recording the location, we divided the breast into four quadrants, including upper inner quadrant, upper outer quadrant, lower inner quadrant and lower outer quadrant, and assessed the location according to the center of the lesion. According to the nipple level, the breast was divided into upper half (upper inner quadrant and upper outer quadrant) and lower half (lower inner quadrant and lower outer quadrant). Upper inner quadrant and lower inner quadrant constituted the inner half, while upper outer quadrant and lower outer quadrant constituted the outer half.

Histopathologic examination

All the lesions enrolled underwent surgical excision, and histopathological outcome was used as the Gold Standard, which was made by a pathologist with 20 years of experience in breast pathology who was blinded to the US results.

Statistical analysis

Statistical analyses were performed by Y.L.C and J.J.C using SPSS, version 19.0 (SPSS, Chicago, IL, USA). Receiver operating characteristic (ROC) curves were analyzed using MedCalc for Windows, version 15.6 (MedCalc Software, Mariakerke, Belgium). The area under ROC curves (AUC) for conventional US, quantitative parameters of SWE and anisotropy coefficients were calculated for diagnostic performance analysis. The optimal cutoff values were determined with the Youden index. Comparison of AUC was performed using the method proposed by DeLong et al. [16]. Anisotropy coefficients were compared between benign and malignant lesions, using the Kruskal-Wallis test. Nonparametric tests for trend were used for analysis across ordered groups. Spearman correlation coefficient (ρ) was used for correlation analysis. A $P < 0.05$ was considered to indicate a statistically significant difference.

Results

The histopathological results of the 276 lesions were shown in Table 1, among which 174 (63.0%) were malignant, and 102 (37.0%) were benign. The average of maximal diameter at conventional US was 15.65 ± 5.57 mm (range, 6–31 mm; median 14.76 mm), with malignant lesions significantly larger than benign lesions (19.70 ± 6.02 mm vs. 15.28 ± 5.24 mm, $P < 0.001$). Except for 32 (11.6%) lesions detected by

imaging, the rest 244 (88.4%) were palpable, among which 104 lesions were movable.

Quantitative elasticity of two orthogonal planes

Both by considering the total lesions together and the benign group alone, the average Emax, Emean, Esd and Eratio were significantly higher in View A than View B ($P < 0.05$). In the malignant group, Emax and Emean were significantly higher in View A than View B ($P < 0.05$), without significant difference for Esd and Eratio Figs. 1, 2.

All the quantitative parameters (Emax, Emean, Esd and Eratio) in View A and View B were significantly higher in malignant group than benign group ($P < 0.001$) Fig. 1.

Anisotropy of quantitative parameters of SWE

We calculated the AD and AF of Emax, Emean, Esd and Eratio between two orthogonal planes. ADs showed positive correlation with quantitative parameters of in View A ($P < 0.001$) while negative correlation with View B ($P < 0.01$). AFs showed positive correlation with quantitative parameters (Emax, Emean, Esd and Eratio) ($P < 0.001$). ADs didn't show significant difference between malignant and benign lesions. However, AFs were significantly higher in malignant lesions than in benign lesions ($P < 0.001$) Fig. 3.

Diagnostic performance of anisotropy coefficient

AUC of conventional US according to BI-RADS was 0.918, with cutoff value between BI-RADS 4A and 4B. AUCs of ADs and AFs were inferior to AUCs of quantitative parameters (Emax: 0.940, Emean: 0.921, Esd: 0.944, Eratio: 0.940) and conventional US ($P < 0.001$), while AUCs of AFs (AFmax: 0.760, AFmean: 0.702, AFsd: 0.802, AFratio: 0.804) were superior to ADs

Table 1 Pathologic Diagnosis of 276 Breast Lesions

Pathologic Diagnosis	No. of Lesions	Percent
Malignant Lesions	174	
Invasive ductal Carcinoma	156	89.7
Invasive lobular Carcinoma	4	2.3
Ductal carcinoma in situ	13	7.5
Mucinous adenocarcinoma	1	0.6
Benign Lesions	102	
Fibroadenoma	59	57.8
Adenosis	19	18.6
Intraductal papilloma	19	18.6
Benign phyllodes tumor	1	1.0
Mastitis	4	3.9

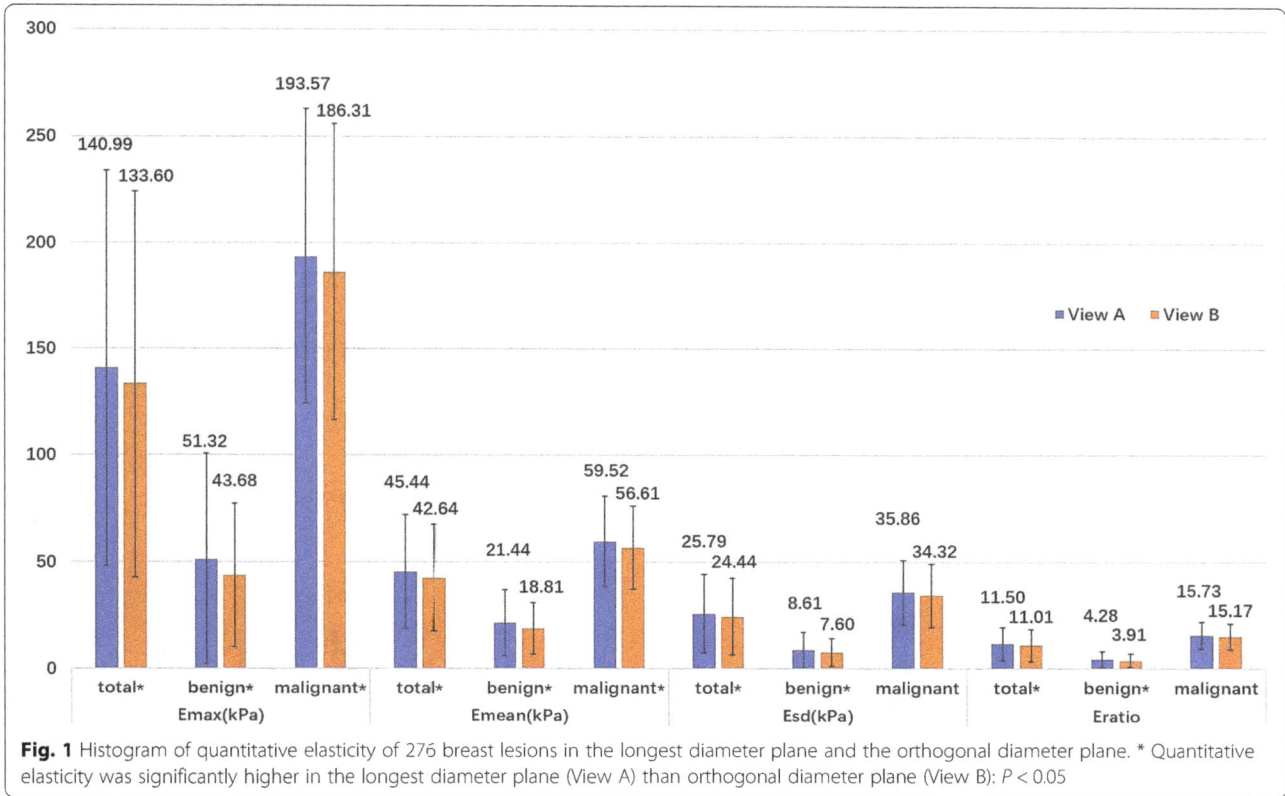

Fig. 1 Histogram of quantitative elasticity of 276 breast lesions in the longest diameter plane and the orthogonal diameter plane. * Quantitative elasticity was significantly higher in the longest diameter plane (View A) than orthogonal diameter plane (View B): $P < 0.05$

(ADmax: 0.525, ADmean: 0.501, ADsd: 0.516, ADratio: 0.512) ($P < 0.001$), with optimal cutoff value higher than 159.52 kPa^2 (AFmax), 21.44 kPa^2 (AFmean), 10.89 kPa^2 (AFsd) and 1.35 (AFratio) Fig. 4.

All the SWE quantitative parameters (Emax, Emean, Esd and Eratio) were significantly higher in high-suspicious group (BI-RADS 4B, 4C & 5) than in low-suspicious group (BI-RADS 3 & 4A) ($P < 0.001$). ADs showed no significant difference between two groups ($P > 0.05$), while AFs were significantly higher in high-suspicious group than in low-suspicious group ($P < 0.001$) Fig. 5.

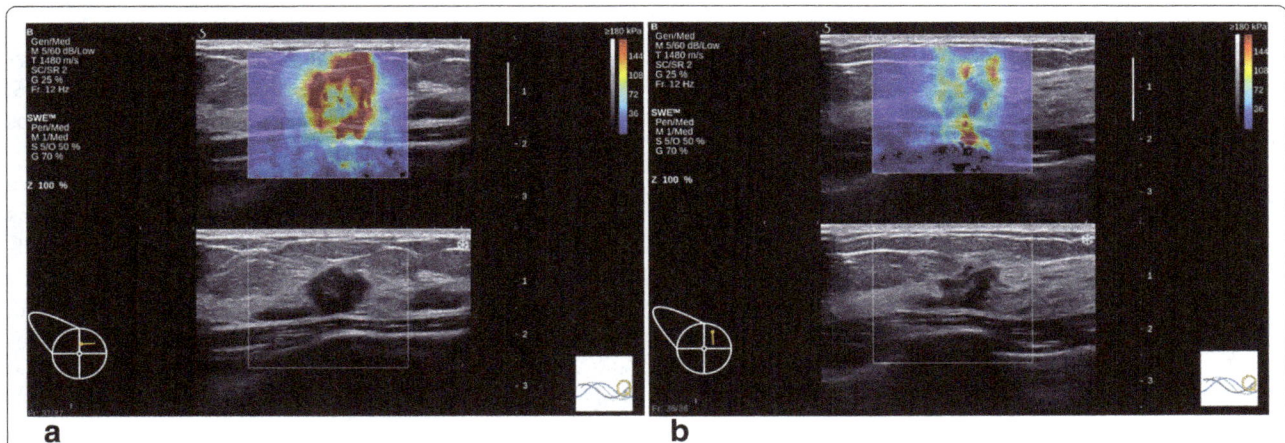

Fig. 2 The longest diameter plane (View A) showed higher elasticity than the orthogonal diameter plane (View B) in a malignant lesion. A mass in the upper-inner quadrant of right breast of a 45-year-old woman was histopathologically confirmed as invasive ductal carcinoma (Grade II). **a** In View A, Emax, Emean and Esd were 300 kPa, 145.4 kPa and 61.9 kPa, respectively. **b** In View B, Emax, Emean and Esd were 164.2 kPa, 70.9 kPa and 25.9 kPa, respectively

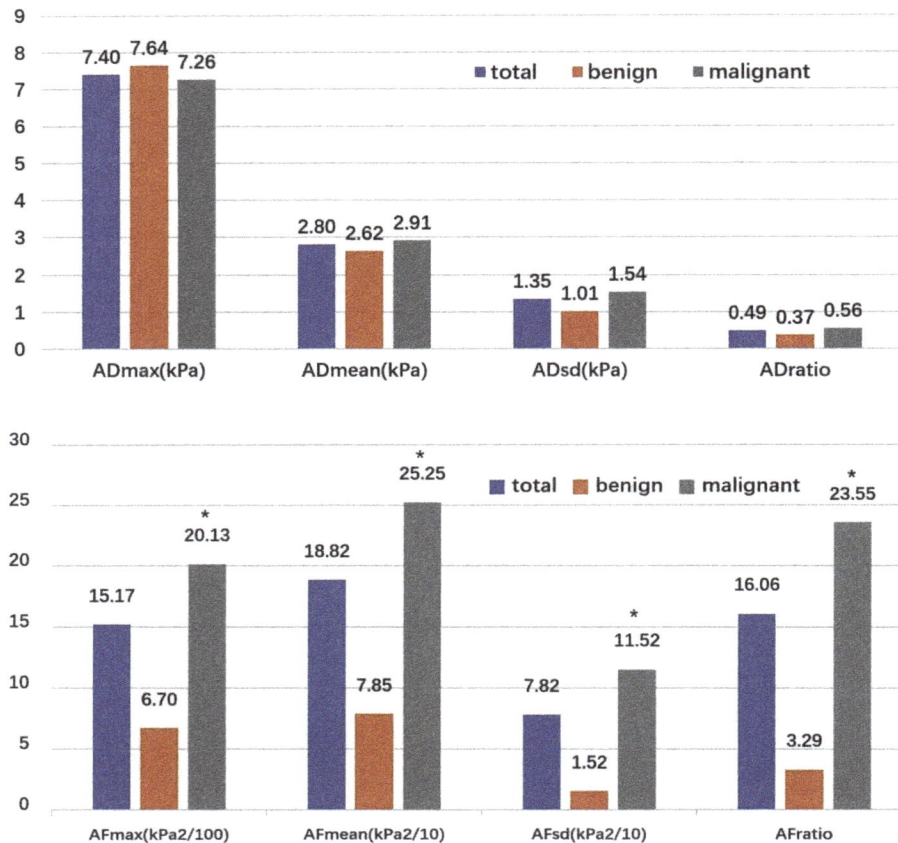

Fig. 3 Anisotropy factor (AF) was significantly higher in malignant lesions than in benign lesions (*P* < 0.001), while anisotropic difference (AD) did not show significant difference. * malignant vs. benign: *P* < 0.05

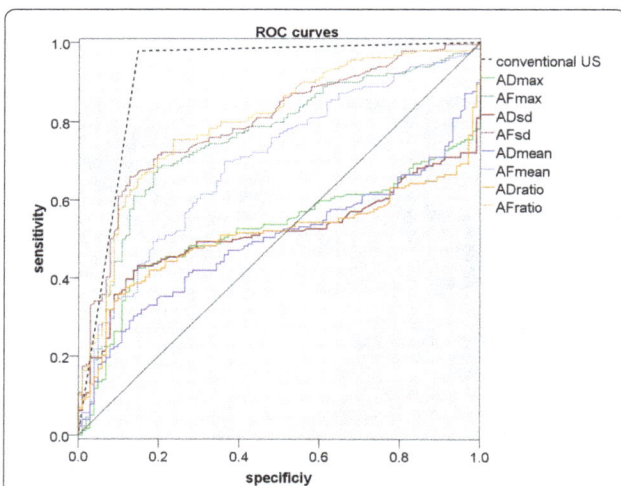

Fig. 4 ROC curves of anisotropic difference (ADs) and anisotropy factor (AFs) compared to conventional US assessment. The diagnostic performance of ADs and AFs was inferior to that of conventional US, while diagnostic performance of AFs was superior to that of ADs

Correlation of anisotropy coefficients with lesion size

The total lesions were divided into large lesions group (≥ 15 mm) and small lesions group (< 15 mm) according to the cutoff value calculated by ROC analysis in our study cohort (≥ 15 mm). A cut-off threshold of 15 mm was used also because it was between the median (14.76 mm) and the mean (15.45 mm) of the lesion size, and therefore, gave groups of similar numbers.

Quantitative parameters Emax, Esd and Eratio were significantly higher in large lesions than small lesions (*P* < 0.001), while Emean did not show significant difference. ADmax, ADmean and ADsd were significantly higher in small lesions than large lesions (*P* < 0.05), while AFsd was significantly higher in large lesions (*P* = 0.042). ADs did not show significant difference between malignant and benign group, either in large lesions or small lesions. AFs were significantly higher in malignant lesions than benign lesions both in large lesions (AFmax, AFmean, AFsd and AFratio: *P* < 0.001) and in small lesions (AFsd: *P* = 0.020; AFratio: *P* = 0.005) Fig. 6.

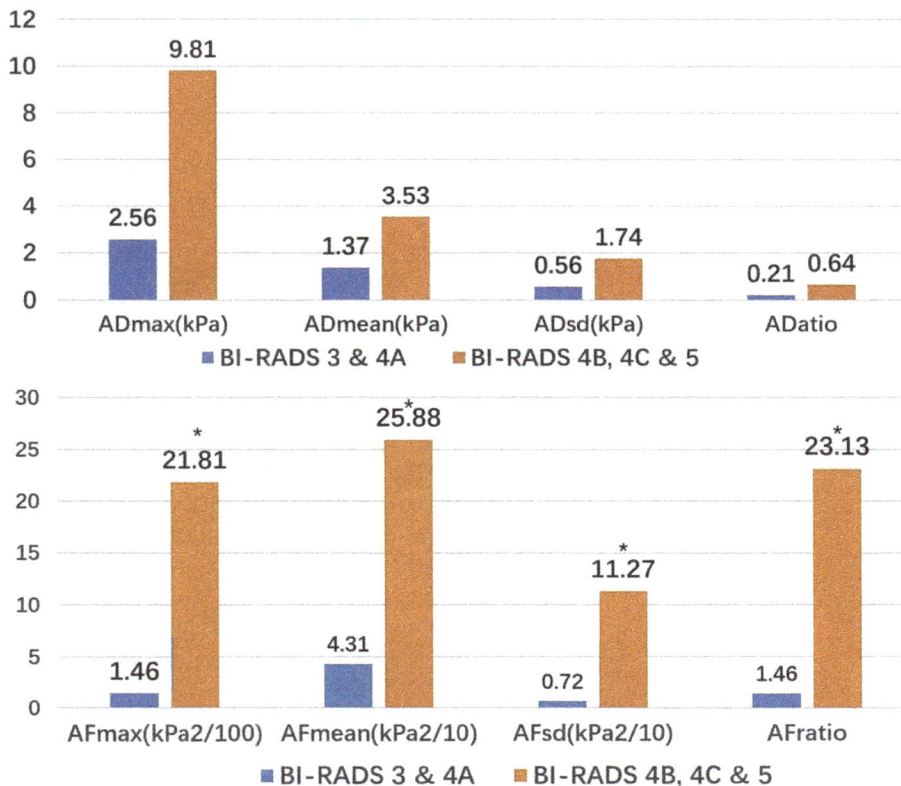

Fig. 5 Correlation between anisotropy and malignancy. Anisotropy factor (AF) was significantly higher in high-suspicious group (BI-RADS 4B, 4C & 5) than in low-suspicious group (BI-RADS 3 & 4A) ($P < 0.001$), while anisotropic difference (AD) showed no significant difference. * high-suspicious group vs. low-suspicious group: $P < 0.05$

Correlation of anisotropy coefficients with clinical findings

All the quantitative parameters (Emax, Emean, Esd and Eratio) were significantly higher in palpable lesions than impalpable lesions ($P < 0.001$), and significantly higher in immovable lesions than movable lesions ($P < 0.001$).

ADs did not show significant correlation with palpability and movability. AFsd and AFratio were significantly higher in palpable lesions than impalpable lesions (AFsd: $P = 0.009$; AFratio: $P < 0.001$), while AFmax, AFmean showed no significant difference between two groups. In palpable group, AFs were significantly higher in immovable lesions than movable ones (AFmax: $P < 0.001$; AFmean: $P = 0.006$; AFsd: $P < 0.001$; AFratio: $P = 0.002$) Table 2.

Correlation of anisotropy coefficients with distance of lesions from the nipple

By analyzing the total lesions together, negative correlation was found between AFmean and distance of lesions from the nipple ($\rho = -0.124$, $P = 0.039$).

In the benign group, all the quantitative parameters (Emax, Emean, Esd and Eratio) and AFs except AFmean showed significantly negative correlation with the distance from the nipple ($P < 0.05$) Table 3.

Correlation of anisotropy coefficients with the depth of lesions

By analyzing the total lesions, negative correlation with the depth of lesions was found in all the quantitative parameters (Emax, Emean, Esd and Eratio) ($P < 0.001$) and also in AFmax and AFmean ($P < 0.05$).

Nevertheless, negative correlation with the depth of lesions was only found in AFmax in the benign group ($\rho = -0.202$, $P = 0.042$), and in quantitative parameters Emean ($\rho = -0.172$, $P = 0.023$) and Eratio ($\rho = -0.217$, $P = 0.004$) in the malignant group Table 3.

Correlation of anisotropy coefficients with quadrant location of lesions

Analyzing the total lesions, none of the quantitative parameters (Emax, Emean, Esd and Eratio) nor anisotropy coefficients (ADs and AFs) showed significant correlation with quadrant location or upper/lower half

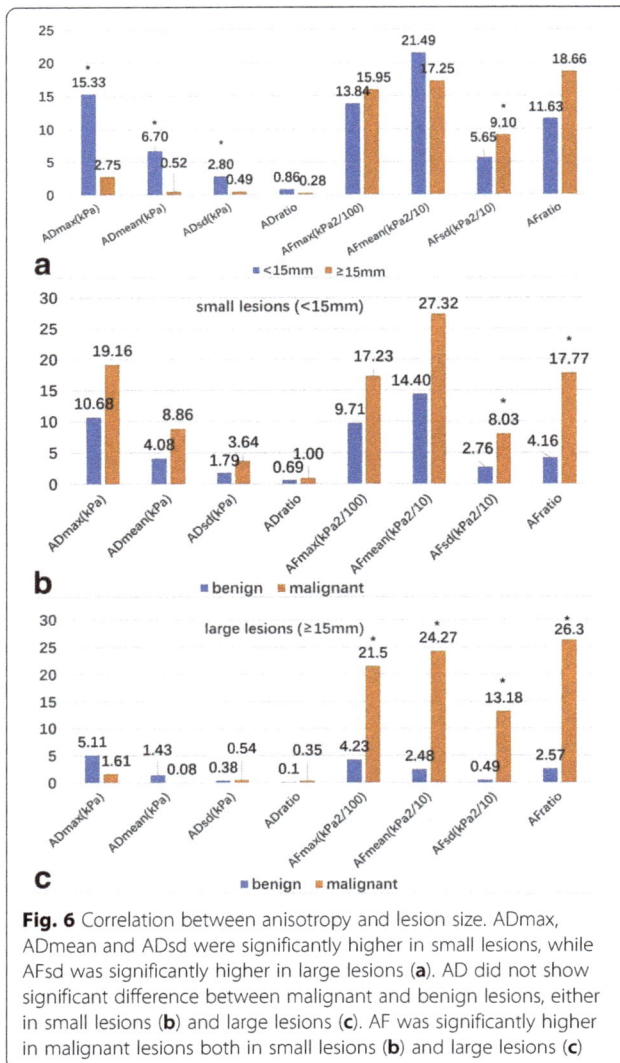

Fig. 6 Correlation between anisotropy and lesion size. ADmax, ADmean and ADsd were significantly higher in small lesions, while AFsd was significantly higher in large lesions (**a**). AD did not show significant difference between malignant and benign lesions, either in small lesions (**b**) and large lesions (**c**). AF was significantly higher in malignant lesions both in small lesions (**b**) and large lesions (**c**)

Correlation of anisotropy coefficients with histopathology

All the quantitative parameters (Emax, Emean, Esd and Eratio) were significantly higher in invasive ductal carcinoma (IDC) lesions than ductal carcinoma in situ (DCIS) lesions ($P < 0.001$).

ADs did not show significant correlation with different tumor types, estrogen receptor (ER)/progesterone receptor (PR), HER2 and Ki-67 expression, and lymph node metastasis ($P > 0.05$).

AFs were significantly higher in IDC lesions than DCIS lesions (AFmax, AFsd, AFratio: $P < 0.01$). AFratio was significantly lower in Grade I IDC than Grade II and Grade III IDC ($P < 0.001$) Table 5.

Some AFs were significantly higher in ER/PR positive lesions than ER/PR negative lesions [ER(+) vs. ER(−): AFsd 13.02 ± 20.28 vs. 7.33 ± 10.96 kPa^2/10, $P = 0.019$; AFmean 29.22 ± 53.32 vs. 14.36 ± 26.72 kPa^2/10, $P = 0.016$; PR(+) vs. PR(−): AFsd 13.59 ± 20.85 vs. 7.28 ± 11.05 kPa^2/10, $P = 0.01$], without significant correlation with HER2, Ki-67 expression and lymph node metastasis.

Discussion

Anisotropy is the property of being directionally dependent, which exists in biological tissues rich in fibers. As the glandular and fatty tissue organized along the ducts leading radially to the nipple, breast tissue is structurally anisotropic with radial orientation in the whole breast [17, 18]. The mechanical anisotropy created by highly aligned collagen fibers facilitates elongation and branching [19]. Recently, anisotropy of elasticity has been demonstrated in normal breast glandular and fatty tissue [13]. Owing to the propagation of shear wave that was roughly parallel to the direction of fibers of Cooper's ligaments and ducts in the radial plane, shear wave velocity in radial plane was significantly higher than anti-radial plane in both glandular tissue and fatty tissue [13]. A previous study has demonstrated the existence of anisotropy of Emean in breast lesions, with a 2 mm ROI focused on the stiffest area of the lesion rather than the measurements of the whole lesions, without analyzing anisotropy of other SWE quantitative parameters such as Emax, Esd and Eratio [15]. The objective of our study was to investigate the anisotropy of

location. Nevertheless, all the quantitative parameters (Emax, Emean, Esd and Eratio) were significantly higher in inner half than outer half ($P < 0.001$), so did the coefficient ADmean ($P = 0.034$). In the benign group, ADmean and AFmean were also significantly higher in inner half than outer half ($P < 0.05$) Table 4.

Table 2 Correlation of anisotropy factor (AF) with Clinical Findings

Clinical Findings	AFmax (kPa^2/100)	AFmean (kPa^2/10)	AFsd (kPa^2/10)	AFratio
Palpable ($n = 244$)	15.71 ± 28.53	19.66 ± 43.56	$8.39 \pm 16.29^*$	$17.54 \pm 37.46^*$
Impalpable ($n = 32$)	11.00 ± 32.46	12.39 ± 20.31	3.52 ± 8.27	4.78 ± 8.13
Movable ($n = 104$)	8.27 ± 21.90	13.82 ± 37.69	4.94 ± 13.06	10.52 ± 28.49
Immovable ($n = 140$)	$21.30 \pm 31.45^\#$	$25.43 \pm 50.92^\#$	$11.43 \pm 18.76^\#$	$23.12 \pm 42.93^\#$

*AFsd and AFratio were significantly higher in palpable lesions than in impalpable ones ($P = 0.009$ and $P < 0.001$; respectively)

#AFmax, AFmean, AFsd and AFratio were significantly higher in immovable lesions than in movable ones ($P < 0.001$, $P = 0.006$, $P < 0.001$ and $P = 0.002$; respectively)

Table 3 Correlation of anisotropy coefficient with distance from the nipple and depth of lesion

Anisotropy Coefficients	Distance from nipple (Spearman's ρ)			Depth of lesions (Spearman's ρ)		
	Total	Benign	Malignant	Total	Benign	Malignant
ADmax	−0.006	−0.101	0.046	−0.082	−0.094	−0.061
ADmean	−0.047	−0.082	−0.031	−0.019	−0.083	−0.006
ADsd	−0.011	−0.111	0.032	−0.069	−0.085	−0.045
ADratio	0.026	−0.193	0.112	−0.026	−0.015	−0.004
AFmax	−0.005	−0.199 *	0.063	−0.125 #	−0.202 #	−0.018
AFmean	−0.124 *	−0.187	−0.131	−0.120 #	−0.089	−0.097
AFsd	−0.010	−0.216 *	−0.003	−0.098	−0.021	−0.087
AFratio	0.013	−0.195 *	0.076	−0.104	−0.102	−0.051

*correlation of AF with the distance from the nipple: Total lesions: AFmean $P = 0.039$. Benign group: AFmax $P = 0.045$; AFsd $P = 0.029$; AFratio $P = 0.049$
#correlation of AFs with the depth of lesions: Total lesions: AFmax $P = 0.039$; AFmean $P = 0.046$. Benign group: AFmax $P = 0.042$

all the quantitative parameters, with large ROI covering as much as the lesion.

In the study by Skerl et al., about half breast lesions were stiffer in radial planes and the other half stiffer in anti-radial planes [15]. Differently in our study, quantitative elasticity of breast lesions was significantly higher in longest diameter plane than orthogonal diameter plane, indicating that anisotropy did exist in elasticity of breast lesions. The different results might due to the different planes chosen for anisotropy analysis between Skerl's study and ours. When assessing breast lesions in conventional ultrasound imaging, the longest diameter and its orthogonal plane were adopted for measurement, as a widely accepted method, rather than always measuring radial/anti-radial planes or anatomically sagittal/axial planes [3]. Because in clinical practice, breast tumors were not always oriented horizontally or vertically but sometimes obliquely within the image. As tumor cells at the tumor boundary contract and align collagen fibers with the assistance of proteolytic cleavage, and then invade along aligned collagen structure to expand the tumor and later metastasize [20]. Previous study

demonstrated that there was an excellent correlation between the mean tumor stiffness value and the maximum diameter ($r = 0.94$, $P < 0.0001$) [21]. The elasticity, represented as Young's modulus E, is positively correlated with the square of propagating speed of shear wave. Therefore, we hypothesized that shear wave propagated faster along the maximum diameter, which could explain the significantly higher elasticity in the longest diameter of the lesions, and was in agreement with that proposed by Skerl et al. [15].

Previous study by Skerl et al. demonstrated that in lesions with higher Esd value (≥ 7 kPa), AFs calculated by radial and anti-radial planes showed no significant difference between malignant and benign lesions, while AFs calculated by two orthogonal planes unrelated to radial orientation (sagittal/axial planes) were significantly higher in malignant lesions than benign lesions [15]. In other words, anisotropy factor calculated by two orthogonal planes unrelated to radial orientation was more predictable for malignancy than that calculated by radial/anti-radial planes for more heterogeneous lesions. In our study, the lesions enrolled were more

Table 4 Correlation of anisotropy coefficient with quadrant location

Anisotropy Coefficients	Quadrant Location					
	Total		Benign		Malignant	
	Inner half	Outer half	Inner half	Outer half	Inner half	Outer half
ADmax (kPa)	12.89 ± 35.95	5.60 ± 38.96	15.92 ± 31.42	6.10 ± 23.35	11.96 ± 37.47	5.25 ± 47.05
ADmean (kPa)	5.96 ± 14.32 *	1.77 ± 13.03	8.15 ± 13.57 *	1.60 ± 6.83	5.29 ± 14.61	1.89 ± 16.05
ADsd (kPa)	2.35 ± 8.39	1.02 ± 8.87	2.11 ± 5.94	0.81 ± 3.24	2.42 ± 9.06	1.16 ± 11.28
ADratio	0.13 ± 3.77	0.61 ± 4.05	0.32 ± 2.53	0.38 ± 1.63	0.07 ± 4.10	0.77 ± 5.12
AFmax (kPa^2/100)	14.40 ± 23.45	15.42 ± 30.63	11.70 ± 27.43	5.76 ± 24.38	15.20 ± 22.32	22.32 ± 32.78
AFmean (kPa^2/10)	23.77 ± 49.40	17.20 ± 38.68	23.97 ± 50.67 *	4.87 ± 12.54	23.72 ± 49.41	25.90 ± 47.58
AFsd (kPa^2/10)	7.49 ± 11.88	7.93 ± 16.71	3.75 ± 6.95	1.10 ± 4.21	8.64 ± 12.86	12.75 ± 20.21
AFratio	14.05 ± 23.30	16.72 ± 38.79	6.10 ± 12.04	2.77 ± 9.64	16.50 ± 25.39	26.56 ± 47.68

*Inner half vs. Outer half:
Total lesions: ADmean $P = 0.034$
Benign group: ADmean $P = 0.004$; AFmean $P = 0.003$

Table 5 Correlation of anisotropy coefficient with histological grades in IDC lesions

	Grade I	Grade II	Grade III
ADmax (kPa)	−12.01 ± 22.33	13.46 ± 44.15	4.20 ± 49.42
AFmax (kPa²/100)	5.72 ± 13.27	21.03 ± 30.09	24.28 ± 33.24
ADmean (kPa)	−1.99 ± 5.64	4.49 ± 17.40	2.11 ± 15.30
AFmean (kPa²/10)	3.13 ± 3.51	31.88 ± 59.04	23.55 ± 42.15
ADsd (kPa)	−3.16 ± 7.46	2.94 ± 11.23	1.23 ± 11.06
AFsd (kPa²/10)	5.77 ± 8.17	13.30 ± 19.15	12.23 ± 19.84
ADratio	−0.57 ± 0.91	0.69 ± 4.69	0.69 ± 5.37
AFratio	1.05 ± 1.32	22.13 ± 38.09 [*]	28.91 ± 48.85 [#]

*AFratio: Grade I vs. Grade II, $P < 0.001$
#AFratio: Grade I vs. Grade III, $P < 0.001$

heterogeneous according to the statistics (Esd ≥ 7 kPa) (longest diameter plane: 25.56 ± 18.49 kPa; orthogonal diameter plane: 24.32 ± 17.93 kPa), and AFs calculated by two orthogonal planes unrelated to radial orientation were significantly higher in malignant lesions than benign lesions, both in small lesions and large lesions, confirming the predictable value for malignancy.

The study by Skerl et al. calculated AF with the ROI on the stiffest 2 mm of the lesion [15], while in our study AF was calculated with elasticity of the whole lesion instead, which could provide more complete information about the elasticity and anisotropy. As mentioned above, the lesions enrolled in our study were more heterogeneous, therefore analyzing the stiffest portion of the lesion alone might lose elastic information of rest part of the lesion. In our study, AUC of AFmax was 0.760, higher than 0.67 reported by Skerl et al. [15], with lower threshold of AFmax (159 kPa² vs 200 kPa²), indicating higher sensitivity. We also found that AFratio yielded the highest AUC (0.804) among all AF parameters, indicating anisotropy of Eratio predictable for malignancy.

This study was the first attempt to our knowledge to fully analyze anisotropy of each quantitative parameter. In previous studies, correlation between quantitative elasticity and histopathological results has been demonstrated [22–26]. Emean of IDC was significantly associated with palpable abnormality, histologic grade, and lymphovascular invasion [22], lymph node involvement and lymphovascular invasion was associated with significantly higher Emean, Emax, and Eratio [23], and higher histologic grade was significantly correlated with higher Emax [24, 25]. According to our results, AF was significantly higher in IDC than DCIS, and AFratio of Grade II and Grade III IDC was significantly higher than Grade I IDC lesions, indicating AF as an effective predictor of histological severity of breast cancer. Previous studies demonstrated that ER (−), PR (−), p53 (+), Ki-67 (−) and high nuclear grade

were associated with a significantly higher Eratio ($P < 0.05$) [25]. Nevertheless in our study, AF was higher in ER (+) and PR (+) lesions, while no significant correlation with HER2, Ki-67 and lymphatic metastasis. The correlation between AF and immunohistochemical factors requires future study.

Correlation between anisotropy and lesion location was analyzed for the first time. Some of the anisotropy factors were higher in lesions located near the nipple and the skin. In other words, lesions located near the nipple and the skin tended to be more anisotropic. That might because compression artifacts more frequently occur near the skin, and the fact that mammary ducts were more convergent near the nipple. Therefore, it may have explained the result in our study that lesions in inner half of the breast tended to be stiffer and more anisotropic, since the breast tissue of inner half is usually thinner than outer half so that lesions located at inner half are likely to be nearer the skin. It reminded us to take anisotropy into account when characterizing lesions near the nipple and skin. When analyzing correlation of anisotropy with palpability, we found that palpable lesions were more anisotropic than impalpable lesions. It might due to the fact that palpable lesions usually tended to be larger or near the skin, and lesions of large size and shallow depth were more anisotropic.

Owing to the existence of anisotropy, it is important to change the transducer orientation to fully assess the lesion when performing SWE. The influence of lesion location should be considered when characterizing breast lesions with the aid of anisotropy.

There were several limitations to our study. First, the two orthogonal planes we compared were longest diameter and orthogonal diameter planes, and therefore uncertain to cover the stiffest portion of the lesions. Second, large lesions which could not be covered by SWE color overlay were excluded in our study. Since large lesions were demonstrated to be more anisotropic, the exclusion of large lesions may cause selection bias. Third, it was a retrospective study, the patients enrolled were scheduled for surgical excision, and the low-suspicious BI-RADS 3 &4A lesions only constituted 32.3% of the lesions. Since high-suspicious group was more anisotropic, statistical results may be affected by the selection bias. Fourth, the small number DCIS cases [7.5% (13/174)] among the malignant group could have statistically influenced the results when comparing anisotropy between IDC and DCIS, and further study of large sample would be needed for validation.

Conclusions

Our study indicated that AF was superior to AD in predicting malignancy. Higher anisotropy was associated with higher suspicion for malignancy and more aggressive breast cancer. Taking anisotropy into account when performing breast SWE may help to characterize breast lesions and predict prognosis of cancer.

Abbreviations

2D: Two-dimensional; ACR: American College of Radiology; AD: Anisotropic difference; AF: Anisotropy factors; AUC: Areas under ROC curves.; BI-RADS: Breast Imaging Reporting and Data System; Emax: Maximal elasticity; Emean: Mean elasticity; Eratio: Ratio between the mean elasticity in the lesion and the fatty tissue; Esd: Standard deviation of elasticity; ROC: Receiver operating characteristic; SWE: Shear wave elastography; US: Ultrasound

Acknowledgements

The study was supported by the Department of Ultrasound of Fudan University Shanghai Cancer Center and Department of Oncology of Fudan University Shanghai Medical College.

Funding

The study was funded by Shanghai Municipal Commission of Health and Family Planning (Grant No. 20174Y0011) and the National Natural Science Foundation of China (Grant No. 81627804).

Authors' contributions

Study concept and design: YLC and CC Imaging data collection: YLC, YG and FW Imaging valuation: CC and WZ Statistical analysis: YLC and JJC Manuscript preparation: YLC All authors have read and approved the final manuscript.

Competing interests

The authors declare that they have no competing interest.

Author details

[1]Department of Ultrasound, Fudan University Shanghai Cancer Center, No. 270 Dong-An Road, Shanghai 200032, China. [2]Department of Oncology, Shanghai Medical College, Fudan University, No. 270 Dong-An Road, Shanghai 200032, China. [3]Department of Breast Surgery, Fudan University Shanghai Cancer Center, No. 270 Dong-An Road, Shanghai 200032, China.

References

1. Berg WA, Bandos AI, Mendelson EB, Lehrer D, Jong RA, Pisano ED. Ultrasound as the Primary Screening Test for Breast Cancer: Analysis From ACRIN 6666. J Natl Cancer Inst. 2015;108(4) https://doi.org/10.1093/jnci/djv367.
2. Taylor KJ, Merritt C, Piccoli C, Schmidt R, Rouse G, Fornage B, et al. Ultrasound as a complement to mammography and breast examination to characterize breast masses. Ultrasound Med Biol. 2002;28(1):19–26.
3. Mendelson EB, Böhm-Vélez M, Berg WA, et al. ACR BI-RADS® ultrasound. In: ACR BI-RADS® atlas, breast imaging reporting and data system. Reston, VA. American college of Radiology. 2013. (see: https://www.acr.org/Clinical-Resources/Reporting-and-Data-Systems/Bi-Rads/Permissions).
4. Gennisson JL, Deffieux T, Fink M, Tanter M. Ultrasound elastography: principles and techniques. Diagn Interv Imaging. 2013;94(5):487–95. https://doi.org/10.1016/j.diii.2013.01.022.
5. Ng WL, Rahmat K, Fadzli F, Rozalli FI, Mohd-Shah MN, Chandran PA, et al. Shearwave Elastography increases diagnostic accuracy in characterization of breast lesions. Medicine (Baltimore). 2016;95(12):e3146. https://doi.org/10.1097/MD.0000000000003146.
6. Cosgrove DO, Berg WA, Dore CJ, Skyba DM, Henry JP, Gay J, et al. BE1 Study Group. Shear wave elastography for breast masses is highly reproducible. Eur Radiol. 2012;22(5):1023–32. https://doi.org/10.1007/s00330-011-2340-y.
7. Berg WA, Cosgrove DO, Doré CJ, Schäfer FK, Svensson WE, Hooley RJ, et al. BE1 investigators. Shear-wave elastography improves the specificity of breast US: the BE1 multinational study of 939 masses. Radiology. 2012; 262(2):435–49. https://doi.org/10.1148/radiol.11110640.
8. Gweon HM, Youk JH, Son EJ, Kim JA. Clinical application of qualitative assessment for breast masses in shear-wave elastography. Eur J Radiol. 2013; 82(11):e680–5. https://doi.org/10.1016/j.ejrad.2013.08.004.
9. Lee SH, Chang JM, Kim WH, Bae MS, Seo M, Koo HR, et al. Added value of shear-wave elastography for evaluation of breast masses detected with screening US imaging. Radiology. 2014;273(1):61–9. https://doi.org/10.1148/radiol.14132443.
10. Klotz T, Boussion V, Kwiatkowski F, Dieu-de Fraissinette V, Bailly-Glatre A, Lemery S, et al. Shear wave elastography contribution in ultrasound diagnosis management of breast lesions. Diagn Interv Imaging. 2014;95(9): 813–24. https://doi.org/10.1016/j.diii.2014.04.015.
11. Giannotti E, Vinnicombe S, Thomson K, McLean D, Purdie C, Jordan L, Evans A. Shear-wave elastography and grayscale assessment of palpable probably benign masses: is biopsy always required? Br J Radiol. 2016;89(1062): 20150865. https://doi.org/10.1259/bjr.20150865.
12. Lee SH, Cho N, Chang JM, Koo HR, Kim JU, Kim WH, et al. Two-view versus single-view shear-wave Elastography: comparison of observer performance in differentiating benign from malignant breast masses. Radiology. 2014; 270(2):344–53. https://doi.org/10.1148/radiol.13130561.
13. Zhou J, Yang Z, Zhan W, Dong Y, Zhou C. Anisotropic properties of breast tissue measured by acoustic radiation force impulse quantification. Ultrasound Med Biol. 2016;42(10):2372–82. https://doi.org/10.1016/j.ultrasmedbio.2016.06.012.
14. Ciurea AI, Bolboaca SD, Ciortea CA, Botar-Jid C, Dudea SM. The influence of technical factors on sonoelastographic assessment of solid breast nodules. Ultraschall Med. 2011;32(Suppl 1):S27–34. https://doi.org/10.1055/s-0029-1245684.
15. Skerl K, Vinnicombe S, Thomson K, McLean D, Giannotti E, Evans A. Anisotropy of solid breast lesions in 2-D shear wave elastography is an indicator of malignancy. Acad Radiol. 2016;23:53–61. https://doi.org/10.1016/j.acra.2015.09.016.
16. DeLong ER, DeLong DM, Clarke-Pearson DL. Comparing the areas under two or more correlated receiver operating characteristic curves: a nonparametric approach. Biometrics. 1988;44(3):837–45.
17. Going JJ. Normal breast. In: O'Malley FP, Pinder SE, Mulligan AM, editors. Breast pathology. 2nd ed. Philadelphia: Elsevier; 2011. p. 53–64.
18. Hassiotou F, Geddes D. Anatomy of the human mammary gland: current status of knowledge. Clin Anat. 2013;26:29–48. https://doi.org/10.1002/ca.22165.
19. Barnes C, Speroni L, Quinn KP, Montevil M, Saetzler K, Bode-Animashaun G, et al. From single cells to tissues: interactions between the matrix and human breast cells in real time. PLoS One. 2014;9:e93325. https://doi.org/10.1371/journal.pone.0093325.
20. Provenzano PP, Eliceiri KW, Campbell JM, Inman DR, White JG, Keely PJ. Collagen reorganization at the tumor-stromal interface facilitates local invasion. BMC Med. 2006;4(1):38.
21. Chamming's F, Latorre-Ossa H, Le Frère-Belda MA, Fitoussi V, Quibel T, Assayag F, et al. Shear wave elastography of tumour growth in a human breast cancer model with pathological correlation. Eur Radiol. 2013;23(8): 2079–86. https://doi.org/10.1007/s00330-013-2828-8.
22. Youk JH, Gweon HM, Son EJ, Kim JA, Jeong J. Shear-wave elastography of invasive breast cancer: correlation between quantitative mean elasticity value and immunohistochemical profile. Breast Cancer Res Treat. 2013; 138(1):119–26. https://doi.org/10.1007/s10549-013-2407-3.
23. Au FW, Ghai S, Lu FI, Moshonov H, Crystal P. Quantitative shear wave elastography: correlation with prognostic histological features and immunohistochemical biomarkers of breast cancer. Acad Radiol. 2015;22(3): 269–77. https://doi.org/10.1016/j.acra.2014.10.007.

24. Cho EY, Ko ES, Han BK, Kim RB, Cho S, Choi JS, et al. Shear-wave elastography in invasive ductal carcinoma: correlation between quantitative maximum elasticity value and detailed pathological findings. Acta Radiol. 2016;57(5):521–8. https://doi.org/10.1177/0284185115590287.

25. Choi WJ, Kim HH, Cha JH, Shin HJ, Kim H, Chae EY, et al. Predicting prognostic factors of breast cancer using shear wave elastography. Ultrasound Med Biol. 2014;40(2):269–74. https://doi.org/10.1016/j.ultrasmedbio.2013.09.028.

26. Berg WA, Mendelson EB, Cosgrove DO, Doré CJ, Gay J, Henry JP, et al. Quantitative maximum shear-wave stiffness of breast masses as a predictor of histopathologic severity. AJR Am J Roentgenol. 2015;205(2):448–55. https://doi.org/10.2214/AJR.14.13448.

23

Identification and characterization of myocardial metastases in neuroendocrine tumor patients using 68Ga-DOTATATE PET-CT

Wolfgang G. Kunz[1]* [ID], Ralf S. Eschbach[1], Robert Stahl[1], Philipp M. Kazmierczak[1], Peter Bartenstein[2], Axel Rominger[2], Christoph J. Auernhammer[3,4], Christine Spitzweg[3,4], Jens Ricke[1] and Clemens C. Cyran[1,4]

Abstract

Background: Focal 68Ga-DOTATATE PET lesions within the myocardium of neuroendocrine tumor (NET) patients are observed in clinical practice. We determined the frequency and characteristics of lesions that are consistent with cardiac metastasis and assessed the lesion detection rate of conventional imaging.

Methods: 629 patients who underwent 68Ga-DOTATATE PET-CT at a supraregional comprehensive cancer center on NET were included from a consecutive registry. Inclusion criteria were: (1) focal 68Ga-DOTATATE tracer uptake within the myocardium in more than two sequential PET exams, and (2) contrast-enhanced CT. To determine the diagnostic accuracy of conventional CT imaging, a case-control cohort with a ratio of 1:3 was used. PET and CT were independently analyzed by two blinded readers. Cohen's κ was assessed for interreader agreement. Descriptive statistics were applied for frequencies and characteristics and group comparisons were analyzed using the Fisher's exact test.

Results: The prevalence of myocardial metastases related to the registry was 2.4% (15 of 629 NET patients fulfilling the inclusion criteria), for a total of 21 myocardial 68Ga-DOTATATE foci detected. Myocardial lesions were most frequently located in the left ventricle (43%) and the septum (43%). No patient demonstrated a pericardial effusion. Patients with myocardial metastases did not differ in demographics, tumor grading, disease stage or circulating tumor markers compared to the overall registry (all $p > 0.05$). Higher Ki67-Indices were observed ($p = 0.049$) for patients with myocardial metastases. Interreader agreement for PET assessment was excellent (Cohen's κ = 1.0). CT reading showed a sensitivity of 19% (95% confidence interval: 6–43%) at a specificity of 100% (95% confidence interval: 90–100%).

Conclusions: 68Ga-DOTATATE PET enables detection of myocardial metastatic lesions in NET patients. In contrast, standard morphologic CT imaging provides very limited sensitivity.

Keywords: Myocardium, Neuroendocrine tumors, Positron-emission tomography, Multidetector computed tomography

* Correspondence: wolfgang.kunz@med.lmu.de
Wolfgang G. Kunz and Ralf S. Eschbach share first authorship.
[1]Department of Radiology, University Hospital, LMU Munich, Marchioninistr. 15, 81377 Munich, Germany
Full list of author information is available at the end of the article

Background

Neuroendocrine tumors (NET) represent a heterogeneous entity of malignant neoplasms that arise from the cells of the endocrine system [1–3]. At initial staging as well as in therapy monitoring, the use of positron emission tomography (PET) has prevailed over conventional imaging assessment due to a significantly higher sensitivity and specificity [4]. In particular for NET, the tracer 68Ga-DOTATATE allows the detection of metastases based on the typical expression of somatostatin receptor 2 (SSTR2) in well-differentiated NET [5].

The heart is a rare but important site of metastasis for many malignant tumors, which can be localized in different cardiac spaces including the myocardium and pericardium [6, 7]. Pericardial metastases often manifest with concomitant pericardial effusion, which facilitates their diagnosis in conventional computed tomography (CT) or magnetic resonance imaging (MRI). Myocardial metastases, however, often remain undetected until autopsy as indicated by the large differences in the frequency of myocardial metastases in autopsies compared to conventional oncologic imaging [7]. Yet, a reliable way of detecting myocardial metastases is of clinical relevance as it may influence treatment decisions [8, 9].

CT as the most frequently used modality in oncologic imaging has limited sensitivity for the detection of myocardial metastases compared to MRI [7]. Moreover, the most frequently applied PET tracer [18F]-fluorodeoxyglucose (18F-FDG) in oncologic imaging shows high physiologic uptake in the myocardium, which masks focal myocardial lesions with altered glucose metabolism. In contrast to 18F-FDG, the tracer 68Ga-DOTATATE only shows a non-specific background-level uptake of the myocardium [10].

We hypothesize that focal myocardial 68Ga-DOTATATE tracer uptake may contribute to the detection of myocardial metastases in patients with NET. We sought to characterize prevalence, clinical and imaging characteristics in these patients based on the registry of a supraregional interdisciplinary comprehensive cancer center on NET.

Methods

Study design and population

The institutional review board of the LMU Munich (Ethikkommission der Medizinischen Fakultät der Ludwig-Maximilians-Universität München) approved this retrospective study, which was conducted according to the Helsinki Declaration of 2013, and waived requirement for informed consent. Based on a prospectively collected NET patient registry at the Interdisciplinary Center for Neuroendocrine Tumors of the Gastroenteropancreatic System (GEPNET-KUM), our initial cohort consisted of 629 consecutive patients who underwent 68Ga-DOTATATE PET-CT between March 2012 and March 2017.

Out of this cohort, we included all subjects with

(1) focal myocardial 68Ga-DOTATATE tracer uptake in at least two sequential PET exams, and
(2) contrast-enhanced CT.

We excluded patients with

(1) non-enhanced CT, and
(2) non-diagnostic quality of PET or CT.

PET-CT and MRI examination protocol

All patients underwent 68Ga-DOTATATE PET-CT (Biograph 64; Siemens Healthcare) 60 min after intravenous injection of a median 223 MBq (standard deviation 22 MBq) of 68Ga-DOTATATE. First, contrast-enhanced CT scans (1.5 mL of iopromide [Ultravist-300; Bayer Healthcare] per kilogram of body weight) were obtained for anatomic localization. Subsequently, the PET scan was acquired by static emission data for 3 min per bed position. PET images were reconstructed using an iterative algorithm (ordered-subset expectation maximization: 4 iterations, 8 subsets). Contrast-enhanced CT data were reconstructed with a slice thickness of 2.0 mm (axial). The reconstructed PET, CT, and fused images were analyzed on the manufacturer's imaging software (syngo.via; Siemens Healthcare; Forchheim, Germany). Liver MRI, which was routinely performed on 1.5- or 3.0-T scanners (MAGNETOM Aera, MAGNETOM Avanto; Siemens Healthcare; Forchheim, Germany) as a part of the complementary NET staging for the detection of liver metastases, was used to crosscheck for possible heart metastases in cases when the heart or parts of it were included in the field of view. The standard liver MRI imaging protocol consisted of T1-w fast spin echo (FSE) sequences in- and opposed phase, a T2-weighted single-shot FSE sequence without fat saturation (fs), and a breath-hold T2-weighted FSE sequence with fs. We intravenously administrated the contrast agent Gd-EOB-DTPA (Primovist; Bayer Healthcare; Leverkusen, Germany) (0.1 mL of a 0.25 mmol/mL solution per kilogram of body weight) and used a dynamic T1-weighted gradient echo sequence (volumetric interpolated breath-hold examination [VIBE]) with fs. This protocol was not optimized for cardiac imaging. Only 5 patients underwent an additional dedicated cardiac MRI protocol.

Definition of myocardial metastasis on 68Ga-DOTATATE PET and prevalence

Focal 68Ga-DOTATATE tracer uptake was considered consistent with myocardial metastasis when clearly located in the myocardium and if the uptake was evident on at least two sequential PET exams. Due to the missing necessity for a myocardial biopsy in the overall management of metastasized NET patients, histopathological validation of the myocardial lesions was not available. In a subgroup of five patients, the myocardial lesions could be confirmed by the use of dedicated cardiac MRI examinations. The prevalence of myocardial lesions on 68Ga-DOTATATE PET in NET patients was calculated in relation to the total number of patients treated at our institution in the given time period of this study.

Diagnostic accuracy of CT for myocardial lesions on 68Ga-DOTATATE PET

To determine the diagnostic accuracy of conventional CT imaging, a case-control-cohort with a ratio of 1:3 was set up including patients without focal myocardial uptake as controls. This design also allows to determine the rate of false-positive findings based on the inclusion of control patients and was chosen to minimize bias during the diagnostic readout [11]. In a randomized and blinded fashion, PET and CT were independently analyzed by two readers, one board-certified in radiology and diagnostic nuclear medicine with 10 years of experience in hybrid imaging (C.C.C.) and one board-certified in nuclear medicine with 15 years of experience in hybrid imaging (A.R.). Interreader agreement was assessed using Cohen's κ.

Statistical analysis

We performed all statistical analyses using SPSS Statistics 23 (IBM; Armonk, NY, USA). For the comparison of categorical variables, the Fisher's exact test was used. Categorical variables are presented as frequency and percentage. All metric and normally distributed variables are reported as mean ± standard deviation; non-normally distributed variables are presented as median (interquartile range, IQR). The Mann-Whitney U test was applied for numeric variables. Normal distribution was assessed using the Kolmogorov-Smirnov test. P-values below 0.05 were considered to indicate statistical significance.

Results

Patient characteristics

The prevalence of myocardial lesions on 68Ga-DOTATATE PET in relation to the overall patient registry was 2.4%. 15 out of 629 NET patients (age: 65 ± 9; male sex: 60%) with a total number of 21 focal myocardial 68Ga-DOTATATE tracer uptakes fulfilled the inclusion criteria. All focal myocardial uptakes detected were reproducible in follow-up PET exams. There was excellent agreement between the two readers (Cohen's κ = 1.0). In NET patients with myocardial lesions, the primary tumor was most frequently located in the small intestine (73%). Regarding initial disease stage, distant metastases were frequently observed (73%). Compared to the overall NET

registry of our comprehensive cancer center, there were no significant differences of patients with myocardial metastases in patient age, patient sex, tumor grading, initial disease stage, or initial levels of NET tumor markers (all $p > 0.05$). Yet, patients with myocardial metastases demonstrated higher expression of the proliferation marker Ki67-Index compared to the overall registry ($p = 0.049$). None of the patients with myocardial metastases suffered from carcinoid heart disease. In one patient, the myocardial metastasis was operatively resected due to its size with histopathological results consistent with a NET metastasis. The patient characteristics at the initial disease stage are shown in Table 1.

Detection of myocardial PET lesions by conventional imaging

CT reading showed a sensitivity of 19% (95% confidence interval: 6–43%) at a specificity of 100% (95% confidence interval: 90–100%) for the detection of myocardial lesions. The diagnostic accuracy measures are shown in Table 2. Liver MRI was part of the complementary NET staging in 14 subjects. Despite the partial field of view and incomplete scanning of the heart, five out of fourteen lesions could be detected with liver MRI. Patient examples are shown in Figs. 1, 2 and 3.

Characteristics and conventional imaging appearance of myocardial PET lesions

Myocardial lesions were already detected at initial staging in five patients (33% of study population). In the remaining patients, myocardial lesions were identified a median of six years after the initial diagnosis. The median myocardial lesion SUVmax was 8.6 (relative to the physiologic spleen uptake: 0.386), the median myocardial lesion SUVmean was 4.3 (relative to the physiologic spleen uptake: 0.225). The lesions were most frequently located in the left ventricle (43%) and the septum (43%), no lesions were located in the left or right atrium. If evident, the myocardial lesions most frequently appeared isodense on CT, hyperintense on T2-weighted MR images and isointense on non-enhanced as well as contrast-enhanced T1-weighted MR images. None of the patients demonstrated a pericardial effusion. The characteristics are shown in Table 3.

Discussion

Myocardial metastases detected by the PET component of 68Ga-DOTATATE PET-CT were present in 2.4% of NET patients in our comprehensive cancer center registry. The sensitivity of conventional CT imaging was very low within our study population while yielding very high specificity. None of the patients demonstrated a pericardial effusion, which might have indicated a cardiac spread of the disease. Aside from higher values of the

Table 1 Characteristics of NET patients with myocardial lesions on 68Ga-DOTATATE PET at the time point of their initial NET diagnosis

	Study population (n = 15)	CCC NET registry[a] (n = 629)	P value
Age (yrs)	65 (± 9)	63 (± 14)	0.915
Male sex	9/15 (60%)	333/616 (54%)	0.795
Location of primary tumor			
Jejunum/Ileum	11/15 (73%)	182/387 (47%)	N/A
Appendix	1/15 (6.7%)	18/387 (4.6%)	
Colon	2/15 (13%)	27/387 (7.0%)	
Undetermined	1/15 (6.7%)	15/387 (3.9%)	
Tumor grading			
G1	5/10 (50%)	126/255 (49%)	0.353
G2	3/10 (30%)	109/255 (43%)	
G3	2/10 (20%)	20/255 (8%)	
Ki67-Index			
≤ 2%	5/12 (42%)	131/292 (45%)	0.049[b]
> 2–20%	4/12 (33%)	142/292 (49%)	
> 20%	3/12 (25%)	19/292 (7%)	
Disease stage			
Localized	2/15 (13%)	44/227 (19%)	0.743
Regional metastasis	11/15 (73%)	N/A N/A	
Regional metastasis only	2/15 (13%)	21/162 (13%)	1.000
Distant metastasis	11/15 (73%)	113/162 (70%)	1.000
Hepatic	6/11 (55%)	N/A N/A	
Peritoneal	4/11 (36%)	N/A N/A	
Osseous	6/11 (55%)	N/A N/A	
Myocardial	5/11 (45%)	N/A N/A	
Other	2/11 (18%)	N/A N/A	
Chromogranin A (ng/mL)	175 (95–9578)	N/A N/A	
Elevated Chromogranin A	7/10 (70%)	178/312 (57%)	0.526
5-HIAA urine secretion (mg/24 h)	26 (10–80)	N/A N/A	
Elevated 5-HIAA urine secretion	4/6 (66%)	178/312 (57%)	0.701
Carcinoid heart disease	0/15 (0%)	N/A N/A	

Values presented are count/available values (percentage) for categorical, mean and standard deviation or median (interquartile range) for continuous variables. Cut-off values for elevated Chromogranin A and 24-h 5-HIAA urine secretion were 98 ng/mL and 9 mg/24 h respectively. 5-HIAA, 5-hydroxyindoleacetic acid; N/A, not available
[a] Data are taken from the registry on neuroendocrine tumors (NET) of the comprehensive cancer center (CCC). [b]Statistical test indicates significant differences between groups

histological proliferation marker Ki67-Index in patients with myocardial metastases compared to the overall registry, no significant differences in patient characteristics were detected. The frequency of myocardial metastases in our patient cohort, the location of metastases,

Table 2 Diagnostic accuracy of contrast-enhanced CT for myocardial lesions detected on 68Ga-DOTATATE PET in NET patients

	Sensitivity	Specificity	PPV	NPV
All lesions (N = 21)				
CT	19 (6–43)	100 (90–100)	100 (40–100)	73 (60–93)

Values presented are percentages with the 95% confidence interval in parentheses. PPV, positive predictive value; NPV, negative predictive value

and the time from initial NET diagnosis to diagnosis of myocardial metastasis are in line with previous echocardiographic studies [12–14], with one study also investigating cardiac MRI [14]. The results of our study demonstrate that patients with myocardial metastases from NET had very similar clinical, histological and serological parameters during the initial tumor evaluation. In particular, the tumor grading and the disease stage showed no difference. In line with Calissendorff et al. we also observed myocardial metastases in patients without hepatic metastases [15].

The first reports on myocardial metastases in NET patients based on somatostatin receptor scintigraphy date back to 1996 [16]. Soon after the introduction of 68Ga-DOTATATE PET imaging, reports followed on the detection of focal myocardial uptakes consistent with metastasis [17–19]. We extend the evidence on the diagnostic value of 68Ga-DOTATATE PET by reporting the interreader agreement for myocardial metastasis detection, which was excellent in our study, further supporting 68Ga-DOTATATE PET as a very accurate and robust technique in staging well-differentiated NET. Additionally, we provide data on the repeated detection of the focal myocardial tracer uptakes, which were evident for every myocardial lesion in every follow-up PET exam analyzed. Besides 68Ga-DOTATATE, studies also investigated 18-Fluoro-dihydroxyphenylalanin (18F-DOPA) for the detection of myocardial metastases [20, 21], demonstrating the value of functional imaging in the detection of myocardial lesions.

Regarding diagnostic accuracy, we report the low sensitivities of CT imaging for myocardial metastasis detection as evaluated by expert reading of a case-control cohort. We characterized the imaging appearance in contrast-enhanced CT, and in MR imaging of the liver whenever the lesions were depicted and evident. In CT, only the mass effect contributed to the diagnosis as all metastases appeared isodense to the surrounding myocardium. For liver MR imaging, which is often performed as a complementary diagnostic exam in NET patients, T2-weighted sequences were occasionally useful for incidental detection of myocardial metastases. This further supports the use of 68Ga-DOTATATE PET in the staging of NET patients, which has been shown to be superior compared to morphologic imaging in the

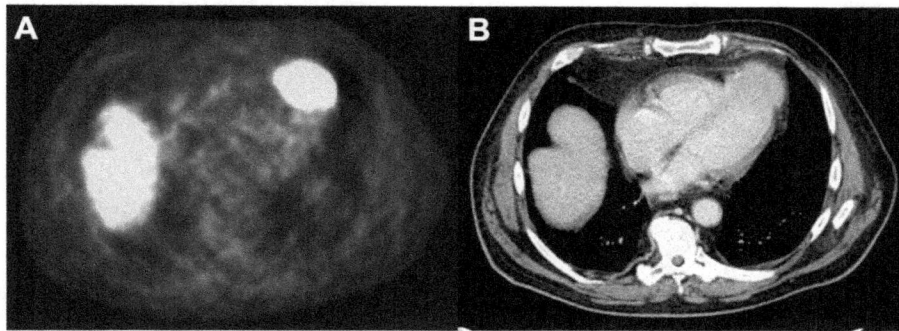

Fig. 1 Patient example with a myocardial metastasis located at the apex evident on 68Ga-DOTATATE PET (**a**) and CT (**b**). A 77-year-old male patient with a G3 neuroendocrine tumor of unknown origin with a myocardial metastasis to the apex of the heart. Strong 68Ga-DOTATATE tracer uptake (**a**) correlates to the morphologic mass detected on CT imaging (**b**)

detection of the primary, the lymphatic as well as the hematogenic spread of the disease [5]. Most importantly, 68Ga-DOTATATE PET significantly impacts therapeutic management in more than 50% of NET patients, including initiation or continuance of peptide receptor radionuclide therapy, medical treatment or referral to surgery. This is primarily driven by improved detection of the primary tumor site or nodal, hepatic and peritoneal metastases [8, 9]. It remains to be determined if the enhanced detection of myocardial metastases impacts patient management.

Carcinoid heart disease (CHD) is a frequent manifestation in NET patients with carcinoid syndrome that has been identified decades earlier than myocardial metastases [22]. CHD significantly contributes to morbidity and mortality of NET patients [13]. It likely results from high levels of circulating vasoactive substances such as serotonin and is characterized by plaque-like, fibrous endocardial thickening involving in particular the right-sided heart valves. This leads to valvular dysfunction and right-sided heart failure. The management of CHD has improved over time,

and its prevalence decreased as a consequence of the use of somatostatin analogues [23]. However, 68Ga-DOTATATE PET appears to have no value in the diagnosis of CHD, which is based on echocardiography and circulating biomarkers [23].

Yet, identifying myocardial metastasis may have clinical implications based on the early reported significant overlap with carcinoid heart disease [12]. However, in our study population, none of the patients suffered from carcinoid heart disease at the time that the myocardial lesions were detected, which is in line with a recent report [20]. In accordance with this observation, we detected no difference in circulating tumor markers Chromogranin A or 5-hydroxyindoleacetic acid (5-HIAA) urine secretion, possible biomarkers for CHD [23], between patients with myocardial metastases compared to the overall registry. This further provides support to the hypothesis that CHD and myocardial metastases are truly distinct pathologies.

There are limitations to this study that need to be considered when interpreting the results. First, histopathological validation of the focal myocardial 68Ga-DOTATA

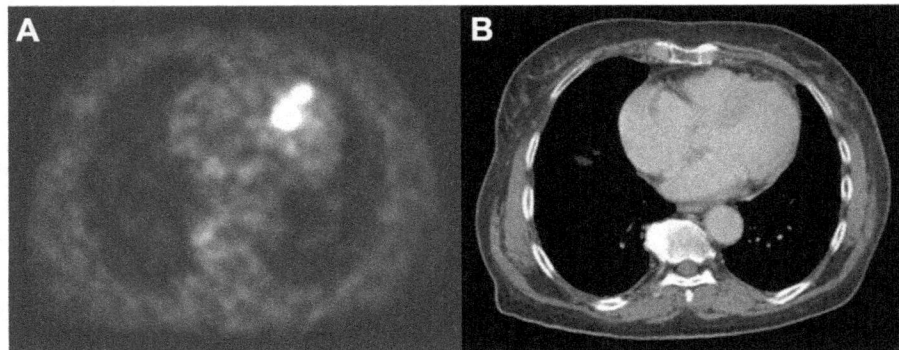

Fig. 2 Patient example with a myocardial metastasis detected using 68Ga-DOTATATE PET (**a**) without evidence on CT (**b**). In a 74-year-old female patient with a G2 neuroendocrine tumor of the small intestine, 68Ga-DOTATATE PET (**a**) demonstrates strong focal uptake in the interventricular septum without a morphologic correlate on CT imaging (**b**). This uptake was observed throughout all follow-up examinations consistent with a myocardial metastasis

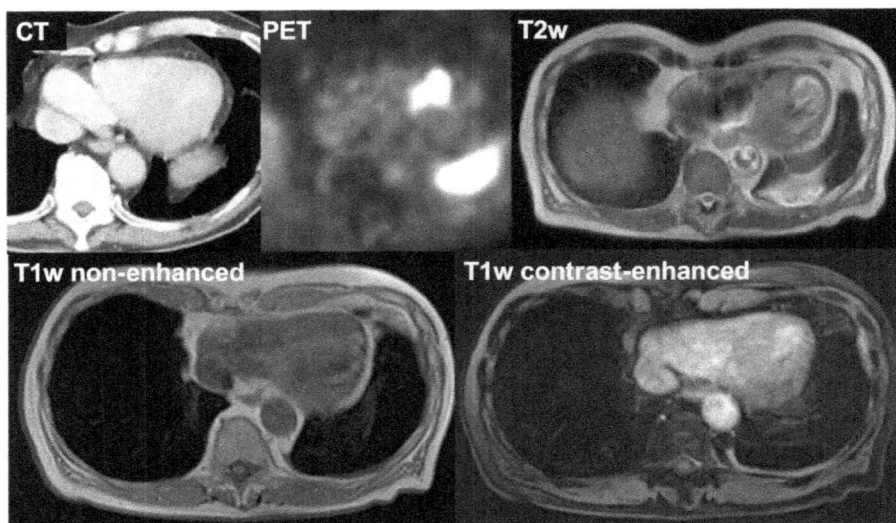

Fig. 3 Appearance of a myocardial metastasis on liver MRI performed as part of the complementary staging of the NET disease. A 72-year-old male patient with a G1 neuroendocrine tumor of the small intestine demonstrates a myocardial metastasis in the interventricular septum (evident on CT imaging) with strong 68Ga-DOTATATE tracer uptake in the PET image. The morphologic appearance in the complementary liver MRI is characterized by an intermediate T2w signal and isointense signal on non-enhanced and contrast-enhanced T1w images

Table 3 Characteristics of myocardial lesions on 68Ga-DOTATA TE PET in NET patients

	Patients ($n = 15$) with myocardial lesions ($n = 21$)
Myocardial lesion at baseline	5 (45%)
Time from initial diagnosis to lesion appearance (yrs)	6 (2–10)
Patients with multiple lesions	3 (20%)
Patients with pericardial effusion	0 (0%)
Location	
Left atrial	0 (0%)
Left ventricular	9 (43%)
Septal	9 (43%)
Right atrial	0 (0%)
Right ventricular	3 (14%)
Lesion SUVmax	8.6 (5.2–17.4)
Lesion SUVmean	4.3 (3.7–11.6)
Spleen SUVmax	22.3 (16.4–27.2)
Spleen SUVmean	19.1 (14.7–25.8)
Lesion appearance on CT imaging[a]	
hyper–/ iso–/ hypodense	0 / 3 / 1
Lesion appearance on liver MR imaging[a]	
T2w-hyper- / iso- / hypointense	5 / 0 / 0
T1w-hyper- / iso- / hypointense	0 / 3 / 0
CE-T1w-hyper- / iso- / hypointense	0 / 4 / 0

Values presented are count (percentage) for categorical and median (interquartile range) for continuous variables. SUV, standardized uptake value; T2w, T2-weighted; T1w, T1-weighted; CE-T1w; contrast-enhanced T1-weighted
[a] If evident on conventional imaging. Liver MRI was only available in 14 subjects

TE uptake was not available as the risks conferred by myocardial biopsies outweigh the diagnostic yield in the context of metastatic NET patient management. However, repeated focal myocardial PET tracer uptakes are consistent with myocardial metastases. Second, our study population had a limited number of patients, reflecting the comparatively low prevalence of myocardial metastases in NET patients.

Conclusions

68Ga-DOTATATE PET imaging provides added diagnostic value compared to morphologic CT imaging in the detection as well as in the follow-up of myocardial metastases in NET patients. Further studies are needed to determine the impact on patient management.

Abbreviations
CT: Computed tomography; MRI: Magnetic resonance imaging; NET: Neuroendocrine tumor; PET: Positron emission tomography; DOTATA TE: 1,4,7,10-tetraaza-cyclododecane-1,4,7,10-tetraaceticacid-[Tyr3] octreotate

Authors' contributions
WGK, RES, AR, RS, PMK, and CCC analyzed and interpreted the patient data. WGK, RES, and CCC drafted the manuscript. All authors reviewed the manuscript draft. All authors read and approved the final version of the manuscript.

Competing interests
The authors declare that they have no competing interests.

Author details

[1]Department of Radiology, University Hospital, LMU Munich, Marchioninistr. 15, 81377 Munich, Germany. [2]Department of Nuclear Medicine, University Hospital, LMU Munich, Munich, Germany. [3]Department of Internal Medicine IV, University Hospital, LMU Munich, Munich, Germany. [4]Comprehensive Cancer Center (CCC LMU) and Interdisciplinary Center for Neuroendocrine Tumors of the Gastroenteropancreatic System (GEPNET-KUM), University Hospital, LMU Munich, Munich, Germany.

References

1. Auernhammer CJ, Spitzweg C, Angele MK, et al. Advanced neuroendocrine tumours of the small intestine and pancreas: clinical developments, controversies, and future strategies. Lancet Diabet Endocrinol. 2017. https://doi.org/10.1016/s2213-8587(17)30401-1.

2. Yao JC, Hassan M, Phan A, et al. One hundred years after "carcinoid": epidemiology of and prognostic factors for neuroendocrine tumors in 35,825 cases in the United States. J Clin Oncol. 2008;26:3063–72.

3. Ramage JK, Ahmed A, Ardill J, et al. Guidelines for the management of gastroenteropancreatic neuroendocrine (including carcinoid) tumours (NETs). Gut. 2012;61:6–32.

4. Sundin A, Arnold R, Baudin E, et al. ENETS consensus guidelines for the standards of Care in Neuroendocrine Tumors: radiological, Nuclear Medicine & Hybrid Imaging. Neuroendocrinology. 2017;105:212–44.

5. Sadowski SM, Neychev V, Millo C, et al. Prospective study of 68Ga-DOTATA TE positron emission tomography/computed tomography for detecting gastro-Entero-pancreatic neuroendocrine tumors and unknown primary sites. J Clin Oncol. 2016;34:588–96.

6. Maleszewski JJ, Anavekar NS, Moynihan TJ, Klarich KW. Pathology, imaging, and treatment of cardiac tumours. Nat Rev Cardiol. 2017;14:536–49.

7. Chiles C, Woodard PK, Gutierrez FR, Link KM. Metastatic involvement of the heart and pericardium: CT and MR imaging. Radiographics. 2001;21:439–49.

8. Ambrosini V, Campana D, Bodei L, et al. 68Ga-DOTANOC PET/CT clinical impact in patients with neuroendocrine tumors. J Nucl Med. 2010;51:669–73.

9. Frilling A, Sotiropoulos GC, Radtke A, et al. The impact of 68Ga-DOTATOC positron emission tomography/computed tomography on the multimodal management of patients with neuroendocrine tumors. Ann Surg. 2010;252: 850–6.

10. Tarkin JM, Joshi FR, Evans NR, et al. Detection of atherosclerotic inflammation by 68Ga-DOTATATE PET compared to [18F]FDG PET imaging. J Am Coll Cardiol. 2017;69:1774–91.

11. Rothman KJ. Epidemiology: an introduction. 2nd ed. USA: Oxford University Press; 2012.

12. Pandya UH, Pellikka PA, Enriquez-Sarano M, Edwards WD, Schaff HV, Connolly HM. Metastatic carcinoid tumor to the heart: echocardiographic-pathologic study of 11 patients. J Am Coll Cardiol. 2002;40:1328–32.

13. Pellikka PA, Tajik AJ, Khandheria BK, et al. Carcinoid heart disease. Clinical and echocardiographic spectrum in 74 patients. Circulation. 1993;87:1188–96.

14. Bhattacharyya S, Toumpanakis C, Burke M, Taylor AM, Caplin ME, Davar J. Features of carcinoid heart disease identified by 2- and 3-dimensional echocardiography and cardiac MRI. Circ Cardiovasc Imaging. 2010;3:103–11.

15. Calissendorff J, Maret E, Sundin A, Falhammar H. Ileal neuroendocrine tumors and heart: not only valvular consequences. Endocrine. 2015;48:743–55.

16. Yeung HW, Imbriaco M, Zhang JJ, Macapinlac H, Goldsmith SJ, Larson SM. Visualization of myocardial metastasis of carcinoid tumor by indium-111-pentetreotide. J Nucl Med. 1996;37:1528–30.

17. Jann H, Wertenbruch T, Pape U, et al. A matter of the heart: myocardial metastases in neuroendocrine tumors. Horm Metab Res. 2010;42:967–76.

18. Carreras C, Kulkarni HR, Baum RP. Rare metastases detected by (68)Ga-somatostatin receptor PET/CT in patients with neuroendocrine tumors. Recent Results Cancer Res. 2013;194:379–84.

19. Calissendorff J, Sundin A, Falhammar H. (6)(8)Ga-DOTA-TOC-PET/CT detects heart metastases from ileal neuroendocrine tumors. Endocrine. 2014;47:169–76.

20. Noordzij W, van Beek AP, Tio RA, et al. Myocardial metastases on 6-[18F] fluoro-L-DOPA PET/CT: a retrospective analysis of 116 serotonin producing neuroendocrine tumour patients. PLoS One. 2014;9:e112278.

21. Fiebrich HB, Brouwers AH, Links TP, de Vries EG. Images in cardiovascular medicine: myocardial metastases of carcinoid visualized by 18F-dihydroxy-phenyl-alanine positron emission tomography. Circulation. 2008;118:1602–4.

22. Roberts WC, Sjoerdsma A. The cardiac disease associated with the carcinoid syndrome (carcinoid heart disease). Am J Med. 1964;36:5–34.

23. Davar J, Connolly HM, Caplin ME, et al. Diagnosing and managing carcinoid heart disease in patients with neuroendocrine tumors: An Expert Statement. J Am Coll Cardiol. 2017;69:1288–304.

Clinical efficacy of chemoembolization with simultaneous radiofrequency ablation for treatment of adrenal metastases from hepatocellular carcinoma

Hongjun Yuan, Fengyong Liu*, Xin Li, Yang Guan and Maoqiang Wang

Abstract

Background: This study investigated the safety and efficacy of transcatheter arterial chemoembolization (TACE) with simultaneous radiofrequency ablation (RFA) as treatment for adrenal metastases (AM) from hepatocellular carcinoma(HCC).

Methods: The records of 63 patients with AM who were treated at our Hospital between February 2013 and August 2016 were retrospectively reviewed. Patients were divided into a TACE+RFA group (n = 38) and a control group that received TACE alone (n = 25) according to different treatment methods. The success rate, tumor control rate, and safety of these groups were compared, and survival was evaluated using the Kaplan-Meier method.

Results: All treatments could be completed technically successful in both groups. The tumor control rate at first imaging after 1 months was 92.1% (35/38) in the TACE+RFA group and 76.0% (19/25) in the TACE group(P = 0.041). The assisted local tumor control rate allowing repeated interventions in case of local recurrence was 70.0% (7/10) in the TACE+RFA group and 30.8% (4/13) in the TACE group (P = 0.039). During the follow up period, the TACE+RFA group had better survival than the TACE group at 1 year (92.1% vs. 88.0%), 2 years (73.7% vs. 64.0%), and 3 years (55.3% vs. 44.0%) (P = 0.040). The mean survival time was 26.8 ± 2.0 months (95% CI, 22.8–30.7) in the TACE+RFA group and 17.5 ± 2.2 months (95% CI, 13.1–21.8) in the TACE group.

Conclusion: TACE+RFA led to better control of local disease progression and longer survival time than TACE alone in the treatment of AM from HCC. Although patients given TACE+RFA had more complications than those given TACE alone, these complications were easily managed.

Keywords: Chemoembolization, Therapy, Radiofrequency ablation, Adrenal metastases

Background

Many primary malignancies metastasize to the adrenal gland, and the risk for adrenal metastasis is as high as 32–73% in some populations of tumor patients [1]. Adrenal metastases (AM) mainly originate from tumors of the lung, liver, kidney, gastrointestinal system, and pancreas, and metastases may be disseminated via hematogenous, lymphatic, or local infiltration [1, 2]. Most patients with AM have no evidence of adrenocortical or medulloadrenal dysfunction, and no clinical symptoms, such as pain. The diagnosis of AM is mainly based on imaging results because there are no specific blood markers for AM [3]. AM may be found in patients with hepatocellular carcinoma (HCC) who undergo regular MRI/CT imaging after treatment. To benefit patient survival, it is necessary to actively treat AMs while treating HCC. If AM are large or there are metastases to major organs, surgical intervention may not be feasible [4]. Chemotherapeutic agents may be given as palliative treatment. Radiotherapy is one of the most established therapies for AM, specially Stereotactic Body Radiation Therapy(SBRT)and cyber knife [5, 6]. However, patients who are unsuitable or unwilling to undergo surgery or

* Correspondence: liufengyong301@163.com
Department of Interventional Radiology, Chinese PLA General Hospital, 28 Fuxing Road, Beijing 100853, People's Republic of China

radiotherapy may be given minimally invasive treatments such as chemoembolization or radiofrequency ablation (RFA) [6, 7]. In transcatheter adrenal arterial chemoembolization (TACE), high-dose chemotherapeutic agents and lipiodol are used to embolize vessels that supply the tumor, in an effort to kill or slow the growth tumor cells. RFA has been widely used in the treatment of liver tumors due to its minimally invasive nature and favorable safety profile, and is also recently used for treatment of adrenal tumors [6–9]. Most studies have focused on TACE or RFA alone, and few studies have examined the combined use of TACE with RFA.

In this study, we retrospectively compared patients who received TACE+RFA with patients who received RFA alone for the treatment of AM to evaluate the safety and efficacy of these treatment methods.

Methods

Study design

The Institutional Review Board approved this retrospective study in August 2017. Written informed consent was obtained from all patients. A total of 63 patients were diagnosed with AM from HCCs at our hospital between February 2013 and August 2016, and the location of the primary tumor was confirmed for each patient. The included patients received simultaneous TACE+RFA ($n = 38$) or TACE alone ($n = 25$). All patients received Computed tomography (CT) or magnetic resonance imaging (MRI) and pathological examinations before treatment. TACE and RFA were performed by the same clinician who had more than 20 years of experience in interventional therapy. One month after the initial treatment, patients received a follow-up CT or MRI exams and had follow-up evaluations every 3 months thereafter. Local tumor progression and survival were evaluated. If residual tumor was observed during a follow-up evaluation, re-treatment was performed.

Patient characteristics

The inclusion criteria were: diagnosis of a primary tumor and confirmation of AM by imaging examinations; contraindication for surgical intervention due to liver or kidney dysfunction or other contradictions such as cardiac or lung dysfunction, and severe diabetes mellitus; refusal of surgical intervention; and no receipt of local chemotherapy or radiotherapy. The exclusion criteria were: coagulation dysfunction and platelet count below $30 \times 10^9/L$; local infection or uncontrollable systemic infection; contraindication for interventional therapy due to severe liver, kidney, or cardiac dysfunction; and Eastern Cooperative Oncology Group (ECOG) score of 0 to 2. The pros and cons of interventional therapy were explained to all patients before treatment, and written informed consent was obtained before treatment. Table 1

Table 1 Baseline characteristics of patients with AM who received TACE+RFA or TACE alone

Variable	TACE+RFA	TACE	χ^2/t	P
Age, years	54.2 ± 9.3	56.8 ± 8.8	1.108	0.272
Gender			0.092	0.762
M	26 (68.4%)	18 (72.0%)		
F	12 (31.6%)	7 (28.0%)		
Child-Pugh grade			0.076	0.783
A	30 (78.9%)	19 (76.0%)		
B	8 (21.1%)	6 (24.0%)		
ECOG			0.406	0.523
0	33 (86.8%)	23 (92.0%)		
1	5 (13.2%)	2 (8.0%)		
Outcome of primary tumor			0.834	0.933
Resection	9 (23.7%)	5 (20.0%)		
CR[a]	17 (44.7%)	12 (48.0%)		
PR	7 (18.4%)	5 (20.0%)		
SD	1 (2.6%)	0		
PD	4 (10.5%)	3 (12.0%)		
Extra-adrenal metastases			1.638	0.440
None	16 (42.1%)	7 (28.0%)		
One organ metastases	14 (36.8%)	13 (52.0%)		
Multiple organ metastases	8 (21.1%)	5 (20.0%)		
AM location			0.118	0.731
Unilateral	29 (76.3%)	20 (80.0%)		
Left	11 (28.9%)	11 (44.0%)		
Right	18 (47.4%)	9 (36.0%)		
Bilateral	9 (23.7%)	5 (20.0%)		
Maximal diameter of AM(cm)			0.414	0.519
≥ 3	11 (23.4%)	9 (30.0%)		
<3	36 (76.6%)	21 (70.0%)		
Tumor size of AM(cm)				
Range	1.5~ 7.3	1.2~ 8.1		
Mean	3.3 ± 1.6	3.5 ± 1.7	0.473	0.637

Abbreviations: *ECOG* Eastern Cooperative Oncology Group, *CR* complete remission, *PR* partial remission, *SD* stable disease, *PD* progressive disease, *AM* adrenal metastasis
Note [a]Assessed according to the mRECIST

shows the baseline characteristics of the 63 patients who received treatment.

Instruments

TACE and RFA were performed under the guidance of an Angio-CT (Miyabi; Siemens Medical Solutions AG, Erlangen, Germany), which combines Artis zee digital subtraction plate angiography and a Somatom Emotion 16-slice spiral CT (Siemens Medical Solutions AG, Erlangen, Germany). RFA was performed using a RITA radiofrequency system (model 1500;RITA Medical System, Mountain View, CA, USA) and a RITA electrode.

Treatments

Angio-CT combines digital subtraction angiography (DSA) and CT. For patients in the TACE+RFA group, TACE was conducted under the guidance of DSA, and then RFA was performed immediately afterwards under the guidance of CT (Figs. 1 and 2). Patients in the TACE group received TACE alone under the guidance of DSA (Fig. 3).

Pre-operative preparation

All patients received comprehensive preoperative examinations that included routine blood tests, detection of coagulation time, and measurement of kidney and liver function, plasma cortisol, and catecholamines. Intravenous access was established, and blood pressure was measured non-invasively. Blood oxygen saturation, pulse, and heart rate were monitored during the procedure, and oxygen was administered via a nasal catheter. Other emergency drugs and a ventilator were also prepared before treatment. Sodium nitroprusside, urapidil, and metoprolol were available for immediate administration during RFA.

TACE treatment

The TACE regimen was identical in the two groups. Each patient's chemotherapeutic protocol was designed according to the primary tumor or pathology, and was prepared for administration by TACE after local sterilization and local anesthesia with 1% lidocaine. A modified Seldinger vascular puncture was performed at the femoral artery, and abdominal aortography was performed under the guidance of DSA (injection rate: 20 mL/s; total volume of contrast: 50–60 mL). The orifice of the adrenal artery was identified, and a 4 Fr Cobra catheter or Rosch hepatic (RH) catheter was used for selective angiography of the arteriae suprarenalis superior, arteriae suprarenalis media, and arteriae suprarenalis inferior to identify blood vessels supplying the tumor and their sources, sizes, and number. Then, a 2.6 Fr microcatheter (Progreat;Terumo Corp, Japan) was used for superselective catheterization of the supplying vessels, followed by chemoembolization. Epirubicin, mitomycin, and platinum-based chemotherapeutics were mixed with lipiodol to form an emulsion before periinterventional; 5-fluurouracil (5-FU), calcium levofolinate, and other chemotherapeutics were mixed with lipiodol, and the mixture was intermittently injected into the target vessels. During periinterventional, the embolization was strengthened with gelatin sponge particles or polyvinyl alcohol (PVA) particles when the target vessels were larger than the catheter; if the target vessels were small and tortuous, superselective catheterization could cause vascular spasm, so local injection of lidocaine before catheterization was performed. If the target vessels became spasmodic during the bolus

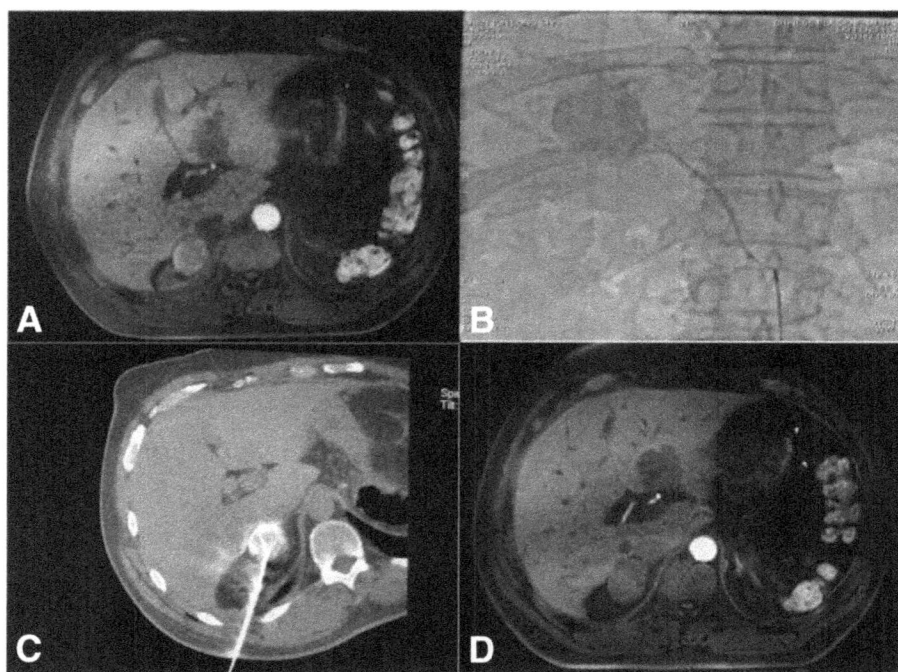

Fig. 1 A 52-year-old male patient with right adrenal metastases from HCC who received TACE+RFA. **a** Enhanced MRI before surgery, indicating adrenal metastases with uneven enhancement. **b** TACE of the adrenal metastases. **c** RFA immediately after TACE. **d** Enhanced MRI 1 month after surgery, indicating no enhancement or coagulation necrosis

Clinical efficacy of chemoembolization with simultaneous radiofrequency ablation for treatment of adrenal...

205

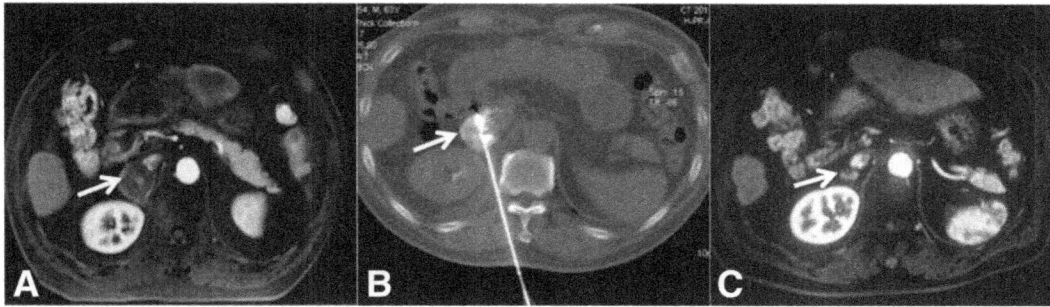

Fig. 2 A 63-year-old male patient with right adrenal metastases from HCC who received TACE+RFA. **a** Pre-operative enhanced MRI, showing right adrenal metastases with uneven enhancement (arrow). **b** RFA immediately after TACE of the adrenal metastases. **c** Enhanced MRI 2 years after treatment, showing no enhancement and a smaller tumor (arrow)

injection of chemotherapeutics, this made the treatment impossible, so injection of the lipiodol emulsion was discontinued after relief of the vascular spasm, and lipiodol alone was injected to avoid chemotherapeutic-induced vascular spasm.

TACE+RFA treatment

For the TACE+RFA group, Patients were changed to the prone position after the TACE, and the C-arm was moved toward the dorsal side to leave a space for CT scanning. According to the preoperative CT or MRI results, the patient's position was determined, and grid locators were placed. The CT parameters were 120 kV and 70 mA, and the slice thickness was 5 mm. After scanning, the puncture site, route, angle, and depth were determined according to the tumor size, location, adjacent structures, intra-operative lipiodol deposition, and peripheral status of the lesion. Then, surface markers were

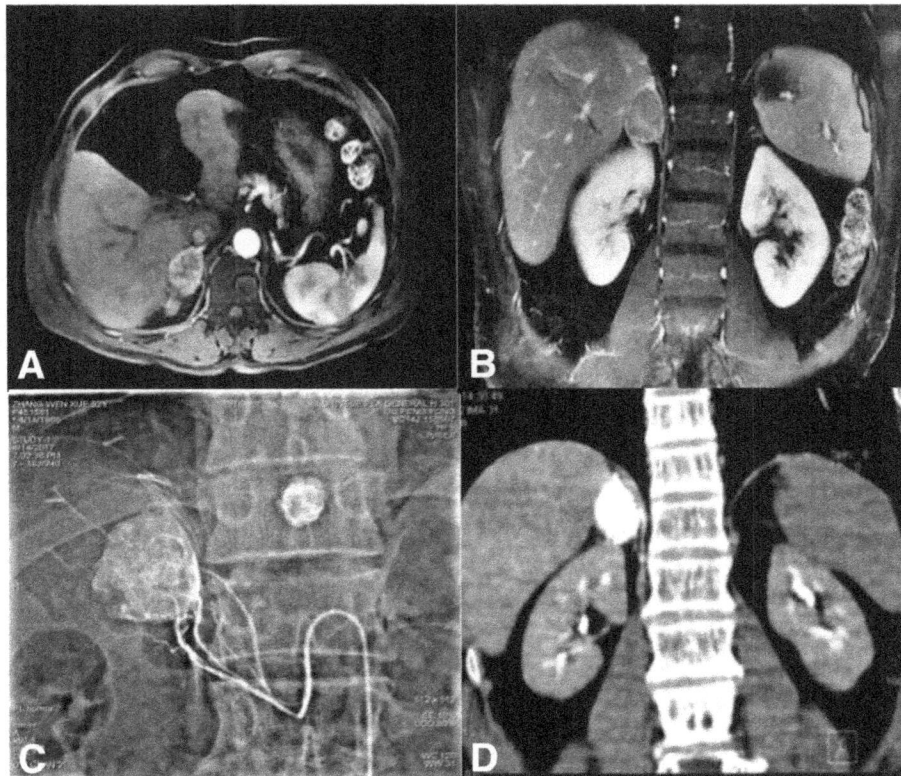

Fig. 3 A 65-year old female patient with right adrenal metastasis of a primary liver tumor who received TACE alone. **a** & **b** Abdominal enhanced MRI, showing uneven enhancement in the arterial phase, and continuous enhancement in the venous phase. **c** TACE of the adrenal metastasis. **d** Abdominal CT at 1 month after treatment, showing favorable lipiodol deposition

placed for the RFA. After skin sterilization, local anesthesia was performed using 1% lidocaine. The puncture needle was placed to avoid the liver, lungs, and major vessels, and CT was performed at least once to confirm its location. Once the needle reached the target, CT was performed again to confirm successful puncture, and this was followed by RFA. Tumor temperature and impedance were monitored in real time, and the output power was adjusted accordingly. The power was 140 to 200 W, the baseline impedance of the tumor was 50 to 70 Ω, and the treatment duration was 10 to 20 min. A multipole RF needle was used for ablation of lesions larger than 3 cm at multiple sites, until the periphery of ablation was 1 cm larger than the lesion size. A unipolar RF needle was used for ablation, except for lesions that were 3 cm or less from important organs. When the needle was withdrawn, ablation at 70–90 °C was performed at the puncture tract to prevent hemorrhage and possible implantation metastasis.

Intra-operative monitoring

Intra-operative monitoring was performed for both groups. In particular, vital signs (especially heart rate and blood pressure) were monitored closely because damage to the adrenal gland could cause release of large amounts of catecholamines, leading to sudden and significant increases in heart rate and blood pressure that could result in a life-threatening hypertensive crisis. If necessary, sodium nitroprusside or Betaloc was injected to reduce the blood pressure and heart rate.

Post-operative management

After treatment, both groups received analgesic therapy, anti-infection treatment, and urine alkalinization. The TACE+RFA group also received hydration therapy to improve the excretion of contrast and prevent renal injury. Vital signs were also closely monitored after interventions, and all side-effects and complications (such as pain, hemorrhage, fever, vomiting, hemoglobinuria, and hypertension) were recorded.

Definitions and follow up

Technical success was defined as superselective catheterization of the supplying artery and puncture of the target lesion. One month after interventions, patients were followed up by CT or MRI, and the local lesion was assessed for evaluation of therapeutic efficacy. The extent of image-guided tumor ablation was defined according to the Standardization of Terminology and Reporting Criteria (2009 and 2014) [10, 11]. In particular, therapeutic efficacy was defined as lesion eradication, lesion shrinkage, or unchanged lesion without enhancement on CT or MRI; residual tumor was defined by enhancement of the lesion on CT or MRI (difference in

CT of at least 20 HU; evident attenuation in MRI). Local tumor progression was defined as the appearance of tumor foci at the edge of the ablation zone, after at least one contrast-enhanced follow-up study documented adequate ablation, and the absence of viable tissue in the target tumor and surrounding ablation margin based on imaging. Survival time was defined as the time from first interventional adrenal treatment (TACE or TACE+RFA) to death or censoring (October 2017). The mean duration of follow up was 26.3 ± 19.3 months (range: 4–66 months). If residual tumor or tumor progression was observed during the follow up, retreatment could be performed.

Statistical analysis

Statistical analysis was performed using SPSS version 24.0 (IBM Corporation, Armonk, NY, USA). Data are expressed as the mean ± standard deviations. A two-sample t-test was used to compare quantitative data between the two groups, and a chi square test was used for comparisons of qualitative data. Survival was analyzed using the Kaplan-Meier method. Curves for overall survival (OS) were compared using the log-rank test. A p-value below 0.05 was considered statistically significant.

Results

Technical success rate

All patients received superselective catheterization for chemoembolization. In the TACE+RFA group, one patient underwent a transhepatic approach and three patients received injections of normal saline to separate the adrenal tumor from adjacent structures, followed by puncture. All patients in both groups were treated successfully, and the technical success rate was 100%.

Tumor control rate and local tumor progression

The tumor control rate at first imaging after 1 months was 92.1% (35/38) in the TACE+RFA group and 76.0% (19/25) in the TACE group(P = 0.041). Three patients in the TACE+RFA group and 6 patients in the TACE group had residual tumors at the edge of the original tumors. At the end of follow up (Figs.4 and 5), 7 patients in the TACE+RFA group and 7 patients in the TACE group had local tumor progression. The assisted local tumor control rate allowing repeated interventions in case of local recurrence was 70.0% (7/10) in the TACE+RFA group and 30.8% (4/13) in the TACE group (P = 0.039). The mean local tumor progression-free survival was 8.6 ± 6.5mo in the TACE+RFA group and 6.4 ± 7.3 mo.

Survival analysis

The overall survival rate was better for the TACE+RFA group than the TACE group at 1 year (92.1% vs. 88.0%), 2 years (73.7% vs. 64.0%), and 3 years (55.3% vs. 44.0%; P = 0.040). The mean survival time was 26.8 ± 2.0 months

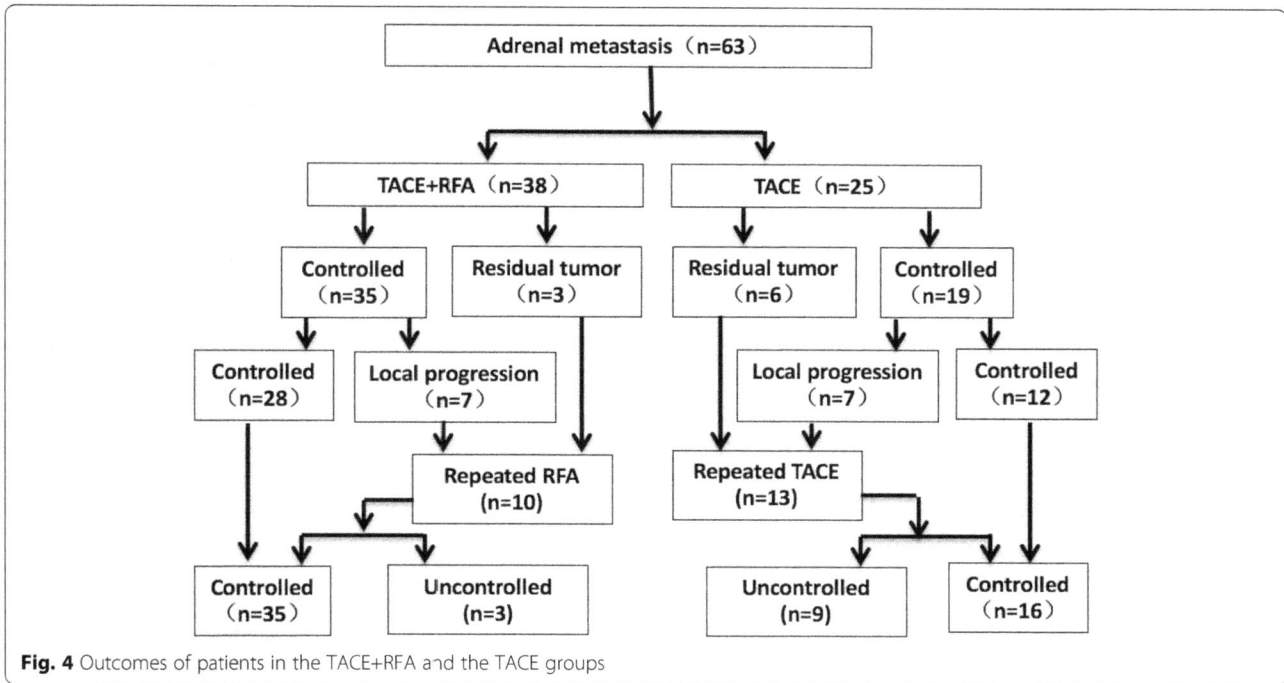

Fig. 4 Outcomes of patients in the TACE+RFA and the TACE groups

in the TACE+RFA group (95% CI, 22.8–30.7 months) and 17.5 ± 2.2 months in the TACE group (95% CI, 13.1–21.8 months).

Complications and side effects

No patients in the TACE+RFA group had serious adverse effects after TACE (Table 2). However, 6 patients in the TACE+RFA group developed hypertensive crisis (blood pressure greater than 220/115 mmHg and heart rate greater than 117 beats/min) after RFA. In each case, ablation was immediately discontinued, a selective alpha-1 blocker was administered, blood pressure and heart rate normalized after 20 min, and ablation was then continued. Two patients in the TACE+RFA group developed mild hemothorax and pneumothorax. Pain was the most common adverse effect in both groups. Morphine was administered upon complaint of pain during surgery, and oxycodone hydrochloride was used as an analgesic after surgery. Twenty-one patients in the TACE+RFA group and 13 patients in the TACE group experienced post-embolization/post-ablation syndrome, characterized by fever (> 38.5 °C), nausea, vomiting,

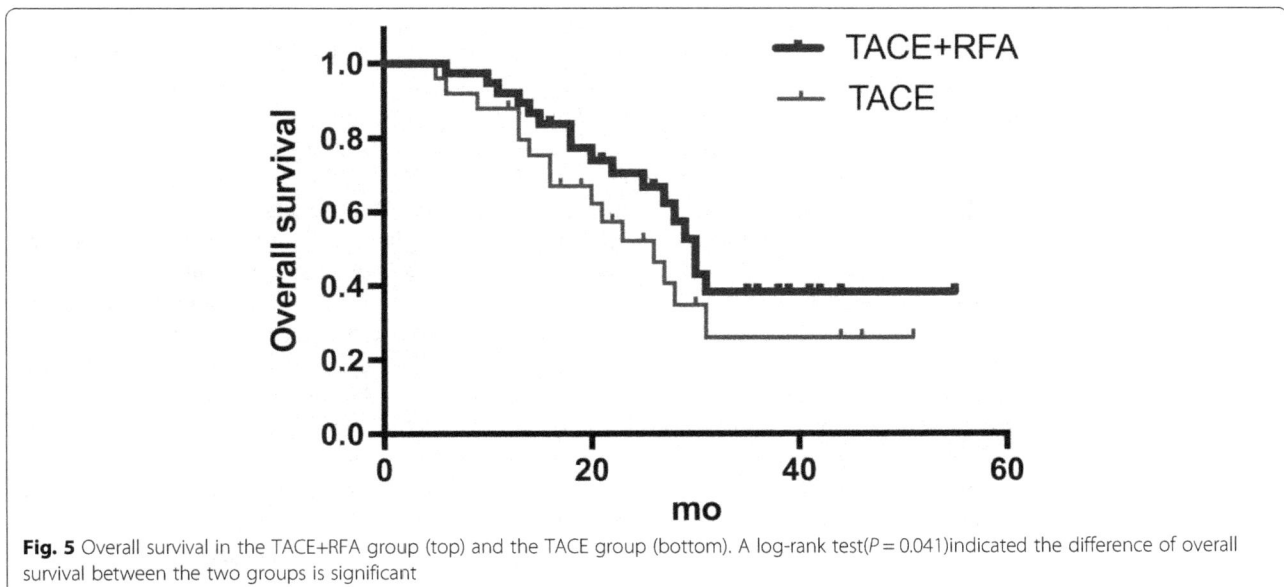

Fig. 5 Overall survival in the TACE+RFA group (top) and the TACE group (bottom). A log-rank test($P = 0.041$)indicated the difference of overall survival between the two groups is significant

Table 2 Complications in the TACE+RFA and TACE groups

Complication	TACE+RFA	TACE
Hypertensive crisis	6	0
Hemothorax and pneumothorax	2	0
Post-embolization/post-ablation syndrome	21	13
Pain		
Mild(VAS ≤ 3)	16	10
Moderate(3<VAS ≤ 7)	10	5
Serious(7<VAS ≤ 10)	7	2

Abbreviations VAS visual analogue scale

fatigue, and general malaise, and were given treatment to manage their symptoms. None of the patients died during surgery. The incidence of postoperative complications was higher in the TACE+RFA group than in the TACE group (presumably due to the RFA), all complications resolved after active management of symptoms, and no patients had life-threatening complications.

Discussion

Sorafenib is recommended as a first-line treatment to systemic treatment of hepatocellular carcinoma metastasis [12], but the effect of the adrenal metastasis of the HCC is rarely reported. In recent years, clinicians have increasingly used TACE and RFA for the treatment of AM due to the minimal invasiveness of these techniques. However, multiple treatment sessions are necessary to obtain complete tumor necrosis with RFA, and can greatly increase the risk of hypertensive crisis [13]. It is difficult to embolize all adrenal arteries because adrenal tumors are fed by several arteries [14, 15]. So we tried a combination treatment of RFA + TACE。The results of our study show that radiofrequency ablation combined with adrenal arterial chemoembolization is safe and effective management of adrenal metastasis of HCC.

Previous studies [16, 17] of patients with AM reported the disease control rate was 77–83% after local surgical intervention and the median survival time was 8–30 months, depending on the pathological type of the primary tumor. Specifically, the survival times was 11–29 months for patients with non-small cell lung tumor (NSCLC), 20–89 months for patients with renal cell carcinoma, 23–29 months for patients with colorectal tumor, and 12–21 months for patients with hepatocellular carcinoma (HCC) [16]. In our study, there was successful control of adrenal metastasis in 75.0% of patients in the TACE+RFA group and in 35.3% of patients in the TACE group at the last follow up evaluation. In addition, the mean survival time was 26.8 ± 2.0 months in the TACE +RFA group and 17.5 ± 2.2 months in the TACE group. The disease control rate and mean survival time after TACE+RFA were similar to those previously reported after adrenalectomy. This finding may be ascribed to a

synergistic interaction of TACE and RFA. Wang et al. [18, 19] speculated that complete lipiodol deposition could provide better heat transduction when RFA is given immediately after TACE, and that this heat had a strong tumoricidal effect, especially for irregular tumors, because RFA alone cannot completely cover the whole lesion in all three dimensions. In other words, angio-CT guided TACE and RFA can transfer heat to surrounding tissues, thereby reducing recurrence and metastasis. Moreover, adrenal artery embolism may also have an anti-tumor effect because it blocks blood flow, reducing the cooling effect of circulation during RFA and decreasing heat loss [20]. In addition, TACE+RFA targets the lesion when the concentration of chemotherapeutics is the highest, possibly providing a synergistic anti-tumor effect [21]. We speculate that TACE+RFA increases the efficacy of treatment due to a synergistic interaction of TACE and RFA.

Our results also indicate that patients given TACE+RFA had better prognosis than those given TACE alone at 6 months (100% vs. 88.2%), 12 months (87.5% vs. 70.6%), and 24 months (68.8% vs. 41.2%). The overall survival rate was significantly better in the TACE+RFA group than in the TACE group. These results suggest the combined therapy is more effective. Yamakado et al. [22] investigated 6 patients with adrenal metastasis from HCC who received adrenal artery chemoembolization and RFA, and reported the median survival time was 24.9 months, similar to that of patients given adrenalectomy.

Six patients in our TACE+RFA group developed transient hypertension during RFA, and required a selective alpha-1 blocker (urapidil) and sodium nitroprusside to lower blood pressure. Urapidil and sodium nitroprusside are commonly used to control peri-operative hypertensive crises. Chini et al. [23] also reported that transient use of a heart-selective beta blocker (esmolol) effectively controlled RFA-induced hypertensive crisis. In addition, the TACE+RFA group had a higher incidence of post-embolization or post-ablation syndrome, a higher incidence of postoperative pain, and more severe post-operative pain. Considering the severity of postoperative pain after TACE+RFA, we recommend analgesic therapy for 3 days. Our results also showed that the incidences of complications and adverse effects were higher in the TACE+RFA group, presumably due to the use of RFA. However, these complications and adverse effects resolved after active management of symptoms, and no patients had severe complications. These findings indicate that TACE+RFA therapy is safe.

There were some limitations in this study. There might have been a selection bias caused by non-randomization. This was a single-center study, the sample size was relatively small, and some of the patients did not have biopsies and pathologic examinations, thus there is a possibility of misdiagnosis from the exclusive use of CT and MRI.

Conclusions

Taken together, our results indicate that TACE+RFA is a feasible and effective treatment for AM from HCC. Although the use of concomitant RFA may increase post-operative complications and adverse effects rate, the complications and adverse effects were shown to resolve after active management of symptoms. Combined TACE+RFA treatment may prolong the survival time and benefit patients with AM from HCC.

Abbreviations

AM: Adrenal metastasis; CR: Complete remission; ECOG: Eastern Cooperative Oncology Group; HCC: Hepatocellular carcinoma; PD: Progressive disease; PR: Partial remission; RFA: Radiofrequency ablation; SD: Stable disease; TACE: Transcatheter arterial chemoembolization; VAS: Visual analogue scale

Funding

This study was supported by grants from The National Natural Science Foundation of China (No. 81671800), and The General Program of Beijing Municipal National Natural Science Foundation(No.7172204).

Authors' contributions

HY performed the data analyses and wrote the manuscript. FL contributed to the conception of the study. XL and YG contributed significantly to analysis and manuscript preparation. All authors read and approved the final manuscript

Competing interests

The Authors declare that they have no competing interests.

References

1. Wagnerova H, Lazurova I, Felsoci M. Adrenal metastases [J]. Bratislava Medical Journal-bratislavske Lekarske Listy. 2013;114(4):237–40.
2. Lombardi CP, Raffaelli M, De CC, et al. Role of laparoscopy in the management of adrenal malignancies [J]. J Surg Oncol. 2006;94(2):128–31.
3. Rajaratnam A, Waugh J. Adrenal metastases of malignant melanoma: characteristic computed tomography appearances [J]. Australas Radiol. 2005;49(4):325–9.
4. Sancho JJ, Triponez F, Montet X, et al. Surgical management of adrenal metastases [J]. Langenbecks Archives of Surgery. 2012;397(2):179–94.
5. Ahmed KA, Barney BM, Macdonald OK, et al. Stereotactic body radiotherapy in the treatment of adrenal metastases [J]. Am J Clin Oncol. 2013;36(5):509–13.
6. Desai A, Rai H, Haas JA, et al. A retrospective review of CyberKnife stereotactic body radiotherapy for adrenal tumors (primary and metastatic): Winthrop University hospital experience [J]. Front Oncol. 2015:185–5.
7. Frenk NE, Daye D, Tuncali K, et al. Local control and survival after image-guided percutaneous ablation of adrenal metastases [J]. J Vasc Interv Radiol. 2017;29(2):276–84.
8. Szejnfeld D, Nunes TF, Giordano EE, et al. Radiofrequency ablation of functioning adrenal adenomas: preliminary clinical and laboratory findings [J]. J Vasc Interv Radiol. 2015;26(10):1459–64.
9. Yamakado K, Anai H, Takaki H, et al. Adrenal metastasis from hepatocellular carcinoma: radiofrequency ablation combined with adrenal arterial chemoembolization in six patients [J]. Am J Roentgenol. 2009;192(6)
10. Ahmed M, Solbiati L, Brace CL, et al. Image-guided tumor ablation: standardization of terminology and reporting criteria—a 10-year update [J]. Radiology. 2014;273(1):241–60.
11. Ahmed M. Image-guided tumor ablation: standardization of terminology and reporting criteria-a 10-year update: supplement to the consensus document [J]. J. Vasc. Interv. Radiol. 2014;25(11):1706–8.
12. Jordi B, Morris S. Management of hepatocellular carcinoma: an update [J]. Hepatology (Baltimore, Md). 2011;53(3):1020–2.
13. Haga H, Saito T, Okumoto K, et al. Successful percutaneous radiofrequency ablation of adrenal metastasis from hepatocellular carcinoma [J]. J Gastroenterol. 2005;40(11):1075–6.
14. Park JS, Yoon DS, Kim KS, et al. What is the best treatment modality for adrenal metastasis from hepatocellular carcinoma? [J]. J Surg Oncol. 2007;96(1):32–6.
15. Momoi H, Shimahara Y, Terajima H, et al. Management of adrenal metastasis from hepatocellular carcinoma [J]. Surg Today. 2002;32(12):1035.
16. Kim SH, Brennan MF, Russo P, et al. The role of surgery in the treatment of clinically isolated adrenal metastasis [J]. Cancer. 2015;82(2):389–94.
17. Bradley CT, Strong VE. Surgical management of adrenal metastases [J]. J Surg Oncol. 2014;109(1):31.
18. Wang ZJ, Wang MQ, Duan F, et al. Clinical application of transcatheter arterial chemoembolization combined with synchronous C-arm cone-beam CT guided radiofrequency ablation in treatment of large hepatocellular carcinoma [J]. Asian Pac J Cancer Prev. 2013;14(3):1649–54.
19. Wang ZJ, Wang MQ, Duan F, et al. Transcatheter arterial chemoembolization followed by immediate radiofrequency ablation for large solitary hepatocellular carcinomas [J]. World J Gastroenterol. 2013;19(26):4192–9.
20. Yasumoto T, Hayashi S, Shimizu J, et al. [Radiofrequency ablation combined with transcatheter arterial chemoembolization for the local recurrent tumor after resection of the adrenal metastasis from hepatocellular carcinoma--a case report] [J]. Gan to Kagaku Ryoho Cancer & Chemotherapy. 2009;36(12):2371.
21. Wood BJ, Abraham J, Hvizda JL, et al. Radiofrequency ablation of adrenal tumors and adrenocortical carcinoma metastases [J]. Cancer. 2003;97(3):554–6.
22. Hasegawa T, Yamakado K, Nakatsuka A, et al. Unresectable adrenal metastases: clinical outcomes of radiofrequency ablation [J]. Radiology. 2015;277(2):142029.
23. Chini EN, Brown MJ, Farrell MA, et al. Hypertensive crisis in a patient undergoing percutaneous radiofrequency ablation of an adrenal mass under general anesthesia [J]. Anesth Analg. 2004;99(6):1867.

Imaging and clinical features of primary hepatic sarcomatous carcinoma

Dongli Shi[1], Liang Ma[2], Dawei Zhao[1], Jing Chang[3], Chen Shao[3], Shi Qi[1], Feng Chen[1], Yunfang Li[1], Xing Wang[1], Yanyan Zhang[1], Jing Zhao[1] and Hongjun Li[1*]

Abstract

Background: Primary hepatic sarcomatous carcinoma (PHSC) is a rare malignancy composed of both carcinomatous (either hepatocellular or cholangiocellular) and sarcomatous components. The purpose of our study was to evaluate the imaging and clinical findings of PHSCs, improving the understanding and diagnosis of tumors.

Methods: We retrospectively reviewed the imaging and clinical findings of ten patients with pathologically proven PHSCs, including two cases of sarcomatous intrahepatic cholangiocarcinoma (S-ICC), seven cases of sarcomatous hepatocellular carcinoma (S-HCC) and one case of sarcomatous combined hepatocellular and cholangiocarcinoma (S-HCC–CC). Six patients underwent computed tomography (CT) scans and five underwent magnetic resonance imaging (MRI) scans with one of them having both CT and MRI scans.

Results: Eight of ten patients had a background of chronic hepatitis or cirrhosis. The elevation of alpha-fetoprotein (AFP) was positive in half of the patients. All the tumors were located near the liver subcapsular area and six of ten cases were massive with round or oval shapes and ill-defined. The lesion textures were mainly heterogeneous in eight tumors for the necrosis or hemorrhage. Eight tumors showed hypo-enhancement and nine tumors exhibited initial peripheral rim (five cases) or heterogeneous (four cases) enhancement, followed by progressive (six cases) and peripheral or partial washout (three cases) on the later phases. Of the seven surgically resected tumors, five showed liver capsular invasion with one of them rupturing into the perihepatic space. Vascular thrombosis (five cases), intrahepatic metastasis (four cases), adjacent organ invasion or seeding (three cases), and lymph node metastasis (four cases) were found on imaging or in pathology. The follow-up period ranged from one to 36 months. Four patients with T3-T4 staging died from recurrence and metastasis between 2 and 5 months, and three patients with T1 staging did not have any recurrence between 16 and 24 months.

Conclusion: PHSC generally presents as a subcapsular mass with hypovascularity and may be characterized by rim-like or heterogeneous enhancement on the arterial phase and a progressive dynamic pattern. These tumors usually coincide with chronic hepatitis or cirrhosis and poor prognosis appears to be associated with TNM staging.

Keywords: Liver, Sarcomatous carcinoma, Combined hepatocellular-cholangiocarcinoma, Cholangiocarcinoma, Hepatocellular carcinoma

* Correspondence: lihongjun00113@126.com
[1]Department of Diagnostic Radiology, Beijing You'an Hospital, Capital Medical University, No.8, Xi Tou Tiao, Youanmen wai, Fengtai District, Beijing 100069, China
Full list of author information is available at the end of the article

Background

Primary hepatic sarcomatous carcinoma (PHSC) is a rare malignancy composed of both carcinomatous (either hepatocellular or cholangiocellular) and sarcomatous components [1]. This entity is differentiated from hepatic carcinosarcoma (CS), which contains both hepatocellular carcinoma and a true heterogonous sarcoma component such as chondrosarcoma, malignant fibrous histiocytoma, osteosarcoma, leiomyosarcoma, fibrosarcoma, rhabdomyosarcoma, and other mesenchymal tumors arising in the liver [1–4]. Various terms have been used to describe these biphasic tumors, including CS, sarcomatoid carcinoma, pseudosarcoma, and spindle cell carcinoma. Sarcomatous carcinoma (SC) and CS, however, are most commonly used and easily confused. Currently, pathologists are still faced with the dilemma of how to distinguish CS from SC when making pathological diagnoses. It is suggested that such mixed tumors should be diagnosed as SC when the sarcomatous component is predominantly composed of spindle cells, but the epithelial cells are still morphologically, immunohistochemically, and ultrastructurally identifiable [1, 5–8].

PHSC is extremely rare, accounting for only 0.2% of the primary malignant liver tumors [1]. The prevalence of sarcomatous hepatocellular carcinoma (S-HCC) and sarcomatous intrahepatic cholangiocarcinoma (S-ICC) is 1.8–9.4% of hepatocellular carcinoma (HCC) and 4.5% of intrahepatic cholangiocarcinoma (ICC) [1, 9, 10], and the sarcomatous combined hepatocellular and cholangiocarcinoma (S-HCC–CC) is rarely published in the literature, with no more than 20 cases [11–14]. It was reported in a previous study that the PHSC carried higher aggressiveness and poorer prognosis [1, 5, 9–11, 15]. However, its prognostic significance remained unclear. Since the literature was restricted to either case reports or small case series [7, 16–20], the cross-sectional imaging features of PHSC were largely ill-defined and clinical diagnosis was difficult. The purpose of our study is to further characterize these tumors by reporting the imaging findings and clinical features of a series of 10 patients, improving the understanding and diagnosis of tumors.

Methods

Patient selection

We retrospectively reviewed the medical records of 13 patients with pathologically proven PHSC by fine-needle aspiration biopsy or liver resection in accordance with the World Health Organization (WHO) definition, in 2000, at our institution from January 2011 to April 2018. One patient was excluded for transcatheter arterial chemoembolization (TACE) intervention prior surgery. Extrahepatic origin of SC with liver metastasis in two patients were also excluded. The remaining 10 patients did not receive any treatment prior to the CT or MR examination. The clinical data (including demographic features, laboratory findings, clinical interventions and treatment outcomes), imaging data and pathology reports were reviewed. The study protocol was reviewed and approved by the Institutional Review Board of our hospital.

Image acquisition

CT protocol

Six patients underwent Computed tomographic (CT) scans. CT scans were obtained with 64-detector row scanner (LightSpeed VCT 64, GE Healthcare, Waukesha, Wisconsin, USA). The imaging study was performed from the diaphragm to the iliac crest. The scanning parameters were as follows: tube voltage, 120 kV; tube current, 189–200 mA; matrix, 512 mm; and section thickness 5 mm. Using Iopromide (Ultravist 370, Bayer Schering Pharma, Berlin, Germany) as CT contrast agent, dose: 1.5 mL/kg, injection flow rate: 3 mL/s. Finally, a 20 mL saline flush was injected at a rate of 3 mL/s. Serial dynamic contrast-enhanced scans were obtained on hepatic arterial phase (HAP) (25–40 s), portal venous phase (PVP) (45–90 s) and equilibrium phase (EP) (2–5 min) after the contrast injection by means of a bolus-triggered technique.

MRI protocol

Five patients underwent magnetic resonance (MR) scans. Upper abdomen MRI studies were performed on 3.0 T whole-body MRI systems (Trio, Siemens Healthineers, Erlangen, Germany) with a torso coil. The MRI protocol consisted of the following sequences and parameters: Breath-hold T1-weighted fast low angle shot sequence: TR, 170 ms; TE, 2.30 [in-phase]/3.67 ms [out-of-phase]; matrix size, 256×205; flip angle, 65°; T2-weighted turbo spin echo (TSE) BLADE sequence: TR, 2200 ms; TE, 103 ms; flip angle, 140°; matrix size, 320×106; a three-dimensional volumetric interpolated breath-hold examination (3D-VIBE) sequence was obtained before (pre-contrast) and serial dynamic contrast-enhanced scans were obtained on HAP (25–40 s), PVP (45–90 s) and EP (2–5 min) after intravenous administration of contrast agent (Gd-BOPTA, MultiHance, Bracco Pharma, Italy) at a rate of 2 mL/s for a dose of 0.1 mmol/kg body weight using a power injector. Diffusion-weighted single-shot echo-planar imaging (DWI) with simultaneous respiratory triggering was performed using TR/TE 1600 ms/76 ms. Scanning parameters were as follows: b value 0, 150, and 800 s/mm; matrix size, 192×144; field of view, 35×35 cm; number of excitations, 2; slice thickness, 5 mm; slice gap, 1 mm; and 26 axial slices.

Image analysis

The imaging findings were evaluated as follows: 1) The location and size; 2) Gross type (nodular, massive, multinodular confluent, and infiltrative) [15]; 3) Contour (round, lobulated or irregular) and margin (sharp and indistinct); 4) Capsule (absent, complete or partial);5) Attenuation or intensity (hypo-, iso-, or hyper- attenuation or intensity relative to the background liver); 6) Lesion texture (homogeneous or heterogeneous); 7) Lesion enhancement characteristics were studied in detail as follows: the distribution in the arterial phase (peripheral rim enhancement, homogeneous enhancement and heterogeneous such as internal only or a mix rim and internal heterogeneous enhancement [21, 22]), enhancement degree of the whole tumor (heterogeneous lesions were evaluated according to the predominant parts more than 50%) [21] and the solid part only (hyperenhancement: increased enhancement compared to the background liver; hypoenhancement: decreased enhancement compared to the background liver), dynamic pattern of enhancement (partial or complete washout, progressive or persistent enhancement, no or minimal enhancement), progressive enhancement was defined as persistent or gradually increased enhancement of a tumor on portal, hepatic venous or equilibrium phase images compared with arterial phase images, as described in a previous report [23]; 8) The presence of capsule was considered positive when portal phase and equilibrium phase images demonstrated a peripheral rim of smooth hyperenhancement around the tumor [14]; and 9) Vascular invasion, intrahepatic metastasis or satellite nodule, adjacent organs invasion or seeding and lymph node metastasis. Based on these findings, image interpretation was performed retrospectively and blindly by two experienced reviewers (12 and 7 years of experience, respectively) in consensus.

Pathology analysis

The reference standard of pathology for PHSC was based on the histopathological examination of surgical specimens for seven patients and percutaneous biopsies for three patients. The tumors were diagnosed based on the histopathologic findings and immunohistochemical results. The histopathological factors that were assessed for each tumor were as follows: gross type; histological type; fibrous capsule; necrosis or hemorrhage; vascular invasion; bile duct invasion; presence of satellite nodule or intrahepatic metastasis; and presence of extrahepatic seeding or lymph node metastasis. Microscopically, the tumors were mostly composed of pleomorphic spindle cells (sarcomatous component), and moderately to poorly differentiated adenocarcinoma or HCC component. The diagnoses and analyses were made by two senior pathologists who were in consensus.

Result

Baseline clinical and histological characteristics

The clinical findings are summarized in Table 1. The majority of patients in our series were male adults (nine cases), with a mean age of 53.8 years (range: 37–62 years old). The hepatitis B virus surface antigen (HBsAg) was found positive in 70% (seven of 10) of the patients and 85.7% (six of seven) of the S-HCC patients. The most common complaints were abdominal discomfort (five of 10) and fever (two of 10). Half of the patients with PHSC were detected incidentally in their routine physical examinations for the hepatitis B. The elevation of alpha-fetoprotein (AFP) was found in 50% (five of 10) of the patients and 57.1% (four of seven) of the S-HCC patients. The carbohydrate antigen 19–9 (CA19–9) was positive in 40% (four of 10) of the patients. Seven patients underwent surgical resection, and five of them were treated in combination with TACE (four cases) and radiofrequency ablation (RFA) (one case). The remaining three patients were treated with TACE (three cases) with one of them having additional percutaneous microwave ablation (PMA). According to the American Joint Committee on Cancer (AJCC) staging system of liver tumors, three patients (30%) had TNM stage I tumor, one patient (10%) had stage II, four patients (40%) had stage III, and two patients (20%) had stage IV. During the follow-up period of two-36 months, three patients with stage I had no tumor recurrence or progression, six patients with stage II-IV underwent progression, four of whom died between 2 and 5 months after diagnosis, and the remaining case with stage III did not experience any progression 1 year after the operation.

Table 2 shows pathologic features of the study population. Of the seven surgically resected tumors, the hemorrhage (three cases) and different degrees of necrosis (six cases) were found (Fig. 1). Complete and partial capsules were identified in S-ICC (Fig. 2) and S-HCC-CC respectively. Five cases involved the liver capsules (Fig. 1) with two of them (S-ICC and S-HCC) rupturing into the perihepatic space. Additional findings were vascular thrombosis (four cases), adjacent organ invasion or seeding (two cases), satellite nodules or intrahepatic metastasis (two cases), and lymph node metastasis (two cases).

CT and MRI findings

The imaging features of PHSC are summarized in Table 3. All of the tumors were located near the liver subcapsular area (Figs. 1, 2, 3, 4, 5, 6 and 7), with an obvious dominance (90%) in the right lobe. Tumors ranged in diameter from 3.4 cm to 22.0 cm with a mean diameter of 8.3 cm. The most common gross morphology was massive (six cases) with round or oval shapes, and the remaining included nodular (two cases), infiltrative (one case) (Fig. 5),

Table 1 Clinical findings of 10 patients with PHSC

NO.	Age (y)	Sex	Histolgic diagnosis	Confirm	Underlying disease	AFP	CA19–9	TNM[a]	Treatment after diagnosis	Follow up result
1	55	M	S-ICC	Resection	CH-A	–	–	T4N0M1	Operation	Progress (1 M) death (2 M)
2	47	M	S-ICC	Resection	CH-A	–	+	T3N0M0	Operation	Progress (2 M) death (6 M)
3	39	M	S-HCC	Resection	CH-B	+	+	T1N0M0	TACE and Operation	Tumor-free (16 M)
4	55	M	S-HCC	Biopsy	Normal	–	–	T1N0M0	TACE and RFA	Tumor-free (21 M)
5	51	M	S-HCC	Resection	CH-B	+	+	T3N1M0	Operation and TACE	Tumor-free (12 M)
6	56	M	S-HCC	Biopsy	CH-B	+	–	T3N1M1	TACE	Death (4 M)
7	56	M	S-HCC	Biopsy	CH-B	–	–	T4N1M1	TACE	Death (5 M)
8	62	F	S-HCC	Resection	CH-B	–	+	T2N0M0	Operation	Recurrence (8 M) alive (10 M)
9	60	M	S-HCC	Resection	CH-B	+	–	T1N0M0	Operation	Tumor-free (24 M)
10	57	M	S-HCC–CC	Resection	CH-B	+	–	T3N1M0	Operation and PMA	Recurrence (6 M) alive (36 M)

+ yes/present/positive, – no/absent/negative

CH-A chronic alcoholic hepatitis, CH-B chronic viral hepatitis B, CH-C chronic viral hepatitis C, AFP alpha-fetoprotein (positive defined as > 7 ng/mL), CA19–9 carbohydrate antigen 19–9 (positive defined as > 27 U/mL), RFA radiofrequency ablation, TACE transcatheter arterial chemoembolization, PMA percutaneous microwave ablation

[a] AJCC TNM Staging of Liver Tumors (7th edition, 2010)

and multinodular confluent patterns (one case) (Fig. 6). Six tumors were poorly defined, especially at CT (five cases) and the rest were demarcated at MRI. The density or signal of the tumors was mainly heterogeneous (eight cases) for hemorrhage or necrosis. The hemorrhage was found in 1S-HCC and 2 S-ICCs, with one S-ICC rupturing into the subcapsular space as shown on MR imaging (Fig. 2). Five complete or partial capsules (Figs. 2 and 4) were found on CT (one case) or MRI (four cases) and two of them were pathologically confirmed in the S-ICC and S-HCC–CC.

All of the five tumors with MR examinations were mainly hypointense on T1WI and hyperintense relative to liver parenchyma on T2WI and DWI. Bright signal intensity similar to that of cyst or hemangioma on T2WI was seen in 1 S-ICC and 2 S-HCCs. The S-ICC presented multiple cystic changes accompanied by fibrous septum and was inhomogeneous restricted with an obviously decreased diffusivity in the center (Fig. 2). The signal with hyperintensity on T1WI and hypointensity on T2WI indicating hemorrhage was found not only inside the center of the tumor but also the subcapsular space (Fig. 2). The 2 S-HCCs showed homogeneous high signal on DWI and T2WI.

Regarding the distribution of enhancement, peripheral enhancement was seen in 2 S-ICCs and 3 S-HCCs (Fig. 3). Mix rim and internal heterogeneous enhancement (Fig. 4) was found in 2 S-HCCs, internal heterogeneous enhancement was shown in 2S-HCCs and 1 S-HCC–CC (Fig. 6), and no homogeneous pattern was observed. Eight tumors including 2 S-ICCs, 5 S-HCCs and 1 S-HCC–CC were hypo-vascular (Figs. 1, 2, 3 and 4) and the remaining 2 S-HCCs mainly presented hyper-intense enhancement on the arterial phase. As to the enhancement degree of the solid part in the tumor, six tumors showed hyper enhancement compared to the background liver.

With respect to the dynamic pattern of enhancement, of the ten tumors, 40% with 2 S-HCCs and 2 S-ICCs showed peripheral enhancement on the arterial phase and progressive enhancement towards the center (Fig. 2) on the later phases, 20% with 2 S-HCCs showed heterogeneous enhancement on the arterial phase and progressive or persistent enhancement on the later phase (Figs. 2, 3, 4 and 5), and 30% with 3 S-HCCs presented obvious peripheral and heterogeneous enhancement on the arterial phase and then wash out peripherally and partially on the later

Table 2 The histopathological findings of 7 patients with PHSC

NO.	Histological type	Fibrous capsule	Necrosis	Hemorrhage	Capsule invasion	Vascular invasion	Intrahepatic metastasis
1	S-ICC	+	+	+	+	–	–
2	S-ICC	–	+	+	+	+	+
3	S-HCC	–	N/A	N/A	–	–	–
4	S-HCC	–	+	–	+	+	+
5	S-HCC	–	+	–	+	+	–
6	S-HCC	–	+	+	+	–	–
7	S-HCC–CC	+	+	–	–	+	–

S-ICC sarcomatous intrahepatic cholangiocarcinoma, S-HCC sarcomatous hepatocellular carcinoma, S-HCC–CC sarcomatous combined hepatocellular and cholangiocarcinoma, N/A not available

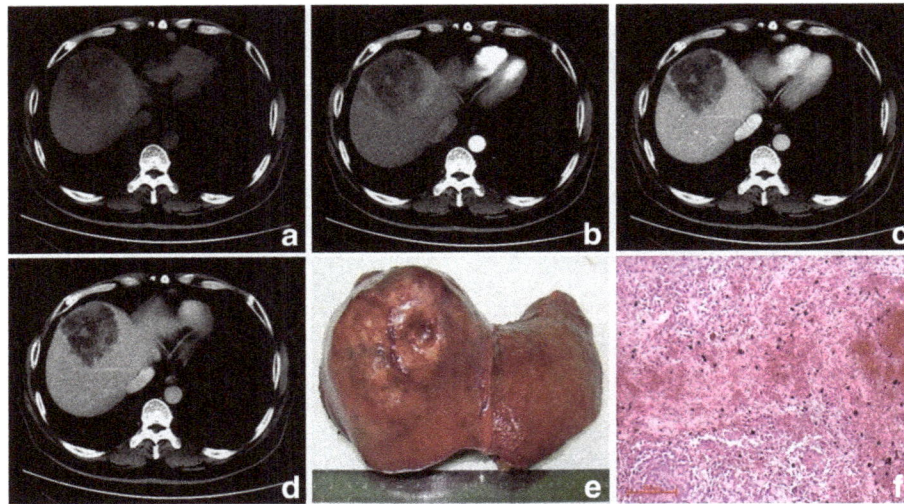

Fig. 1 Sarcomatous intrahepatic cholangiocarcinoma in a 47 year-old man. The axial CT scans display a hypovasular mass with intratumoral hemorrhage (**a-d**). The bisected specimen displays a large solid tan mass with hemorrhage and necrosis breaching the liver capsule without complete penetration (**e**). Hematoxylin and eosin (H & E) stain shows multifocal hemorrhage and necrosis. Hemosiderosis is found (**f**)

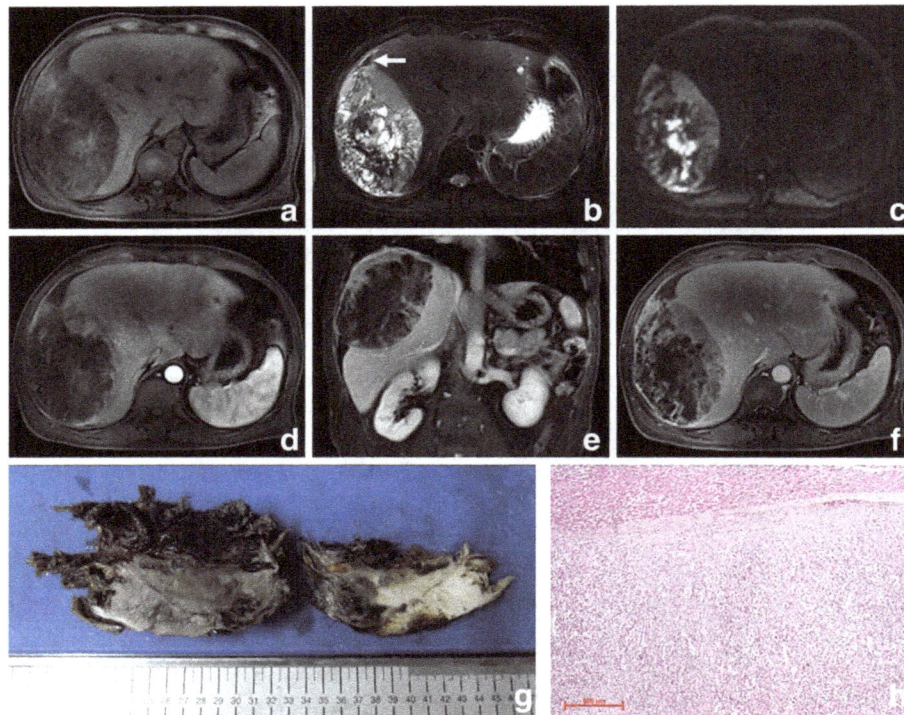

Fig. 2 Sarcomatous intrahepatic cholangiocarcinoma in a 55 year-old man. Pre-contrast T1WI and T2WI weighted images exhibit a subcapsular mass with multilocular cystic changes and hemorrhage (**a**, **b**). The mass is inhomogeneous restricted with an obviously decreased diffusivity in the center ©. The hypo-vascular mass mainly shows irregular peripheral rim enhancement on the arterial phase (**d**), followed by centrally progressive enhancement with septa on the equilibrium phase (**e**), and capsule formation is found (**f**). The tumor is ruptured with hemorrhage found in the subcapsular space (white arrow) (**b**) and invades the diaphragm (**d**). The bisected specimen shows a fragile solid and partially necrotic white to tan mass with massive hemorrhage inside and around the tumor (**f**). H & E stain shows a fibrous capsule, separating the normal liver from tumor cells. The neoplastic cells with pleomorphism have a poor cell adhesion (**g**)

Table 3 The imaging findings of 10 patients with PHSC

NO.						Enhancement characteristics		
	Histological type	Imaging protocol	Radiological gross type	Capsule	Lesion texture	Distribution	Degree	Dynamic pattern
1	S-ICC	MR	Massive	+	Hetero	Peripheral rim	Hypo	Progressive enhancement
2	S-ICC	CT	Massive	–	Hetero	Peripheral rim	Hypo	Progressive enhancement
3	S-HCC	MR/ CT	Nodular	–	Hetero	Internal heterogeneous	Hyper	Wash out
4	S-HCC	MR	Nodular	+	Hetero	Rim and internal	Hypo	Progressive enhancement
5	S-HCC	MR	Massive	+	Homo	Internal heterogeneous	Hyper	Wash out
6	S-HCC	CT	Massive	–	Hetero	Peripheral rim	Hypo	Progressive enhancement
7	S-HCC	CT	Infiltrative	–	Homo	Peripheral rim	Hypo	Progressive enhancement
8	S-HCC	CT	Massive	–	Hetero	Peripheral rim	Hypo	Wash out
9	S-HCC	MR	Massive	+	Hetero	Rim and internal	Hypo	Progressive enhancement
10	S-HCC–CC	CT	Multinodular confluent	+	Hetero	Internal heterogeneous	Hypo	Unclassified

S-ICC sarcomatous intrahepatic cholangiocarcinoma, *S-HCC* sarcomatous hepatocellular carcinoma, *S-HCC–CC* sarcomatous combined hepatocellular and cholangiocarcinoma.Hetero heterogeneous, Homo homogeneous, Hypo hypoenhancement, Hyper hyperenhancement

phase, mimicking ordinary HCC. The remaining S-HCC–CC exhibited a variable enhancement character for its multinodular change (Fig. 6). The tumor showed mild inhomogeneous enhancement on the arterial phase, and the portion near the subcapsular area of the tumor showed persistent thin rim enhancement accompanied by an mural nodular on the portal and equilibrium phase, next to the cyst change was the mild to moderate progressive fill-in enhancement, and the upper portion presented washout on the equilibrium phase.

Taking the pathology and imaging results together, five (50%) tumors including 3 S-HCCs, 1 S-ICC and 1 S-HCC–CC were accompanied by vascular invasion or thrombosis. Intrahepatic metastasis or satellite nodule was founded in 40% (4/10) tumors with 3 S-HCCs and 1 S-ICC. Extrahepatic involvement including adjacent organs invasion or seeding was observed in 1 S-ICC (Fig. 2) and 2 S-HCCs (Fig. 5), and the subcapsular rupture occurred in the S-ICC. Lymph node metastasis was found in 3 S-HCCs and 1 S-HCC–CC.

Discussion

In agreement with previous reports, most patients (70%) in this study were found to be positive for HBsAg and negative for hepatitis C virus antigen (HCVAg), suggesting that hepatitis B virus infection might be related to PHSC [1, 5], especially to the S-HCC. Unlike S-HCCs, S-ICCs were reported to show a relatively high incidence in patients with HCV-related hepatitis as the "normal" ICCs [24, 25]. Nevertheless, the two patients with S-ICCs in our study had history of alcoholic cirrhosis without any viral hepatitis or cirrhosis. The elevation of AFP was found in 57.1% of the patients with S-HCCs, which was slightly lower than that in "normal" HCC ones. As reported in some previous studies, S-HCC was characterized by lower serum AFP level [9, 15]. Meanwhile, the opposite conclusion came from the other studies [1, 5]. Therefore, further research about the relationship among AFP, hepatitis or cirrhosis and PHSC needs to be done with a larger sample in the future.

Our study demonstrated that PHSC generally presented hypovascularity seen as peripheral enhancement on the arterial phase imaging. The PHSC was characterized by the peripheral viable cancerous tissue with fibrous stroma and central necrosis or hemorrhage [14, 26]. Similar to prior results [6, 15], the necrosis was more frequently seen with a high frequency of 85.7% (six of seven) in the surgically resected tumors in our study.

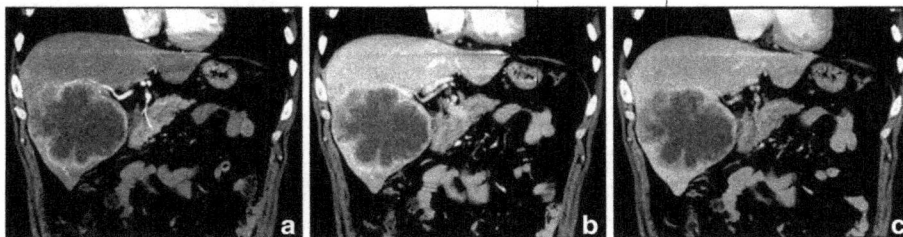

Fig. 3 Sarcomatous hepatocellular carcinoma in a 56 year-old man. The heterogeneous mass with a large area of cystic change exhibits rim enhancement on the arterial phase (**a**) with a slight progression towards the center on the later phases (**b**, **c**)

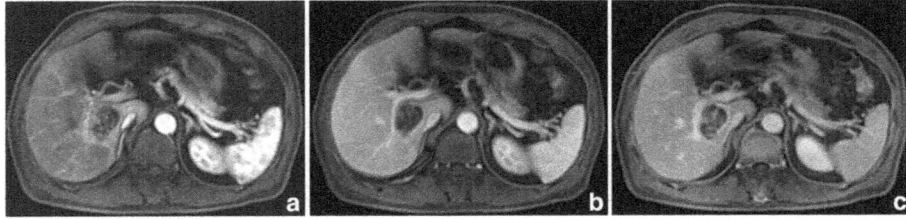

Fig. 4 Sarcomatous hepatocellular carcinoma in a 55 year-old man. The mass shows a mix rim and internal enhancement in the arterial phase (**a**) and progressive or persistent enhancement on the portal venous and equilibrium phase (**b**, **c**). An incomplete capsule is found (**c**)

The poorly differentiated cells of the sarcomatoid component grew so rapidly that the neovasculature could not adequately supply the fast-growing malignant cells, resulting in the central necrosis. In additional to the peripheral ring enhancement, when the necrosis was accompanied by fibrous septum or was scattered, the tumors might exhibit heterogeneous enhancement distribution such as a mix of rim and internal or internal only heterogeneous enhancement as shown in our study.

In the present study, the most common dynamic pattern of enhancement was progressive enhancement with persistent enhancement included in S-ICCs and S-HCCs. Additionally, the washout could also be found in S-HCCs. It was concluded in a previous radiologic–pathologic correlation study of S-HCC-CC that areas of arterial phase enhancement and later phase wash out were suggestive of HCC, progressive enhancements suggestive of CC, persistent and slight hypoenhancement in the subcapsular region suspicious for sarcomatoid transformation and hypodensity with little or no enhancement in keeping with the tumor necrosis [12]. Histologically, pleomorphic spindle shaped cells having loose mutual contact and fibrous stroma showed persistent or progressive enhancement, viable cells displayed a trabecular pattern with little or without fibrous stroma in the periphery of the tumor exhibited typical HCC enhancement washout, and a definite glandular pattern with fibrous stroma also showed progressive enhancement [11, 26]. Similar to the result, the S-HCC-CC in our study also presented as a lobulated multinodular confluent tumor with different dynamic enhancement

patterns (Figs. 6 and 7). It was supposed that the diverse tissue composition might determine the various enhancement patterns. However, even the S-HCC exhibited different dynamic enhancement characters. So we inferred that the diverse imaging findings of the sarcomatous carcinoma not only depended on the tissue composition but also the proportion. The manifestations varied when certain histopathological components ranged from focal to prominent. Therefore, it may be necessary to further sub-classify PHSC not only using morphological criteria that define biologically distinct subgroups but also the amount of certain component, which may be related not only to the imaging findings but sometimes even the biologic behavior of these cancers [11].

On the MR imaging of five patients, bright signal intensity similar to that of cyst or hemangioma on T2WI might be explained by necrosis [14] and the signal might be attributed to hemorrhage seen as hypointensity or hyperintensity on T1WI and hypointensity on T2WI not only inside the center of the tumor but also in the subcapsular area. The other S-HCCs showed inhomogeneous high signals on DWI and T2WI, similar to the "normal" type. Five tumor capsules were observed on imaging, and only two of them were confirmed in pathology. It was reported that a high incidence was correlated with well differentiated HCC and the tumor capsules were much more common in ordinary HCC when compared with the S-HCC [5]. Similar to the result, we did not find capsules in S-HCCs, except for a complete capsule in the S-ICC and a partial one in the S-HCC-CC pathologically.

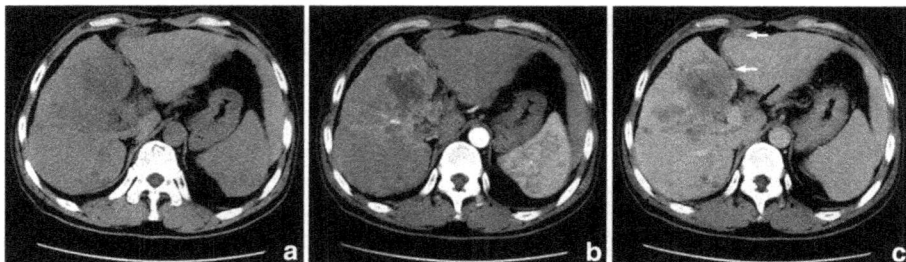

Fig. 5 Sarcomatous hepatocellular carcinoma in a 56 year-old man. An ill-defined infiltrative mass with punctate calcification is located in the left lobe of the liver (**a**). Intrahepatic metastasis, peritoneal seeding (white arrow) and lymph node metastasis (black arrow) are found (**b**, **c**)

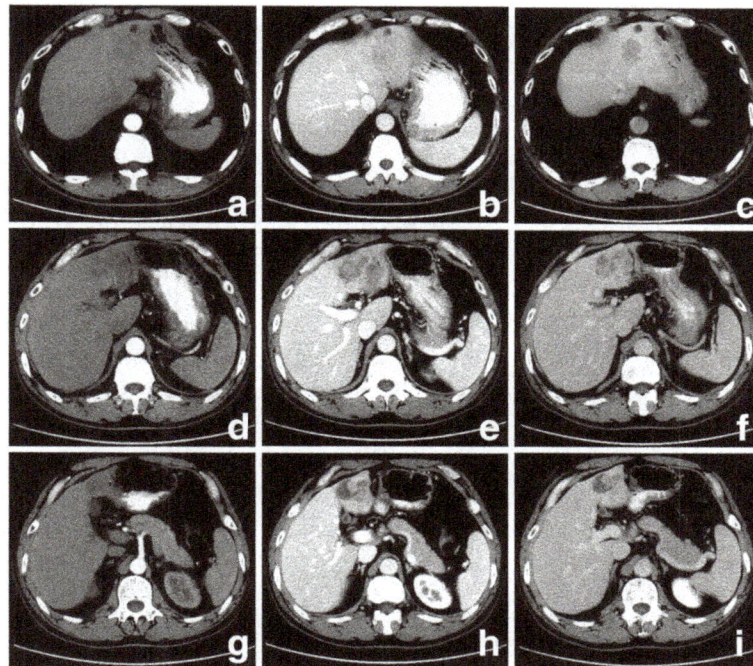

Fig. 6 Sarcomatous combined hepatocellular and cholangiocarcinoma in a 57 year-old man. A multinodular confluent mass shows mild inhomogeneous enhancement on the arterial phase (**a**, **d**, **g**). The upper nodular shows iso-hypo enhancement on the portal venous phase (**b**) and wash out on the equilibrium phase (**c**). The lower nodular shows persistent ring enhancement with mural nodular (**h**, **i**) and the middle area shows progressive enhancement (**e**, **f**)

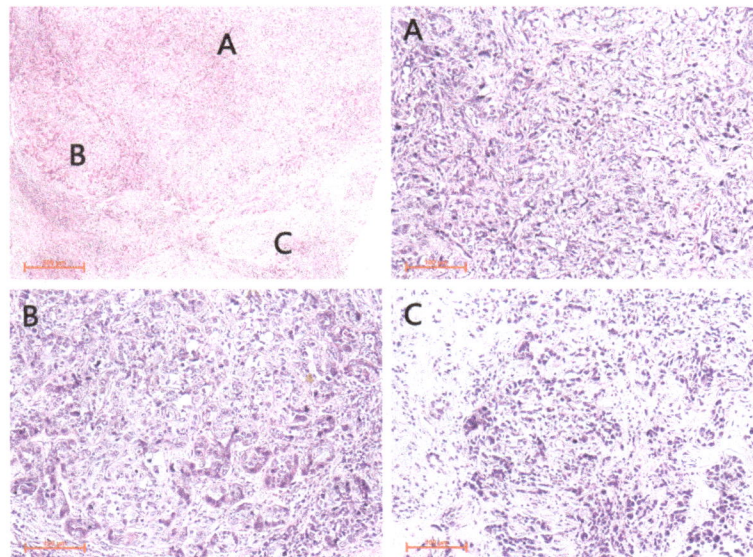

Fig. 7 H & E stain showing tumor was composed of poor differentiated or undifferentiated sarcomatoid combined HCC and CCC (×40). The area of sarcomatous transformation in part **a** is composed of spindle and epithelioid cells that were intensively distributed, and clumped chromatin and nucleolus can be seen (×200); some neoplastic cells in part **b**, which are arranged in gland trabecular, strands with distinct nuclei and prominent nucleoli, are keeping with cholangiocarcinoma (×200); some carcinoma cells with hyperchromatic nuclei and no prominent nucleoli in part **c** were arranged in sheets and strands, indicating HCC (×200)

All of the PHSCs in our study located near the liver subcapsular area where the liver capsules were frequently involved (five of seven) and sometimes subcapsular metastasis or peritoneal seeding (three of 10) occurred. The invasion of the liver capsular in sarcomatous carcinoma was more common than that in the "normal" type, which might be explained by the sarcomatoid component [20]. It was found that one of mass-forming S-ICCs with a subcapsular rupture in our study protruded out of the liver contours, involve diaphragm and resulted in multifocal tumor seeding. To the best of our knowledge, four of the 30 S-ICCs reported in the English literature presented with spontaneous rupture thus far [14, 27]. The spontaneous rupture of hepatic tumor was the result of a complex interaction of various factors such as location, composition or pressure and so on [28–30]. The "normal" cholangiocarcinoma seldom ruptured spontaneously as a hard tumor with abundant fibrous stroma. Nevertheless, the S-ICC in our study presented as multiple cysts indicating more necrosis and less fibrous stroma, resulting in a fragile tumor. In comparison to the "normal" cholangiocarcinoma, the S-ICC was prone to rupture.

In additional to the liver capsular involvement found in our study, we also observed that the vascular invasion or thrombosis (50%), intrahepatic metastasis or satellite nodule (40%) were relatively common, similar to prior results [9, 16]. As for the treatment of the tumor, it was reported that radical resection at an early stage may contribute to a relatively favorable prognosis. Nevertheless, its treatment protocols and effects were still controversial. Sometimes surgical removal of the tumor alone seemed to be insufficient. The sarcomatous carcinoma was thought to be associated with aggressive tumor biology, frequent metastasis, low resectability and frequent recurrence after curative resection, segmentectomy and even liver transplantation [1, 5, 31]. The TNM stage was revealed to be one of independent risk factors for overall survival [5], which had been partially proved in our study that all deaths occurred in PHSC patients with stage III-IV between 2 and 5 months and no tumor recurrence or progression happened in the patients with stage I between 16 and 24 months.

We acknowledge several limitations to our study. The major one was its retrospective nature make the complete section-by-section matching between imaging and pathologic findings technically unfeasible. Thus, to some extent our explanations for the imaging findings might be considered speculative. Due to the retrospective nature, we were unable to categorize the amount of the certain component such as sarcomatous component and evaluated its radiological findings and prognostic significance. The second limitation was relatively small sample size, which had inherent shortcomings but was unavoidable because of the rare incidence of these tumors. The last one was that

our study was only descriptive for a selected case without control group and no statistical data on differential features between them were obtained.

Conclusion

In summary, PHSC typically manifests as subcapsular mass with hypovascularity and initial rim or heterogeneous enhancement with a dynamic progressive enhancement on later phases. They generally have a history of chronic hepatitis or cirrhosis and the treatment protocols and effect were still controversial. As a highly aggressive malignancy with more frequent vascular invasion and intrahepatic metastasis, the prognosis of PHSC was extremely poor. Given the very heterogeneous appearance of these tumors, a prospective non-invasive diagnosis based on imaging findings alone is not possible at present. Further prospective studies are warranted to enlarge the sample size, categorize the amount of certain component of the tumor and further evaluate its radiological findings and prognostic significance. Furthermore, preoperative combination therapies and postoperative adjuvant therapies in recurrent cases need to be evaluated.

Abbreviations
AFP: Alpha-fetoprotein; CA 19–9: Carbohydrate antigen 19-9; CH-A: Chronic alcoholic hepatitis; CH-B: Chronic viral hepatitis B; CH-C: Chronic viral hepatitis C; CS: Carcinosarcoma; CT: Computed tomography; EP: Equilibrium phase; HAP: Hepatic arterial phase; MRI: Magnetic resonance imaging; PHSC: Primary hepatic sarcomatous carcinoma; PMA: Percutaneous microwave ablation; PVP: Portal venous phase; RFA: Radiofrequency ablation; RFA: Radiofrequency ablation; SC: Sarcomatous carcinoma; S-HCC: Sarcomatous hepatocellular carcinoma; S-HCC–CC: Sarcomatous combined hepatocellular and cholangiocarcinoma; S-ICC: Sarcomatous intrahepatic cholangiocarcinoma; TACE: Transcatheter arterial chemoembolization

Acknowledgements
This work was supported in part by the Department of Interventional Radiology and Department of Interventional pathology of Affiliated Youan Hospital of Capital Medical University.

Funding
Beijing Municipal Administration of Hospitals Clinical Medicine Development of Special Funding Support (ZYLX201511).

Authors' contributions
DIS: data acquisition and analysis, manuscript preparation. LM: collection of clinical data, manuscript editing. JC and CS: pathological data analysis. Jing Zhao: manuscript editing. The others: collected and review the data. All authors read and approved the final manuscript.

Competing interests
The authors declare that they have no competing interests.

Author details

[1]Department of Diagnostic Radiology, Beijing You'an Hospital, Capital Medical University, No.8, Xi Tou Tiao, Youanmen wai, Fengtai District, Beijing 100069, China. [2]Center of Interventional Oncology and Liver Diseases, Beijing You'an Hospital, Capital Medical University, No.8, Xi Tou Tiao, Youanmen wai, Fengtai District, Beijing 100069, China. [3]Department of pathology, Beijing You'an Hospital, Capital Medical University, No.8, Xi Tou Tiao, Youanmen wai, Fengtai District, Beijing 100069, China.

References

1. Wang QB, Cui BK, Weng JM, Wu QL, Qiu JL, Lin XJ. Clinicopathological characteristics and outcome of primary sarcomatoid carcinoma and carcinosarcoma of the liver. J Gastroint Surg. 2012;16:1715–6.
2. Lee JW, Kim MW, Choi NK, Cho IJ, Hong R. Double primary hepatic cancer (sarcomatoid carcinoma and hepatocellular carcinoma): a case report. Mol Clin Oncol. 2014;2:949–52.
3. Nishi H, Taguchi K, Asayama Y, Aishima S, Sugimachi K, Nawata H, et al. Sarcomatous hepatocellular carcinoma: a special reference to ordinary hepatocellular carcinoma. J Gastroenterol Hepatol. 2003;18:415–23.
4. Li J, Liang P, Zhang D, Liu J, Zhang H, Qu J, et al. Primary carcinosarcoma of the liver: imaging features and clinical findings in six cases and a review of the literature. Cancer Imaging. 2018;18:7.
5. Lu J, Zhang J, Xiong XZ, Li FY, Ye H, Cheng Y, et al. Primary hepatic sarcomatoid carcinoma: clinical features and prognosis of 28 resected cases. J Cancer Res Clin Oncol. 2014;140:1027–35.
6. Nakajima T, Tajima Y, Sugano I, Nagao K, Kondo Y, Wada K. Intrahepatic cholangiocarcinoma with sarcomatous change. Clinicopathologic and immunohistochemical evaluation of seven cases. Cancer. 1993;72:1872–7.
7. Murata M, Miyoshi Y, Iwao K, Wada H, Shibata K, Tateishi H, et al. Combined hepatocellular/cholangiocellular carcinoma with sarcomatoid features: genetic analysis for histogenesis. Hepatol Res. 2001;21:220–7.
8. Rossi G, Cavazza A, Sturm N, Migaldi M, Facciolongo N, Longo L, et al. Pulmonary carcinomas with pleomorphic, sarcomatoid, or sarcomatous elements: a clinicopathologic and immunohistochemical study of 75 cases. Am J Surg Pathol. 2003;27:311–24.
9. Lu J, Xiong XZ, Li FY, Ye H, Lin YX, Zhou RX, et al. Prognostic significance of Sarcomatous change in patients with hepatocellular carcinoma after surgical resection. Ann Surg Oncol. 2015;22(Suppl 3):1048–56.
10. Watanabe G, Uchinami H, Yoshioka M, Nanjo H, Yamamoto Y. Prognosis analysis of sarcomatous intrahepatic cholangiocarcinoma from a review of the literature. Int J Clin Oncol. 2014;19:490–6.
11. Aishima S, Kuroda Y, Asayama Y, Taguchi K, Nishihara Y, Taketomi A, et al. Prognostic impact of cholangiocellular and sarcomatous components in combined hepatocellular and cholangiocarcinoma. Hum Pathol. 2006; 37:283–91.
12. Pua U, Low SC, Tan YM, Lim KH. Combined hepatocellular and cholangiocarcinoma with sarcomatoid transformation: radiologic-pathologic correlation of a case. Hepatol Int. 2009;3:587–92.
13. Yin X, Zhang BH, Qiu SJ, Ren ZG, Zhou J, Chen XH, et al. Combined hepatocellular carcinoma and cholangiocarcinoma: clinical features, treatment modalities, and prognosis. Ann Surg Oncol. 2012;19:2869–76.
14. Gu KW, Kim YK, Min JH, Ha SY, Jeong WK. Imaging features of hepatic sarcomatous carcinoma on computed tomography and gadoxetic acid-enhanced magnetic resonance imaging. Abdom Radiol (NY). 2017;42: 1424–33.
15. Koo HR, Park MS, Kim MJ, Lim JS, Yu JS, Jin H, et al. Radiological and clinical features of sarcomatoid hepatocellular carcinoma in 11 cases. J Comput Assist Tomogr. 2008;32:745–9.
16. Chin S, Kim Z. Sarcomatoid combined hepatocellular-cholangiocarcinoma: a case report and review of literature. Int J Clin Exp Pathol. 2014;7:8290–4.
17. Bilgin M, Toprak H, Bilgin SS, Kondakci M, Balci C. CT and MRI findings of sarcomatoid cholangiocarcinoma. Cancer Imaging. 2012;12:447–51.
18. Inoue Y, Lefor AT, Yasuda Y. Intrahepatic cholangiocarcinoma with sarcomatous changes. Case Rep Gastroenterol. 2012;6:1–4.
19. Malhotra S, Wood J, Mansy T, Singh R, Zaitoun A, Madhusudan S. Intrahepatic sarcomatoid cholangiocarcinoma. J Oncol. 2010;2010:701476.
20. Kaibori M, Kawaguchi Y, Yokoigawa N, Yanagida H, Takai S, Kwon AH, et al. Intrahepatic sarcomatoid cholangiocarcinoma. J Gastroenterol. 2003;38: 1097–101.
21. Kim SA, Lee JM, Lee KB, Kim SH, Yoon SH, Han JK, et al. Intrahepatic mass-forming cholangiocarcinomas: enhancement patterns at multiphasic CT, with special emphasis on arterial enhancement pattern—correlation with clinicopathologic findings. Radiology. 2011;260:148–57.
22. Kim SJ, Lee JM, Han JK, Kim KH, Lee JY, Choi BI. Peripheral mass-forming cholangiocarcinoma in cirrhotic liver. AJR Am J Roentgenol. 2007;189: 1428–34.
23. Jeong HT, Kim MJ, Chung YE, Choi JY, Park YN, Kim KW. Gadoxetate disodium-enhanced MRI of mass-forming intrahepatic cholangiocarcinomas: imaging-histologic correlation. AJR Am J Roentgenol. 2013;201:603–11.
24. Donato F, Gelatti U, Tagger A, Favret M, Ribero ML, Callea F, et al. Intrahepatic cholangiocarcinoma and hepatitis C and B virus infection, alcohol intake, and hepatolithiasis: a case-control study in Italy. Cancer Causes Control. 2001;12:959–64.
25. Kobayashi M, Ikeda K, Saitoh S, Suzuki F, Tsubota A, Suzuki Y, et al. Incidence of primary cholangiocellular carcinoma of the liver in japanese patients with hepatitis C virus-related cirrhosis. Cancer. 2000;88:2471–7.
26. Honda H, Hayashi T, Yoshida K, Takenaka K, Kaneko K, Fukuya T, et al. Hepatocellular carcinoma with sarcomatous change: characteristic findings of two-phased incremental CT. Abdom Imaging. 1996;21:37–40.
27. Jung GO, Park DE, Youn GJ. Huge subcapsular hematoma caused by intrahepatic sarcomatoid cholangiocarcinoma. Korean J Hepatobiliary Pancreat Surg. 2012;16:70–4.
28. Watanabe Y, Matsumoto N, Ogawa M, Moriyama M, Sugitani M. Sarcomatoid hepatocellular carcinoma with spontaneous intraperitoneal bleeding. Intern Med. 2015;54:1613–7.
29. Hung Y, Hsieh TY, Gao HW, Chang WC, Chang WK. Unusual computed tomography features of ruptured sarcomatous hepatocellular carcinoma. J Chin Med Assoc. 2014;77:265–8.
30. Chong RW, Chung AY, Chew IW, Lee VK. Ruptured peripheral cholangiocarcinoma with hemoperitoneum. Dig Dis Sci. 2006;51:874–6.
31. Hwang S, Lee SG, Lee YJ, Ahn CS, Kim KH, Park KM, et al. Prognostic impact of sarcomatous change of hepatocellular carcinoma in patients undergoing liver resection and liver transplantation. J Gastrointest Surg. 2008;12:718–24.

Permissions

The contributors of this book come from diverse backgrounds, making this book a truly international effort. This book will bring forth new frontiers with its revolutionizing research information and detailed analysis of the nascent developments around the world.

We would like to thank all the contributing authors for lending their expertise to make the book truly unique. They have played a crucial role in the development of this book. Without their invaluable contributions this book wouldn't have been possible. They have made vital efforts to compile up to date information on the varied aspects of this subject to make this book a valuable addition to the collection of many professionals and students.

This book was conceptualized with the vision of imparting up-to-date information and advanced data in this field. To ensure the same, a matchless editorial board was set up. Every individual on the board went through rigorous rounds of assessment to prove their worth. After which they invested a large part of their time researching and compiling the most relevant data for our readers.

The editorial board has been involved in producing this book since its inception. They have spent rigorous hours researching and exploring the diverse topics which have resulted in the successful publishing of this book. They have passed on their knowledge of decades through this book. To expedite this challenging task, the publisher supported the team at every step. A small team of assistant editors was also appointed to further simplify the editing procedure and attain best results for the readers.

Apart from the editorial board, the designing team has also invested a significant amount of their time in understanding the subject and creating the most relevant covers. They scrutinized every image to scout for the most suitable representation of the subject and create an appropriate cover for the book.

The publishing team has been an ardent support to the editorial, designing and production team. Their endless efforts to recruit the best for this project, has resulted in the accomplishment of this book. They are a veteran in the field of academics and their pool of knowledge is as vast as their experience in printing. Their expertise and guidance has proved useful at every step. Their uncompromising quality standards have made this book an exceptional effort. Their encouragement from time to time has been an inspiration for everyone.

The publisher and the editorial board hope that this book will prove to be a valuable piece of knowledge for researchers, students, practitioners and scholars across the globe.

List of Contributors

Rebecca S. M. Lim
Department of Otolaryngology and Head & Neck Surgery, Monash Medical Centre, 823-865 Centre Rd, Bentleigh East, VIC 3165, Australia

Rebecca S. M. Lim, Julian A. Smith, Adnan Safdar and Elizabeth Sigston
Department of Surgery, School of Clinical Sciences, Monash University, 246 Clayton Rd, Clayton, VIC 3168, Australia

Shakher Ramdave and Paul Beech
Department of Nuclear Medicine & PET, Monash Medical Centre, 823-865 Centre Rd, Bentleigh East, VIC 3165, Australia

Paul Beech
Department of Nuclear Medicine, The Alfred, First Floor, East Block, Commercial Road, Melbourne, VIC 3004, Australia

Baki Billah
School of Public Health, Monash University, The Alfred Centre, 99 Commercial Road, Melbourne, VIC 3004, Australia

Rebecca S. M. Lim
Department of Radiology, Westmead Hospital, Cnr Hawkesbury Road and Darcy Road, Westmead, NSW 2145, Australia

Yoshiyuki Ozawa, Ritsuko Suzuki and Yuta Shibamoto
Department of Radiology, Nagoya City University, Graduate School of Medical Sciences, 1 Kawasumi, Mizuho-cho, Mizuho-ku, Nagoya 467-8601, Japan

Masaki Hara
Department of Radiology, Nagoya City West Medical Center, Nagoya, Japan

Sabrina Segreto, Sara Pellegrino and Silvana Del Vecchio
Department of Advanced Biomedical Sciences, University of Naples Federico II, Via Pansini 5, Edificio 10, 80131 Naples, Italy

Rosa Fonti and Silvana Del Vecchio
Institute of Biostructures and Bioimaging, National Research Council, Via T. De Amicis 95, 80145 Naples, Italy

Margaret Ottaviano, Vincenzo Damiano and Giovannella Palmieri
Rare Tumors Reference Center, University of Naples Federico II, Via S. Pansini 5, 80131 Naples, Italy

Leonardo Pace
Department of Medicine and Surgery, University of Salerno, Via S. Allende, 84081 Baronissi, Salerno, Italy

Hui Yu, Jing Liu and Ming-Ming Huang
Department of Radiology, Affiliated Hospital of Guizhou Medical University, Guiyang 550004, People's Republic of China

Bo Gao
Department of Radiology, Yantai Yuhuangding Hospital, Yantai 264000, Shandong, People's Republic of China

Yong-Cheng Yu
Department of Neurology, the second affiliated Hospital of Guizhou Medical University, Kaili 556000, People's Republic of China

Mark S. Shiroishi
Department of Radiology, Keck School of Medicine, University of Southern California, Los Angeles, CA, USA

Wen-Xiu Yang and Zhi-Zhong Guan
Department of Pathology, Affiliated Hospital of Guizhou Medical University, Guiyang 550004, People's Republic of China

Gabrielle C. Colleran, Neha Kwatra, Leah Oberg, Frederick D. Grant, Laura Drubach, Michael J. Callahan, Robert D. MacDougall, Frederic H. Fahey and Stephan D. Voss
Department of Radiology, Boston Children's Hospital, Harvard Medical School, 300 Longwood Avenue, Boston, MA 02115, USA

Tomohisa Moriya, Kazuhiro Saito, Yu Tajima, Taiyo L. Harada, Yoichi Araki and Koichi Tokuuye
Department of Radiology, Tokyo Medical University, 6-7-1 Nishishinjuku, Shinjuku-ku, Tokyo 160-0023, Japan

Katsutoshi Sugimoto
Department of Gastroenterology and Hepatology, Tokyo Medical University, Tokyo, Japan

Ralf S. Eschbach, Philipp M. Kazmierczak, Maurice M. Heimer, Heidrun Hirner-Eppeneder, Moritz J. Schneider, Georg Keinrath, Olga Solyanik, Wolfgang G. Kunz, Maximilian F. Reiser, Jens Ricke and Clemens C. Cyran
Department of Radiology, Laboratory for Experimental Radiology, University Hospital, Ludwig-Maximilians-University Munich, Marchioninistr. 15, 81377 München, Germany

Andrei Todica, Jessica Olivier and Peter Bartenstein
Department of Nuclear Medicine, University Hospital, Ludwig-Maximilians-University Munich, Marchioninistr. 15, 81377 München, Germany

Moritz J. Schneider
Comprehensive Pneumology Center, German Center for Lung Research, Munich, Germany

Feng Duan, Li Cui, Yanhua Bai, Xiaohui Li, Jieyu Yan and Xuan Liu
Department of Interventional Radiology, the General Hospital of Chinese People's Liberation Army, Beijing 100853, China

Martin H. Cherk, Grace Kong, Rodney J. Hicks and Michael S. Hofman
Centre for Cancer Imaging, Peter MacCallum Cancer Centre, 305 Grattan Street, Melbourne, VIC 3000, Australia

Rodney J. Hicks
Department of Medicine / Sir Peter MacCallum Department of Oncology, University of Melbourne, Melbourne, Australia

Martin H. Cherk
Department of Medicine, Monash University, Melbourne, Australia
Department of Nuclear Medicine, The Alfred, 55 Commercial Rd, Prahan, VIC 3181, Australia

Mette S. van Ramshorst, Sjoerd Rodenhuis and Gabe S. Sonke
Department of Medical Oncology, Netherlands Cancer Institute, Plesmanlaan 121, 1066 CX Amsterdam, The Netherlands

Suzana C. Teixeira and Bas B. Koolen
Department of Nuclear Medicine, Netherlands Cancer Institute, Plesmanlaan 121, 1066 CX Amsterdam, The Netherlands

Bas B. Koolen, Emiel J. Rutgers and Marie-Jeanne T. Vrancken Peeters
Department of Surgical Oncology, Netherlands Cancer Institute, Plesmanlaan 121, 1066 CX Amsterdam, The Netherlands

Kenneth E. Pengel
Department of Radiology, Netherlands Cancer Institute, Plesmanlaan 121, 1066 CX Amsterdam, The Netherlands

Kenneth G. Gilhuijs
Department of Department of Radiology/Image Sciences Institute, University Medical Centre Utrecht, Heidelberglaan 100, 3584 CX Utrecht, The Netherlands

Jelle Wesseling
Department of Pathology and Division of Molecular Pathology, Netherlands Cancer Institute, Plesmanlaan 121, 1066 CX Amsterdam, The Netherlands

H. Malikova, E. Koubska, J. Weichet and A. Rulseh
Department of Radiology, Na Homolce Hospital, Roentgenova 2, Prague 15000, Czech Republic

H. Malikova and J. Weichet
Department of Radiology, Third Faculty of Medicine, Charles University in Prague and Faculty Hospital Kralovske Vinohrady, Ruska 87, Prague 10000, Czech Republic

J. Klener
Department of Neurosurgery, Na Homolce Hospital, Roentgenova 2, Prague 15000, Czech Republic

A. Rulseh
Department of Radiology, 1st Faculty of Medicine and General University Hospital, Charles University, Prague, Czech Republic

R. Liscak
Department of Stereotactic and Radiation Neurosurgery, Na Homolce Hospital, Roentgenova 2, Prague 15000, Czech Republic

Z. Vojtech
Department of Neurology, Na Homolce Hospital, Roentgenova 2, Prague 15000, Czech Republic
Department of Neurology, Third Faculty of Medicine, Charles University in Prague, Ruska 87, Prague 10000, Czech Republic

Masatoshi Hotta and Ryogo Minamimoto
Division of Nuclear Medicine, Department of Radiology, National Center for Global Health and Medicine, 1-21-1, Shinjuku-ku, Toyama, Tokyo 162-8655, Japan

Hideaki Yano, Yoshimasa Gohda and Yasutaka Shuno
Department of Surgery, National Center for Global Health and Medicine, 1-21-1, Shinjuku-ku, Toyama, Tokyo 162-8655, Japan

Ronald L. Korn
Imaging Endpoints Core Lab, 9700 N 91st St, B-200, Scottsdale, AZ 85258, USA

Daniel D. Von Hoff
Translational Genomics Research Institute and HonorHealth, 445 North Fifth St, Suite 600, Phoenix, AZ 85004, USA

Mitesh J. Borad and Ramesh K. Ramanathan
Mayo Clinic, 13400 E Shea Blvd, Scottsdale, AZ 85259, USA

Markus F. Renschler and Desmond McGovern
Celgene Corporation, 86 Morris Ave, Summit, NJ 07901, USA

R. Curtis Bay
Department of Interdisciplinary Health Sciences, A. T. Still University, 5850 E Still Circle, Mesa, AZ 85206, USA

Masoom A. Haider and Farzad Khalvati
Department of Medical Imaging, Sunnybrook Health Sciences Center, University of Toronto, Rm AG-46, 2075 Bayview Ave, Toronto, Onatrio M4N 3M5, Canada

Alireza Vosough
Department of Radiology, North Bristol NHS Trust, Southmead Hospital, Bristol, UK

Alexander Kiss
Sunnybrook Health Sciences Center, Toronto, Canada

Balaji Ganeshan
Institute of Nuclear Medicine, University College London, London, UK

Georg A. Bjarnason
Sunnybrook Odette Cancer Centre, Division of medical Oncology, University of Toronto, Toronto, ON, Canada

Jing Li, Jinrong Qu, Hongkai Zhang, Yingshu Wang, Lin Zheng, Xiang Geng, Yan Zhao and Hailiang Li
Department of Radiology, the Affiliated Cancer Hospital of Zhengzhou University, Henan Cancer Hospital, 127 Dongming Road, Jinshui District, Zhengzhou, Henan Province 450008, China

Laird B Cameron
Department of Medical Oncology, Peter MacCallum Cancer Centre, Grattan Street, Melbourne, Australia

Damian H S Jiang, Kate Moodie and Bimal Kumar Parameswaran
Department of Cancer Imaging, Peter MacCallum Cancer Centre, Grattan Street, Melbourne, Australia

Catherine Mitchell
Department of Pathology, Peter MacCallum Cancer Centre, Grattan Street, Melbourne, Australia

Benjamin Solomon
Department of Medical Oncology, Peter MacCallum Cancer Centre; Sir Peter MacCallum Department of Oncology, University of Melbourne, Melbourne, Australia

Asem Mansour and Hussein Abuali
Department of Radiology, King Hussein Cancer Center, Amman, Jordan

Nayef Abdel-Razeq
Istishari Hospital, Amman, Jordan

Mohammad Makoseh, Nouran Shaikh-Salem, Kamelah Abushalha and Samer Salah
Department of Internal Medicine, King Hussein Cancer Center, Amman, Jordan

Li-ming Li, Xiao-hua Chen, Pan Liang, Jing Li and Jian-bo Gao
Department of Radiology, The First Affiliated Hospital of Zhengzhou University, Zhengzhou 450052, Henan Province, China

Lei-yu Feng
Department of Internal Medicine, The First Affiliated Hospital of Zhengzhou University, Zhengzhou 450052, Henan Province, China

Tanja Zitzelsberger, Roland Syha, Gerd Grözinger, Konstantin Nikolaou and Ulrich Grosse
Department of Diagnostic and Interventional Radiology, University of Tuebingen, Hoppe-Seyler-Straße 3, 72076 Tuebingen, Germany

Sasan Partovi
Department of Radiology, Section of Interventional Radiology, University Hospitals Cleveland Medical Center, Case Western Reserve University, Cleveland, OH, USA

Feng Duan, Yan-hua Bai, Li Cui, Jie-yu Yan, Xiao-hui Li and Xiu-qi Wang
Department of Interventional Radiology, the General Hospital of Chinese People's Liberation Army, Beijing 100853, China

Antti Salminen, Otto Ettala and Peter J. Boström
Department of Urology, University of Turku and Turku University hospital, Kiinamyllynkatu 4-8, 20520 Turku, Finland

Ivan Jambor and Johanna Virtanen
Department of Radiology, University of Turku and Turku University Hospital, Turku, Finland

Ilmari Koskinen and Jukka Sairanen
Department of Urology, University of Helsinki and Helsinki University hospital, Helsinki, Finland

Erik Veskimae
Department of Urology, University of Tampere and Tampere University hospital, Tampere, Finland

Pekka Taimen
Department of Pathology, Institute of Biomedicine, University of Turku and Turku University hospital, Turku, Finland

Jukka Kemppainen
Department of Clinical Physiology and nuclear imaging, University of Turku and Turku University hospital, Turku, Finland

Heikki Minn
Department of Oncology and Radiotherapy, University of Turku and Turku University hospital, Turku, Finland

Antti Salminen, Ivan Jambor, Harri Merisaari, Jukka Kemppainen and Heikki Minn
Department of Radiology, Icahn School of Medicine at Mount Sinai, New York, USA

Ya-ling Chen, Yi Gao, Cai Chang, Fen Wang and Wei Zeng
Department of Ultrasound, Fudan University Shanghai Cancer Center, No. 270 Dong-An Road, Shanghai 200032, China
Department of Oncology, Shanghai Medical College, Fudan University, No. 270 Dong-An Road, Shanghai 200032, China

Jia-jian Chen
Department of Breast Surgery, Fudan University Shanghai Cancer Center, No. 270 Dong-An Road, Shanghai 200032, China

Wolfgang G. Kunz, Ralf S. Eschbach, Robert Stahl, Philipp M. Kazmierczak, Jens Ricke and Clemens C. Cyran
Department of Radiology, University Hospital, LMU Munich, Marchioninistr.15, 81377 Munich, Germany

Peter Bartenstein and Axel Rominger
Department of Nuclear Medicine, University Hospital, LMU Munich, Munich, Germany

Christoph J. Auernhammer and Christine Spitzweg
Department of Internal Medicine IV, University Hospital, LMU Munich, Munich, Germany
Comprehensive Cancer Center (CCC LMU) and Interdisciplinary Center for Neuroendocrine Tumors of the Gastroenteropancreatic System (GEPNET-KUM), University Hospital, LMU Munich, Munich, Germany

Hongjun Yuan, Fengyong Liu, Xin Li, Yang Guan and Maoqiang Wang
Department of Interventional Radiology, Chinese PLA General Hospital, 28 Fuxing Road, Beijing 100853, People's Republic of China

Dongli Shi, Dawei Zhao, Shi Qi, Feng Chen, Yunfang Li, Xing Wang, Yanyan Zhang, Jing Zhao and Hongjun Li
Department of Diagnostic Radiology, Beijing You'an Hospital, Capital Medical University, No.8, Xi Tou Tiao, Youanmen wai, Fengtai District, Beijing 100069, China

Liang Ma
Center of Interventional Oncology and Liver Diseases, Beijing You'an Hospital, Capital Medical University, No.8, Xi Tou Tiao, Youanmen wai, Fengtai District, Beijing 100069, China

Jing Chang and Chen Shao
Department of pathology, Beijing You'an Hospital, Capital Medical University, No.8, Xi Tou Tiao, Youanmen wai, Fengtai District, Beijing 100069, China

Index